T0248984

Essentials in Immunology:
Infections, Cancer and Inflammations

Essentials in Immunology: Infections, Cancer and Inflammations

Edited by **Jim Wang**

New Jersey

Published by Foster Academics,
61 Van Reypen Street,
Jersey City, NJ 07306, USA
www.fosteracademics.com

Essentials in Immunology: Infections, Cancer and Inflammations
Edited by Jim Wang

International Standard Book Number: 978-1-63242-184-5 (Hardback)

Contents

Permissions

List of Contributors

Preface

The purpose of the book is to provide a glimpse into the dynamics and to present opinions and studies of some of the scientists engaged in the development of new ideas in the field from very different standpoints. This book will prove useful to students and researchers owing to its high content quality.

Immunology is a branch of biomedical sciences to study the immune system physiology in both diseased and healthy states. Some aspects of autoimmunity enable us to understand that it is not always related to pathology. For example, autoimmune reactions are effective in clearing off the unwanted, excess or aged tissues from the body. Also, autoimmunity occurs after the exposure of the non-self-antigen which is structurally similar to the self, assisted by the stimulatory molecules such as cytokines. Therefore, it can be said that there's a minor difference between immunity and auto-immunity. The question of how physiologic immunity changes to pathologic autoimmunity continue to interest researchers. Answer to such questions can be found by understanding physiology of the immune system. This book covers various topics about immunology, its related aspects and pathologies under two sections namely, Immunology of Viruses & Cancers and Basics of Autoimmunity & Multiple Sclerosis. The contributors of this book have carefully selected topics which would be of reader's interests.

At the end, I would like to appreciate all the efforts made by the authors in completing their chapters professionally. I express my deepest gratitude to all of them for contributing to this book by sharing their valuable works. A special thanks to my family and friends for their constant support in this journey.

Editor

Section 1

Immunology of Viruses and Cancer

Cytokines and Markers of Immune Response to HPV Infection

Jill Koshiol[2] and Melinda Butsch Kovacic[1]
[1]Cincinnati Children's Hospital Medical Center
[2]National Cancer Institute
USA

1. Introduction

Cervical cancer is the third most commonly diagnosed cancer in women worldwide (Ferlay, Shin et al. 2010) and is a result of infection with cancer-causing types of human papillomavirus (HPV) (Bouvard, Baan et al. 2009). HPV is a very common infection, although in most circumstances, infection does not usually result in cervical disease (Trottier and Franco 2006). In fact, the natural history of HPV infection suggests that additional factors are required to drive progression from infection to the development of cancer. Most women are thought to clear their HPV infections within two years, but in approximately 10% of women, infection persists (Schiffman, Castle et al. 2007). Persistent HPV infection is, in effect, the strongest risk factor for progression to cervical precancer and cancer (Koshiol, Lindsay et al. 2008), and a dysfunctional immune response is likely to underlie the amplified risk that leads to HPV persistence and cervical cancer. Although efficacious prophylactic vaccines against the two types of HPV (16 and 18) that cause about 70% of cervical cancers (Munoz, Castellsague et al. 2006) are available, these vaccines are expensive, difficult to administer in poorer countries and will not protect women who have already been exposed to the virus (FUTURE II Study Group 2007; Hildesheim, Herrero et al. 2007) (Su, Wu et al. 2010). Thus, it is important to understand factors that predispose some women infected with a carcinogenic HPV infection to persist and progress.

HPV uses a variety of methods to avoid immune detection, such as maintaining an unobtrusive infectious cycle (e.g., non-viremic and non-cytolytic since replication occurs in cells already destined for natural cell death), suppressing interferon response, and down-regulating toll-like receptor (TLR)-9 (Stanley 2010). By employing such immune evasion tactics, HPV infection itself does not lead to a direct or obvious inflammatory response. Rather, inflammation due to other co-factors such as smoking, parity, oral contraceptive use, co-infection with other sexually transmitted diseases, multiple sexual partners etc. have long been hypothesized to lead to HPV incidence, persistence, and progression to cervical pre-cancer and cancer (Castle and Giuliano 2003). Studies that directly evaluate women's immune response to HPV infection may provide better insights into the role of inflammation and immunity in HPV persistence and cervical carcinogenesis.

Although humoral response to HPV infection has been well-characterized (Bhat, Mattarollo et al. 2011), cell-mediated response has not been well established. Numerous approaches have been used to characterize cell-mediated immune responses to HPV. Such approaches include measurement of cytokines and other immune markers that commonly lead to infiltration of immune cells. Cytokines are pleiotropic glycoproteins that regulate cell survival, proliferation, differentiation and activation at both local and systemic levels. During inflammation, their excessive release may lead to both chronicity and pathogenicity. The purpose of this review is to describe the current state of knowledge regarding these important regulators or other important immune markers of cell-mediated immune response in HPV infection. To this end, we have evaluated studies in plasma or serum from peripheral blood, in cervical secretions, in unstimulated and stimulated PBMCs (and cellular subsets thereof), and in cervical tissues themselves. Importantly, this chapter will highlight not only the large amount of knowledge gained from these studies, but also the many scientific gaps in knowledge that remain.

2. Methods

Relevant studies were identified by searching MEDLINE (via PubMed) using broad search term categories for cervix and immunity (Appendix 1). The search included studies identified through 3 November 2011. Studies that evaluated cell-mediated immune response immune response by HPV status (positivity, persistence, or clearance) were included if there were at least 10 women in each comparison group (usually HPV-positive versus HPV-negative; sometime HPV persistence versus clearance or difference by HPV type). To focus on more functional aspects of immune response, only studies of immune-related proteins and mRNA (evidence of expression) and studies with HPV DNA detection were included. Studies were excluded if the HPV status and disease status of the referent group was unclear or if they focused on DNA polymorphisms alone. Given the focus on HPV infection, studies were also excluded if they include cervical cancer patients, but no other groups [i.e. normal women, women with low-grade squamous intraepithelial lesions (LSIL) or cervical intraepithelial neoplasia (CIN)]. Studies that included some cervical cancer patients along with CIN or normal patients were retained. Post-treatment studies or studies involving mice, cell lines, or HPV at extra-cervical anatomical sites were excluded as well.

Data were abstracted on the study characteristics, HPV measurement, immune marker measurement, and results pertinent to this review. Study characteristics included the country in which the study was conducted, the method of cervical secretion collection, and descriptions of comparison groups relevant for this review (e.g., women with incident HPV versus no HPV). The assay used to detect HPV was also noted. Immune marker-related data included the assay used to measure the immune marker and the specific markers measured, along with the results. Approximately 50% of studies were double abstracted.

3. Literature review

In total, 35 studies met our inclusion criteria. These studies fell into four broad categories (Tables 1 to 4): circulating immune markers in plasma or serum (N = 7), those secreted locally in the cervix (N = 7), immune responses in patient-derived PBMCs (N = 10), and tissue-based immune markers (N = 12). One study contributed to both the circulating and PBMC-based immune marker categories.

Circulating Immune Markers in Plasma/Serum. Cytokines and soluble immune markers are increasingly being measured in readily accessible plasma and serum in the hope that they will provide useful diagnostic and prognostic information, as well as insight into the pathogenesis of numerous diseases. Further, the availability of inexpensive enzyme-linked immunosorbent assays (ELISAs), radioimmunoassays (RIAs), and other bioassays to reliably measure cytokines in these samples make them enticing targets for discovery. Currently, seven studies that met our inclusion criteria have directly examined HPV-infection-related immune responses in either serum or plasma (Table 1). All of these studies have focused on associations with carcinogenic infection using a Hybrid Capture assay. Hildesheim et al. (Hildesheim, Schiffman et al. 1997) was among the first to use plasma to evaluate markers of immunity. However, their comparison of carcinogenic HPV positive women with low-grade lesions to carcinogenic negative women with low-grade lesions failed to find a statistical difference in the soluble IL-2 receptor (sIL-2R; p=0.63). Adam et al. (Adam, Horowitz et al. 1999) similarly compared 10 women with high risk HPV infection to 10 HPV negative women and reported that high risk HPV infection was indeed associated with higher mean serum CSF-1 levels. Abike et al. (Abike, Engin et al. 2011) measured neopterin, often considered a marker of immune activation, and found lower concentrations in HPV-positive versus HPV-negative women with normal through high-grade histology. Unlike the earlier studies, Bais et al. (Bais 2005) measured numerous cytokines simultaneously (IL-2, IL-4, IL-10, IL-12, IFN-γ, TNF-α), as well as soluble markers (sTNFRI and sTNFRII) in plasma. They discovered that higher mean IL-2 levels alone were associated with carcinogenic HPV positivity. Baker et al. (Baker, Dauner et al. 2011) evaluated eleven circulating markers (adiponectin, resistin, tPAI-1, HGF, TNF-α, leptin, IL-8, sVCAM-1, sICAM-1, sFas, MIF) and found elevated levels of resistin [odds ratio(OR) for 3rd versus 1st tertile, 103.3; 95 confidence interval (CI), 19.3–552.8; P < 0.0001], sFas (OR, 4.2; 95% CI, 1.5–11.7; P = 0.003), IL-8 (OR, 59.8; 95% CI, 11.4–312.5; P < 0.0001), and TNA-α (OR, 38.6; 95% CI, 9.1–164.3, P < 0.0001) were in women with persistent HPV infection compared to HPV-negative women. Kemp et al. (Kemp, Hildesheim et al. 2010) evaluated an even broader spectrum of cytokines in their comparison of 50 HPV-positive women older than 45 years and 50 HPV-negative similarly aged women from their population-based cohort study in Guanacaste, Costa Rica. Plasma levels of IL-2, IL-4, IL-5, IL-6, IL-8, IL-10, IL-13, IL-17, IL-1α, IFN-γ, GM-CSF, TNF-α, MCP-1, MIP-1α, IP-10, RANTES, eotaxin, G-CSF, IL-12, IL-15, IL-7, and IL-1β were measured by Lincoplex assay, IFN-α was measured by bead array, and TGF-β1 was measured by ELISA. Their analysis revealed statistically significant differences between cases and controls in levels of IL-6, IL-8, TNF-α, and MIP-1α, GM-CSF, IL-1β (all P < 0.0001) and IL-1α (P = 0.02). However, it should be noted that this study was intentionally designed to explore differences between the extremes of the immunological spectrum. Thus, differences between these groups are likely to be biased away from the null (upward) in comparison to the general population. All six of these studies failed to concurrently evaluate potential confounders, and with the possible exception of TNF-α, none of their findings have been confirmed by other studies.

Unlike the other studies, Hong et al. (Hong, Kim et al. 2010) evaluated several potential confounders (parity, menopausal status, smoking, oral contraceptive use, histological findings of colposcopic-directed biopsy) in their recently published report of HPV persistence and clearance among 160 carcinogenic HPV positive Korean women (normal women or women with histologically confirmed mild dysplasia). While their univariate analysis revealed that the number of women who were serum negative for TNF-α was significantly higher in the carcinogenic HPV clearance group (N=107) than their persistence group (N=53, P = 0.0363), their multivariate logistic regression analysis indicated that none of the four cytokines measured (IFN-γ, TNF-α, IL-6, and IL-10) had a significant association with clearance of the carcinogenic HPV infection, pointing to the importance of these factors in future study design. In fact, they found that only age was significantly associated with clearance of carcinogenic HPV infections (OR, 0.95; 95% CI, 0.92- 0.98; P = 0.001).

Author & Year	Study source (Origin Country)	Immune Marker	HPV -/+ N (Measurement Method)	Major Conclusions
Hildesheim 1997	Kaiser Permanente clinics (US)	CellFree IL-2R test kits for sIL-2R from plasma recovered by centrifugation of peripheral blood	45/60 (Hybrid Capture)	No statistically significant association between sIL-2R and high risk HPV positivity in plasma.
Adam 1999	Centers for Disease Control collection (United States and Panama)	ELISA for Macrophage colony-stimulating factor (CSF-1) in serum	10/10 (ViraPap + ViraType dot blot hybridization assay for screen positives)	High-risk HPV infection is associated with higher mean serum CSF-1 levels.
Bais 2005	Outpatient GYN clinic (The Netherlands)	ELISA for IL-2, IL-4, IL-10, IL-12, IFN-γ, TNF-α, sTNFRI, sTNFRII in plasma and leucoctye count for leucocytes, neutrophils, monocytes, and lymphocytes in peripheral venous blood	11/10 (GP5+/GP6+ PCR)	High-risk HPV infection is associated with higher mean plasma IL-2 levels.
Hong 2010	University hospital and women's health center (Korea)	ELISA for IFN-γ, IL-6, IL-10, TNF-α in serum	0/160* (Hybrid Capture 2)	Based on univariate analysis, the number of women that were serum negative for TNF-α was significantly higher in the high risk HPV clearance group than the persistence group (P = 0.0363). Based on multivariate logistic regression, none of the 4 cytokines had a significant association with clearance of the high risk HPV infection. Only age was significantly associated with clearance of the high risk HPV infection (OR, 0.950; 95% confidence interval, 0.92-0.98; P = 0.001).**
Kemp 2010	Population-based cohort (Costa Rica)	Linco-plex assay for IL-2, IL-4, IL-5, IL-6, IL-8, IL-10, IL-13, IL-17, IL-1α, IFN-γ, GM-CSF, TNF-α, MCP-1, MIP-1α, IP-10, RANTES, eotaxin, G-CSF, IL-12, IL-15, IL-7, and IL-1β; ELISA for TGF-β1; single analyte in a bead array for IFN-α.	50/50 (MY09/11 PCR, dot blot hybridization for genotyping)	Persistent HPV infection in older women with evidence of immune deficit is associated with an increase in systemic inflammatory cytokines and weak lymphoproliferative responses.
Abike 2011	GYN Department (Turkey)	ELISA for neopterin in serum	78/44 (Amplisense HPV multiplex PCR typing kit)	Neopterin levels were lower in women with HPV than women without HPV.
Baker 2011	Population-based cohort (Costa Rica)	Millipore Multiplex Bead Assay for adiponectin, resistin, tPAI-1, HGF, TNF-α, leptin, IL-8, sVCAM-1, sICAM-1, sFas, MIF in PBMCs from heparinized blood	50/50 (MY09/11 PCR, dot blot hybridization for genotyping)	Resistin, sFas, IL-8, and TNA-α were elevated in women with persistent HPV infection compared to HPV-negative women.

* Compared HPV persistence and clearance. Thus, all were HPV-positive at baseline. **Adjusted for age, parity, menopause, oral contraception, histological findings of colposcopic-directed biopsy, and cytokines. Abbreviations: US = United States, HPV = human papillomavirus, DNA = deoxyribonucleic acid, GYN = Gynecology, PCR = polymerase chain reaction, ELISA = enzyme-linked immunosorbent assay, PBMCs = peripheral blood mononuclear cells

Table 1. Studies of circulating immune markers in plasma and serum.

Local Immune Marker Secretions in the Cervix. It is believed that measurement of cytokines in cervical secretions may better reflect local cytokine production relevant to cervical carcinogenesis than circulating cytokines. Currently, seven studies that met our inclusion criteria have measured immune responses in cervical secretions (Table 2). Unlike the studies of circulating cytokines above, most of these studies have tested for a broad range of HPV types, although one (Guha and Chatterjee, 2009) only tested for carcinogenic HPV types using the Hybrid Capture 2 assay, and another only analyzed results for women with carcinogenic HPV infection compared to women without carcinogenic HPV infection (Marks, Viscidi et al. 2011). Scott et al. (Scott, Stites et al. 1999) evaluated RNA expression of IL-4, IL-12, IFN-γ, and TNF and found that a T-helper type 1 (TH1) cytokine expression pattern (as defined by IFN-γ and TNF positivity and IL-4 negativity, with variable IL-12 expression) preceded HPV clearance. Crowley-Nowick et al. (Crowley-Nowick, Ellenberg et al. 2000) measured IL-2, IL-10, and IL-12 cytokine levels in HIV-positive and HIV-negative adolescents recruited from 16 clinical care settings in 13 US cities. Crowley-Nowick et al. found that HPV-positive girls had higher IL-12 concentrations compared to HPV-negative women (P = 0.01). Race, age, SIL status, smoking, other vaginal infections, and CD4 count were considered as potential confounders, but all were dropped out of the backwards regression model. Tjiong van der Vange et al. (Tjiong 2001) evaluated IL-12p40, IL-10, TGF-β1, TNF-α, and IL-1β levels by HPV status in CIN patients referred to an outpatient gynecology department. Similar to Crowley-Nowick et al., Tjiong van der Vange et al. found higher levels of IL-12 in HPV-positive compared to HPV-negative patients (P=0.04) (Tjiong 2001). However, no attempts were made to adjust for potential confounders. Unlike Crowley-Nowick et al. (Crowley-Nowick, Ellenberg et al. 2000) and Tjiong van der Vange et al. (Tjiong 2001), Gravitt et al. (Gravitt, Hildesheim et al. 2003) found no statistical differences in IL-10 and IL-12 concentrations by HPV-positivity versus HPV-negativity in women selected from a population-based cohort study in Guanacaste, Costa Rica, after adjusting for stage of menstrual cycle, recent oral contraceptive use secretion volume, and pH. Lieberman et al. (Lieberman, Moscicki et al. 2008) used a multiplex immunoassay kit to measure IL-1β, IL-2, IL-4, IL-5, IL-6, IL-8, IL-10, IL-12 (p40/p70), IL-13, IFN-γ in young women attending a family-planning clinic or university health center, or their friends. Although no significant differences were observed for women with incident or persistent HPV infections compared to women without HPV, there was some suggestion that IL-1β and IL-13 levels were reduced in women with incident or persistent HPV infections and that IL-6 and IL-2 levels were reduced in women with incident infections. Guha et al. (Guha and Chatterjee 2009) measured IL-1β, IL-6, IL-10, and IL-12 cytokine levels in commercial sex workers or spouses of HIV-positive men coming in for an HIV test. After taking HIV status into account, IL-1β, IL-10, and IL-12 seemed to be elevated in HPV-positive women compared to HPV-negative women. IL-6 was also higher in HPV-positive women compared to HPV-negative women (P ≤ 0.0004). After stratifying by HIV status, however, IL-6 was only notably elevated in in women positive for both HPV and HIV, making the association with HPV less clear. This study also evaluated cytokine levels by abnormal versus normal cervical cytology and found that only IL-6 was related to abnormal cytology (P = 0.03). Finally, a recent study by Marks et al. (Marks, Viscidi et al. 2011) evaluated 27 different cytokines in a multiplex assay in cervical secretions from 35–60-year-old women attending outpatient obstetrics and gynecology clinics for routine examination. Similar to Gravitt et al. (Gravitt, Hildesheim et al. 2003) and Lieberman et al. (Lieberman, Moscicki et al. 2008), this study found no association between IL-12p70 and HPV status. However, IL-5 (p = 0.03), IL-9 (p = 0.04), IL-13 (p = 0.01), IL-17 (p = 0.003), EOTAXIN (p = 0.04), GM-CSF (p = 0.01), and MIP-1α (p = 0.005) levels were elevated in women with carcinogenic HPV infection compared to those without carcinogenic HPV. In addition, T-cell and pro-inflammatory cytokines tended to be correlated with EOTAXIN in women with carcinogenic HPV, while they were correlated with IL-2 in women without carcinogenic HPV. The authors conclude that this shift from IL-2 to EOTAXIN may reflect a shift away from antigen-specific adaptive responses toward innate responses.

Author & Year	Study source (Origin Country)	Immune Marker Measurement	HPV -/+ N (Measurement Method)	Major Conclusions
Scott 1999	Family planning clinics (US)	RT-PCR of cDNA from total RNA for IL-4, IL-12, IFN-γ, TNF	13/22 (MY09/11 PCR)	HPV-positive subjects (especially those who cleared) tended to be IFN-γ positive, TFN positive, and IL-4 negative ("Th1 cytokine pattern").
Crowley-Nowick 2000	16 clinical care settings in 13 cities (United States)	ELISA for IL-2, IL-10, IL-12 in Weck-cel sponges	18/20 (PCR)	"Coinfection with HIV, human papillomavirus, and other STIs predicted the highest IL-12 concentrations."*
Tjiong 2001	GYN department (The Netherlands)	ELISA for IL-12p40, IFN-γ, IL-10, TGF-β1, TNF-α and IL-1β in cervical washes	13/50 (HPV-16-specific PCR; negative samples confirmed by CPI and CPIIG)	IL-12 was more often detected than in the HPV-DNA negative CIN patients (P=0.04, Chi Square test). No other significant associations between cytokine levels and the detection of HPV-DNA were found.
Gravitt 2003	Population-based cohort (Costa Rica)	ELISA for IL-10 & IL12 in Weck-cel sponges	194/51 (MY09/11 + reverse-blot hybridization	No significant association between HPV and IL-10 or IL-12.**
Lieberman 2007	Family-planning clinic or university health center or friends (US)	Protein Multiplex Immunoassay kits for IL-1β, IL-2, IL-4, IL-5, IL-6, IL-8, IL-10, IL-12 (p40/p70), IL-13, IFN-γ in Merocel sponges	34/33 (PGMY09/11 PCR)	Although there were no significant differences between groups, IL-1β and IL-13 seemed to be depressed in women with incident or persistent HPV infections. IL-6 and IL-2 also seemed to be depressed in women with incident infections.
Guha 2009	Commercial sex workers or spouses of HIV+ men (India)	ELISA for IL-1β, IL-6, IL-10, IL-12 in lavage samples	28/17 (Hybrid Capture 2)	Taking HIV status into account, IL-1β, IL-10, and IL-12 seemed elevated in HPV+ vs. HPV- women. IL-6 seemed elevated when HIV was not taken into account (16.6 vs. 4.5 pg/ml, p≤0.0004), but otherwise was only notably elevated in women positive for both HPV and HIV.†
Marks 2011	Outpatient OB/GYN clinics (US)	Bio-Rad multiplex assay for BASICFGF, EOTAXIN, GCSF, GMCSF, IFN-γ, IL-1β, IL-1ra, IL-2, IL-4, IL-5, IL-6, IL-7, IL-8, IL-9, IL-10, IL-12p70, IL-13, IL-15, IL-17, IP-10, MCP-1, MIP-1α, MIP-1β, PDGF-BB, RANTES, TNF-α, VEGF in Merocel sponges	44/34 (Roche HPV Linear Array)	Carcinogenic HPV associated with elevated IL-5, IL-9, IL-13, IL-17, EOTAXIN, GM-CSF, and MIP-1α levels and a shift from IL-2 to EOTAXIN compared to no carcinogenic HPV, possibly reflecting a shift away from antigen-specific adaptive responses toward innate responses.

*Considered potential confounders, but all were dropped through backwards modeling. †Stratified by HIV status, but did not evaluate additional confounders. Abbreviations: US = United States, HPV = human papillomavirus, HIV = human immunodeficiency virus, CIN = cervical intraepithelial neoplasia, GYN = gynecology, OB/GYN = obstetrics and gynecology, PCR = polymerase chain reaction, qRT-PCR = quantitative reverse transcriptase PCR, STI = sexually transmitted infection

Table 2. Studies of immune markers in cervical secretions.

There is little consistency in the cytokines evaluated in these seven studies, but where there is overlap, the results tend to be contradictory. For example, one study found evidence that IL-6 levels were reduced in women with incident HPV infections (Lieberman, Moscicki et al. 2008), while another found that IL-6 levels tended to be elevated in HPV-positive women (Guha and Chatterjee 2009). Similarly, one study found no evidence that IL-12 levels varied by HPV status (Gravitt, Hildesheim et al. 2003), while two others (Crowley-Nowick, Ellenberg et al. 2000; Tjiong, van der Vange et al. 2001) observed higher levels of IL-12 in HPV-positive versus HPV-negative women. In addition, results from the study by Guha et al. (Guha and Chatterjee 2009) suggested a tendency toward increased levels of IL-1β in HPV-positive women versus HPV-negative women, while the results from Lieberman et al. (Lieberman, Moscicki et al. 2008) showed a trend toward decreased levels of IL-1β in women with incident or persistent HPV infection compared to HPV-negative women. These inconsistencies are not yet resolved.

Cytokine Responses in Patient-derived PBMCs. There is evidence that cell-mediated immune responses play an important role in the control of HPV infections. Cell-mediated immune responses are regulated by T lymphocytes [T-helper (Th) lymphocytes and cytotoxic lymphocytes (CTLs)] in cooperation with antigen-presenting cells such as monocytes and dendritic cells. These cells all are modulated by and release cytokines that can influence one another's synthesis. Characterization (including quality and quantity) of lymphocytes directed against HPV epitopes has been examined with the goal of providing insights into the clinical outcomes of HPV-positive patients. To this end, analyses of cytokines and concurrent lymphoproliferative and CTL responses in patient-derived peripheral blood mononuclear cells (PBMCs), T-cell fractions isolated from PBMCs or whole blood cultures after stimulation with several antigens and/or HPV peptides has been evaluated in 10 publications (Table 3).

Tsukui et al. (Tsukui, Hildesheim et al. 1996) was one of the first to measure IL-2 levels in culture supernatants of PBMCs stimulated with predominantly 15mer overlapping peptides from HPV-16 E6 and E7 oncoproteins. The HPV early proteins E2, E6 and E7 are among the first of proteins that are expressed in HPV-infected epithelia. Stimulation with influenza served as a specificity control, and stimulation with phytohemagglutinin (PHA) served as a positive control since it is known to activate lymphocytes and induce rapid cell proliferation as well as lead to the release of inflammatory and immune cytokines. While the report itself focused on associations with IL-2 and disease progression, the study included both HPV typing data and IL-2 response data for each subject included in the study. Interestingly, by using the data presented in the paper for statistical calculation, we found that IL-2 levels were significantly increased in a group of 32 HPV positive healthy women and women with LSIL compared to a group of 51 HPV negative healthy women and women with LSIL (P=0.006). Among 18 women with HSIL with HPV typing and adequate IL-2 data, only 2 women had positive IL-2 levels (1 HPV positive, 1 HPV negative).

Several other studies also attempted to evaluate IL-2 levels in a similar manner. deGruijl et al. (de Gruijl, Bontkes et al. 1998) examined IL-2 reactivity in PBMCs stimulated with HPV16 E7 and sorted by anti-CD4 or anti-CD8 antibodies. They found that positive CD4+ T helper cell IL-2 reactivity was restricted to patients infected by HPV16 and related types and that reactivity was strongly associated with HPV persistence. Further, women with cervical carcinoma showed IL-2 responses at a significantly reduced rate [7 of 15 (47%); P = 0.014].

Author & Year	Study source (Origin Country)	Immune Marker Measurement	HPV -/+ N (Measurement Method)	Major Conclusions
Tsukui 1996	Kaiser Permanent or Simmons Cancer Center (US)	IL-2 was measured by radioimmunoassay in culture supernatants of PBMCs from whole blood that were stimulated with 15mer HPV16 peptides to E6 and E7, or stimulated with FLU or PHA	56/40 (ViraPap: Hybrid Capture with HPV-16-specific Hybrid Capture for + samples. Tumors: GP5+/GP6+ PCR)	IL-2 is signficantly increased in healthy HPV+ women and HPV+ women with LSIL. Few women with HSIL or cancer have detectable IL-2 levels.
Kadish 1997	Colposcopy clinic (US)	Measured lymphocyte proliferation in HPV16 E6 and E7 peptide stimulated cultures of PBMCs from heparinized blood	26/51 (PCR and Southern Blot assay; typing by dot blot for 39 types)	Lymphoproliferative responses to specific HPV16 E6 and E7 peptides are significantly associated with the clearance of HPV infection.
de Gruijl 1998	Non-intervention cohort follow-up study of patients with cervical dysplasia plus follow-up study of HPV-positive women with normal cervical cytology (Netherlands)	IL-2 was measured by IL-2 bioassay in culture supernatants of PBMCs from heparinized blood that were stimulated with 14 different 20mer HPV16 peptides to E7, or stimulated with PHA; T cell subsets were depleted by magnetic bead sorting and anti-CD4 and anti-CD8 antibodies	15/51 (GP5+/GP6+ PCR)	Positive CD4+ T helper cell IL-2 reactivity was restricted to patients infected by HPV-16 and related types and showed a strong association with viral persistence. Women with cervical carcinoma showed IL-2 responses at a significantly reduced rate [7 of 15 (47%); P = 0.014].
Bontkes 1999	Non-intervention cohort follow-up study of patients with cervical dysplasia (Netherlands)	IL-2 was measured by IL-2 bioassay in culture supernatants of PBMCs from heparinized blood that were stimulated with HPV16 N-terminal and C-terminal E2 protein fragments or with PHA.	22/52 (GP5+/GP6+ PCR)	HPV16 infection was not associated with IL-2 responsiveness against the N-terminal domain of E2, but HPV clearance was associated with IL-2 responsiveness against the C-terminal E2 domain
de Gruijl 1999	Non-intervention cohort follow-up study of patients with cervical dysplasia (Netherlands)	IL-2 was measured by IL-2 bioassay in culture supernatants of PBMCs from heparinized blood that were stimulated with HPV16 L1-VLP or synthetic L1-derived 15-mer peptides P1 (amino acids 311-325) and P2 (amino acids 321-335), or stimulated with PHA; T cell subsets were depleted by magnetic bead sorting and anti-CD4 or CD8 antibodies. HPV-16 L1-VLP-specic plasma IgG was measured by ELISA.	15/49 (GP5+/GP6+ PCR)	IgG responses were significantly associated with HPV16 persistence but CD4 T helper IL-2 responses were significantly associated with both HPV clearance and persistence. Neither cell-mediated nor humoral immune responses against HPV16 L1 seemed adequate for viral control.

Abbreviations: US = United States, HPV = human papillomavirus, DNA = deoxyribonucleic acid, GYN = Gynecology, PCR = polymerase chain reaction, ELISA = enzyme-linked immunosorbent assay, PBMCs = peripheral blood mononuclear cells, FLU = influenæ, PHA = phytohemagglutinin, LSIL = low grade squamous intraepithelial lesion, HSIL = high grade squamous intraepithelial lesion, mCTLp = memory cytotoxic T-cell precursor

Table 3. Part 1. Cytokine Responses in Patient-derived PBMCs.

Author & Year	Study source (Origin Country)	Immune Marker Measurement	HPV -/+ N (Measurement Method)	Major Conclusions
Bontkes 2000	Non-intervention cohort follow-up study of patients with cervical dysplasia (Netherlands)	HPV16-specific mCTLp activity was measured in cultured PBMCs from heparinized blood stimulated with both HPV16 E6 and E7 peptides. IL-2 was measured by IL-2 bioassay in culture supernatants of PBMCs that were stimulated with 14 different 20mer HPV16 peptides to E7, or stimulated with PHA.	11/20 (GP5+/GP6+ PCR)	mCTLp activity was significantly associated with persistent HPV16 infection but not observed in HPV negative women or women with viral clearance. HPV16 E7-specific mCTLp activity was associated with previously published IL-2 release in response to HPV 16 E7-derived peptides at the end of follow-up.
Molling 2007	Non-intervention cohort follow-up study of patients with cervical dysplasia (Netherlands)	Cultured PBMCs taken from heparinized blood were stimulated with 14 different 20mer HPV16 E7 peptides or with PHA. IL-2 levels were determined by bioassay. CTL activity determined by chromium release assay. iNKT and Treg counts were measured by FACS. FoxP3 staining was performed using an available kit. Lymphocytes were characterized by staining with monoclonal antibodies.	2458 (GP5+/GP6+ PCR and type specific PCR for 27 types)	Treg frequencies significantly increased in women with persistent HPV16 infection. Treg frequencies were increased in patients who had detectable HPV16 E7 specific IL-2 producing T-helper cells, suggesting HPV may affect Treg development. No evidence that iNKT cells affect persistence of HPV16 infection.
Seresini 2007	Healthy donors and women with cervical lesions (Italy)	CD4+ T cells were purified from cultured PBMCs from peripheral blood stimulated with HPV18 E6 peptides or PHA and CTL activity was measured by chromium release assay as well as IL-4, IL-5, IL-10 and IFN-γ levels using cytometric bead array kits. The immune infiltrates in cervical lesions were also evaluated.	25/37 (Hybrid Capture 2 and typing by reverse hybridization assay)	One or more HPV18 E6 peptides were observed to be able to induce a response in 40-50% of the women evaluated. Response percentages increased to 80-100% when HPV18+ women alone were considered. Levels of IFN-γ released were shown to predict HPV persistence and/or disease relapse after surgery. A higher number of infiltrating CD4(+) and T-bet(+) T cells were observed in the lesions which correlated with favorable clinical outcomes.
Sharma 2007	Outpatient department or cancer clinic (India)	IL-2, IFN-γ, IL-4, and IL-10 was measured by ELISA in cultured PBMCs from heparinized blood stimulated with PHA	30/84 (HPV16 and HPV 18 PCR)	Increasing levels of IL-4 and IL-10 levels were significantly associated with HPV infection. Decreasing levels of IL-2 and IFN-γ were associated with HPV status.
Kemp 2010	Population-based cohort (Costa Rica)	Linco-plex assay for IL-6, IL-8, TNF-α, MIP-1α in unstimulated and PHA stimulated PBMCs	50/50 (MY09/11 PCR, dot blot hybridization for genotyping)	IL-6, TNF-α, MIP-1α levels were significantly higher in unstimulated PBMCs from HPV+ and HPV- women; IL-6, IL-8, TNF-α and MIP-1α levels were significantly lower in PHA stimulated PBMCs between HPV+ and HPV- women

Abbreviations: US = United States, HPV = human papillomavirus, DNA = deoxyribonucleic acid, GYN = Gynecology, PCR = polymerase chain reaction, ELISA = enzyme-linked immunosorbent assay, PBMCs = peripheral blood mononuclear cells, FLU = influenza, PHA = phytohemagglutinin, LSIL = low grade squamous intraepithelial lesion, HSIL = high grade squamous intraepithelial lesion, mCTLp = memory cytotoxic T-cell precursor

Table 3. Part 2. Cytokine Responses in Patient-derived PBMCs.

These findings are consistent with Tsukui et al. (Tsukui, Hildesheim et al. 1996) and suggest that IL-2 responsiveness may differ by cytological and/or disease stage. In 1999, deGruijl et al. (de Gruijl, Bontkes et al. 1999) again evaluated IL-2 levels, as well as IgG responses, in this same population. This time, they used HPV16 L1-VLP or synthetic L1-derived 15-mer peptides P1 (amino acids 311-325) and P2 (amino acids 321-335) to stimulate the PBMCs and sorted them as before. Importantly, they found IgG responsiveness was significantly associated with HPV16 persistence alone, but that CD4 T helper IL-2 responsiveness was significantly associated with both HPV clearance and persistence. Further, they reported that neither cell-mediated nor humoral immune responses against HPV16 L1 seemed adequate for viral control. In another publication, this group took their study one step further and measured IL-2 levels in response to HPV E2 N-terminal and C-terminal protein fragments (Bontkes, de Gruijl et al. 1999). They reported that HPV16 infection was not associated with IL-2 responsiveness against the N-terminal domain of E2, but HPV clearance was associated with IL-2 responsiveness against the C-terminal E2 domain. The following year, Bontkes et al. (Bontkes, de Gruijl et al. 2000) evaluated HPV 16 E6- and E7-specific memory cytotoxic T-cell precursor (mCTLp) activity in the same cohort of patients with cervical dysplasia. They found that activity was significantly associated with persistent HPV16 infection but not observed in HPV negative women or women with viral clearance. Kadish et al. (Kadish, Ho et al. 1997) had previously observed a similar phenomenon. Subjects with positive lymphoproliferative responses to E6 and/or E7 peptides were more likely to be HPV negative at the same clinic visit than were nonresponders (P = 0.039). Subjects who were negative for HPV and those with a low viral load were also more likely to respond than were those with a high viral load (P for trend = 0.037). These data suggest that lymphoproliferative responses to specific HPV 16 E6 and E7 peptides appear to be associated with the clearance of HPV infection.

In 2007, three additional reports evaluating patient-derived PBMCs were published. Sharma et al. (Sharma, Rajappa et al. 2007) focused on IL-2, IFN-g, IL-4, and IL-10 levels in PBMCs stimulated with PHA. They observed that increasing levels of IL-4 and IL-10 levels were significantly associated with HPV infection and that decreasing levels of IL-2 and IFN-γ were associated with HPV status. Seresini et al. (Seresini, Origoni et al. 2007) measured lymphoproliferative responses and IL-2, IFN-g, IL-4, and IL-10 levels in PBMCs stimulated not with HPV16 peptides, but rather with HPV18-specific E6 peptides. Their analyses revealed that one or more HPV18 E6 peptides were able to induce a response in 40-50% of the women evaluated. Response percentages increased to 80-100% when HPV18-positive women alone were considered. Levels of IFN-γ released were also shown to predict HPV persistence and/or disease relapse after surgery. In addition, they showed that a higher number of infiltrating CD4(+) and T-bet(+) T cells in lesions correlated with favorable clinical outcomes. Finally, Molling et. al. (Molling, de Gruijl et al. 2007) evaluated cultured PBMCs again stimulated with 14 different 20mer HPV16 E7 peptides or with PHA and measured both IL-2 levels and CTL activity. Importantly, they also measured invariant natural killer T-cells (iNKT) and FoxP3+ regulatory T cells (Tregs) levels by flow cytometry (FACSCalibur). While iNKT cells did not appear to be associated with HPV persistence, Treg frequencies were significantly increased in women with persistent HPV16 infection; and the Tregs were significantly more common in women who had detectable HPV16 E7 specific IL-2 producing T-helper cells. These data suggest that HPV infection may affect Treg development – a finding that opens the door for a whole new avenue of research related to HPV-related immune research.

Immune Markers in Cervical Tissues   PBMC responses and circulating or secreted cytokines can be useful indicators of immune response, but the best indications may come from the actual site of interaction between HPV infection and the immune system: tissue. A number of studies have attempted to measure immune markers in HPV-positive compared to HPV-negative women in different ways. Among studies included in this review, these markers fall into three major categories: immune presentation molecules, cytokines or cytokine receptors, and immune cells.

Several studies used immunohistochemistry (IHC) to stain for major histocompatibility complex (MHC) proteins in cervical tissue (Table 4). MHC class I molecules present endogenous antigens (cytoplasmic proteins) to cytotoxic (CD8+) T cells and are typically present on all nucleated cells (Murphy, Travers et al. 2011). In contrast, MHC class II molecules present exogenous antigens from outside the cell to helper (CD4+) T cells and are typically present only on antigen presenting cells, such as dendritic cells and macrophages. Thus, normal cervical epithelial cells should be MHC class I positive and MHC class II negative. In humans, MHC class I consists of major human leukocyte antigens (HLA) A, B, and C and minor antigens E, F, and G, while MHC class II consists of HLA-DM, -DO, -DP, -DQ, and -DR.

Using a polyclonal stain specific for HLA-A, -B and -C heavy chains in formalin-fixed, paraffin-embedded (FFPE) tissue from biopsies and resection specimens from women with CIN1-3 or cancer, Cromme et al. (Cromme, Meijer et al. 1993) found that normal MHC class I expression, defined positive staining in ≥75% of cells, was reduced in women with HPV16, 18, or 31 infection versus HPV-negative women (p=0.04). MHC class II expression, as measured through a polyclonal HLA-DR antigen stain, was also altered, with normal staining (<25% positively stained cells) in 42% of women with HPV16, 18, or 31 infection versus 64% of HPV-negative women. This alteration was not statistically significant, however (p=0.14). Gonclaves el al (Goncalves, Le Discorde et al. 2008) also examined MHC class I expression in FFPE biopsy blocks, but in women with normal through cancerous histology. They found that HLA-A/B/C expression was not significantly elevated in HPV-positive compared to HPV-negative women (OR, 2.29; 95% CI, 0.77- 11.00; P = 0.14). Strangely, HPV16/18 infection was inversely associated with HLA-A/B/C expression (OR, 0.12; 95% CI, 0.02- 0.79; P = 0.04), but as reported, it was unclear whether this association was based on comparison to HPV-negative women, or a combination of both HPV-negative women and women with HPV infections other than HPV16 and 18. HLA-E expression tended to be increased in HPV-positive versus HPV-negative women (OR, 3.83; 95% CI, 0.49-30.10; P = 0.22), especially for HPV16/18 infections (OR, 11.25; 95% CI: 2.32-55.47; P = 0.003). Similarly, Dong et al. (Dong, Yang et al. 2010) stained for HLA-G in FFPE blocks from CIN1-3 patients and found higher HLA-G expression in HPV16/18-positive patients than HPV16/18-negative patients (P = 0.02).

In addition to interaction with an antigen MHC complex, T-cells require costimulation with an antigen nonspecific molecule to be full activated. T cells that encounter antigen MHC complex without costimulation may be come anergic and thus tolerant to the presence of HPV. To investigate this possibility, Ortiz-Sanchez et al. (Ortiz-Sanchez, Chavez-Olmos et al. 2007) evaluated expression of the CD80 and CD86 MHC class II costimulatory molecules through immunohistochemistry (IHC), quantitative reverse transcriptase PCR (qRT-PCR), and RNA in situ hybridization (ISH) in FFPE biopsies from histologically normal HPV-negative women and HPV16-positive women with LSIL. They found that CD86, but not CD80, was expressed in all HPV-negative normal cervical epithelial samples, while CD86

Author & Year	Study source (Origin Country)	Immune Marker Measurement	HPV-/+ N (Measurement Method)	Major Conclusions
Cromme 1993	Oncological GYN ouapatient department (Netherlands)	IHC for MHC-I & MHC-II expression in FFPE tissue from biopsies & resection specimens	14/107 (GP 5/6 PCR + TS PCR for HPV6, 11, 16, 18, 31, 33; RNA ISH for HPV16 E7)	Normal MHC-I expression reduced in women with HPV16, 18, or 31 vs. HPV-negative women (p=0.04). MHC-II expression was also altered with HPV16/18/31, but not significantly.
Fernandes 2005	Outpatient GYN Clinic (Brazil)	Double-sandwich ELISA for IFN-γ, TNF-α, IL-10 in snap frozen cervical biopsies	0/42 (GP5/6, MY09/11, HPV16E7.667/HPV16E7.774, HPV18E7.696/HPV18E7.799 PCRs)*	HPV16 associated with higher IL-10 and IFN-γ intralesional levels than other HPV types, but HPV18 was associated with reduced TNF-α and INF-γ levels. Thus, immune response may vary by HPV type.
Ortiz-Sanchez 2007	Women undergoing a routine hysterectomy due to uterine myomatosis and women with LSIL (Mexico)	IHC, qRT-PCR, ISH for CD80 and 86; IHC for IL10 in FFPE biopsies	30/30 (MY09/11 and p16-1 and p16-2R primer PCR. HPV typing by sequence comparison. Only the HPV-16 samples included in CD86 expression analysis.)	CD86 expression was decreased in patients with HPV16 positive LSIL versus normal women, independent of IL-10. Expression of CD86 on normal cervical keratinocytes could indicate the ability to activate cytotoxic T cells, while the shut-off of this molecule in HPV-16 positive lesions could be a mechanism for evading host immune surveillance, resulting in the persistent HPV infection and probable progression of cervical lesions.
Song 2007	OB/GYN clinic (Republic of Korea)	qRT-PCR for IL-6, IL-10, IFN-γ, TNF-α in frozen tissue biopsies	0/67 (Hybrid Capture 2 + HPV DNA Chip)*	IFN-γ was significantly associated with HPV-16 E6, E7, and high-risk HPV viral load among HPV-positive women.**
Bermudez-Morales 2008	Instituto Nacional de Cancerologia (National Cancerology Institute, Mexico)	RT-PCR for IL-10 in cervical scraping and biopsies (storage not specified)	28/47 (PCR-RFLPs)	Strong association between HPV positivity and IL10 mRNA levels
Butsch Kovacic 2008	The ASCUS/LSIL Triage Study for Cervical Cancer (ALTS) trial (US)	Visual counting of lymphocytes, neutrophils, macrophages, plasma cells, and eosinophils in 3 H&E sections per biopsy (stromal and epithelial sections of hematoxylin and eosin stain slides from FFPE biopsy tissue evaluated)	228/288 (Hybrid Capture 2 and PCR)	These data suggest that cervical inflammation varies with type of human papillomavirus infection, risk of persistence and progression and HPV cofactors.**

*Evaluated cytokine expression by HPV type in HPV-positive women. **Study adjusted for confounding factors in regression models. †Compared HPV persistence and clearance. Thus, all were HPV-positive at baseline. Abbreviations: HPV= human papillomavirus, CIN= cervical intraepithelial neoplasia, FFPE= formalin-fixed paraffin-embedded, GYN= gynecology, ISH= in situ hybridization, IHC= Immunohistochemistry, OB/GYN= obstetrics and gynecology, qRT-PCR= quantitative reverse transcriptase PCR, STI= sexually transmitted infection, TIL= tumor infiltrating lymphocytes, RFLPs= Restriction Fragment Length Polymorphisms, ASCUS = Atypical Squamous Cells of Undetermined Significance, LSIL= low grade squamous intraepithelial lesion, HSIL= high grade squamous intraepithelial lesion, US = United States

Table 4. Part 1. Immune Markers in Cervical Tissues.

Author & Year	Study source (Origin Country)	Immune Marker Measurement	HPV -/+ N (Measurement Method)	Major Conclusions
Gonclaves 2008	GYN Reference Services (Brazil)	IHC for HLA-A/B/C and HLA-E in RNA from FFPE biopsy blocks	19/55 (GP5+/6+, MY09/11, HPV16E7.667/ HPV16E7.774, HPV18E7.696/ HPV18E7.799)	Some evidence that HPV infection was associated with increased HLA-E expression, especially HPV16/18 infection. Association with HLA-A/B/C was less clear.
Song 2008	OB/GYN clinic (Republic of Korea)	qRT-PCR for IL-6, IL-10, IFN-γ, TNF-α from frozen tissue biopsies	0/57 (Hybrid Capture 2)†	IFN-γ correlated with high-risk HPV clearance.**
Tirone 2009	Women with CIN or normal women with hysterectomies due to uterine myoma (Brazil)	RT-PCR for IFNAR 1, IFNAR 2, 2'5OAS, IFN-α from cervical tissue biopsies	31/14 (Hybrid Capture 2)	Lower IFN-α receptor expression with HPV infection.
Brismar Wendel 2010	Healthy volunteers at Karolinska Division of Obstetrics and Gynecology (Sweden)	qRT-PCR for CD3, CD4, CD8, CD19, CD27, CCR5, CCL5/Rantes, IL-2, IL-4, IL-10, IL-12a, IL-17a, IL-7R, HLA-DRα, IFN-γ, TNF-β, PD-1, CTLA-4, LAG3, IgA, IgG from frozen biopsy of ectocervix outside the transformation zone	13/11 (Roche Linear Array)	HPV not associated with a local inflammatory immune response as measured by qRT-PCR
Dong 2010	Department of Pathology (China)	IHC for HLA-G and visual counting of TILs in 5 high-power fields from FFPE blocks	22/33 (ISH for HPV16 & 18 in FFPE tissue section)	HLA-G elevated in HPV16/18+ lesions and associated with lower TIL counts, suggesting inhibition of immune response against HPV.
Øvestad 2011	Women refered to a hospital for abnormal Papanicolaou tests (Norway)	IHC for CD4, CD8, CD25, from RNA isolated from paraffin blocks of punch biopsies CD138, FOXp3	0/45 (AMPLICOR and Linear Array)*	HPV16 and related types were correlated with lower CD8-positive cell counts in the stroma compared to other HPV types.**

*Evaluated cytokine expression by HPV type in HPV-positive women. **Study adjusted for confounding factors in regression models. †Compared HPV persistence and clearance. Thus, all were HPV-positive at baseline. Abbreviations: HPV=human papillomavirus, CIN=cervical intraepithelial neoplasia, FFPE=formalin-fixed paraffin-embedded, GYN=gynecology, ISH=in situ hybridization, IHC=Immunohistochemistry, OB/GYN= obstetrics and gynecology, qRT-PCR=quantitative reverse transcriptase PCR, STI=sexually transmitted infection, TIL=tumor infiltrating lymphocytes, RFLPs=Restriction Fragment Length Polymorphisms, ASCUS=Atypical Squamous Cells of Undetermined Significance, LSIL=low grade squamous intraepithelial lesion, HSIL=high grade squamous intraepithelial lesion, US=United States

Table 4. Part 2. Immune Markers in Cervical Tissues.

expression was lower (73% by IHC) in HPV16-positive LSIL samples. This decrease in CD86 expression in HPV-positive women could represent and immune evasion mechanisms through the down-regulation of costimulatory molecules.

The next major category of immune markers measured in cervical tissue includes cytokines and their receptors. In addition to testing for MHC costimulatory molecules, Ortiz-Sanchez et al. (Ortiz-Sanchez, Chavez-Olmos et al. 2007) used IHC to stain for IL-10, which inhibits CD86 expression. IL-10 detection was likewise poor in both HPV-negative normal tissue and HPV16-positive LSIL tissue, but detection was higher in a high-grade SIL (HSIL) control sample. Fernandez et al. 2005 tested for IFN-γ, TNF-α, and IL-10 protein from snap frozen cervical biopsies from HIV-positive or HIV-negative LSIL and HSIL patients infected with HPV using a double-sandwich ELISA approach. They reported that HPV16 was associated with higher IL-10 (P = 0.03) and IFN-γ (P = 0.04) intra-lesional levels than other HPV types, but HPV18 was associated with reduced TNF-α (P = 0.009) and INF-γ levels (P = 0.01) suggesting that immune responses may vary by the infecting HPV type.

The majority of studies measured cytokines with quantitative reverse transcriptase PCR (qRT-PCR). Bermudez-Morales et al. (Bermudez-Morales, Gutierrez et al. 2008) found a strong association between HPV positivity and IL10 mRNA levels, especially for HPV16. Song et al. evaluated IL-6, IL-10, IFN-γ, and TNF-α and both HPV16 positivity (Song, Lee et al. 2008.) and HPV clearance versus persistence (Song 2008) among women positive for carcinogenic HPV. They found that IFN-γ was associated with HPV-16 *E6* (OR, 28.20; 95% CI, 2.66-299.11) and *E7* (OR, 19.62; 95% CI, 2.14-180.25) expression (Song, Lee et al. 2007), as well as with clearance of carcinogenic HPV (OR, 8.26; 95% CI: 1.24-54.94) (Song, Lee et al. 2008.). Tirone et al. (Tirone, Peghini et al. 2009) found some evidence that the IFN-α receptor subunits IFNAR 1 and IFNAR 2 were under-expressed in HPV-positive women with CIN1-3 compared to HPV-negative women with normal through CIN3 histology. Brismar Wendel et al. (Brismar Wendel, Kaldensjo et al. 2010) measured a number of different cytokines and other immune markers and found no difference between HPV-positive and HPV-negative healthy volunteers (22/24 with normal cytology).

Another major category of immune markers is the immune cells themselves. Two studies in this review evaluated infiltrating immune cells in cervical tissue by visually counting the cells. Butsch Kovacic et al. (Butsch Kovacic, Katki et al. 2008) counted lymphocytes, neutrophils, macrophages, plasma cells, and eosinophils among women with typical squamous cells of undetermined significance or LSIL and found that cervical inflammation varies with type of HPV infection, as well as risk of persistence and progression. Women with carcinogenic HPV infections also had more severe epithelial inflammation and less severe stromal inflammation than HPV-negative women. These associations were limited to carcinogenic and not the non-carcinogenic HPV types. Dong et al. (Dong, Yang et al. 2010) determined that among HPV16/18-positive CIN lesions, moderate to strong HLA-G expression was associated with weak immune response, as measured by few tumor infiltrating lymphocytes (TIL), whereas weak HLA-G expression was associated with strong immune response (high numbers of TIL). HLA-G expression was not associated with TIL in HPV-negative women, suggesting that the increased HLA-G expression in HPV-positive lesion may reflect an inhibition of immune response against HPV. Brismar Wendel et al. (Brismar Wendel, Kaldensjo et al. 2010) used qRT-PCR to measure CD3, CD4, CD8, CD19, and CD27 expression but found no difference by HPV status. Finally, Øvestad et al. (Ovestad, Vennestrom et al. 2011) used IHC to stain for cell surface marker in biopsies from CIN2-3 patients and found that HPV16 and related types were correlated with lower CD8-positive cell counts in the stroma compared to other HPV types (P = 0.02).

4. Conclusions and future perspectives

Taken together, these studies support the role of cell-mediated immune response in HPV-related carcinogenesis although their findings, particularly for those measuring cytokines, are largely inconsistent. There are many potential explanations. There has been a real lack of consistency in sample collection methods, cytokine measurement methods and even the outcome definitions used for analyses.

For example, some studies assessed HPV positivity, regardless of timing and/or disease state, while others evaluated incident HPV infection or HPV persistence or clearance. Further, these studies more than often focused on HPV 16, on carcinogenic HPV types, or any HPV type infection together. However, those few studies that did evaluate immune markers by individual HPV type found evidence that immune responses vary by HPV type (Fernandes, Gonçalves et al. 2005; Butsch Kovacic, Katki et al. 2008; Ovestad, Vennestrom et al. 2011). Thus, HPV type is an important consideration. Moreover, while we chose to focus on immune markers' associations with HPV infection, most of the studies reviewed in this chapter predominantly assessed associations between immune markers and disease state (LSIL, HSIL, cancer or CIN1-3 and cancer). Ideally, future studies would evaluate differences by individual HPV type and better consider the timing of disease.

There are also other notable differences in the study populations considered by these studies (e.g., sample size, young versus old women, inclusion of HIV-positive women). Many studies used convenience samples of women. In fact, there is a general lack of consideration for factors that could confound or modify both cytokine production and the infectious outcomes. Only eight of the 35 studies made any attempt to account for co-factors that may influence cytokine level. The importance of adjusting for such potential confounders was recently highlighted at an international workshop that addressed best practices for sampling techniques and assessment of mucosal immune responses. The workshop identified a number of characteristics that should be considered when studying female genital tract immunity, including age, race, body mass index, sexually transmitted infections, other genital tract infections, vaginal flora, alcohol or substance use, recent immunization, pregnancy, phase of menstrual cycle, genital inflammation, recent douching, gynecologic procedures, recent intercourse/semen, and contraception (Anderson and Cu-Uvin 2011). The number of women included in each study is another important consideration in the evaluation of these studies. Twenty-two of the 32 (69%) studies meeting our criteria included less than 30 women in one or more groups (e.g., the HPV-positive or HPV-negative group). Fifteen (47%) included less than 20 in one or more groups. Small numbers of women in the comparison groups can lead to unstable results and may help explain why results for individual immune markers are so inconsistent.

Most studies have measured only a few cytokines, and few have evaluated infiltrating immune cells concurrently with cytokines, making it challenging to explore the activation pathways of cells involved in the immune response against HPV. One research group has made extensive use of their study population to characterize several aspects of immune response as measured in PBMCs (de Gruijl, Bontkes et al. 1998; Bontkes, de Gruijl et al. 1999; de Gruijl, Bontkes et al. 1999; Bontkes, de Gruijl et al. 2000; Molling, de Gruijl et al. 2007). However, few studies have been so thorough. In fact, more than half of the studies of PBMCs (five of nine studies), have come from this same research group with the same study population. Additional studies characterizing many aspects of immune response in different study populations would help clarify whether the results are broadly applicable.

Many studies focused on T-helper type 1 (TH1) versus T-helper type 2 (TH2) polarization, using a single cytokine (or small group of cytokines) to characterize the T-helper phenotype. However, advances in immunology have led to the shift of the TH1/TH2 paradigm to the TH1/TH2/TH17/T-reg hypothesis, a multi-lineage commitment from the same T-helper precursor cells. TH17 cells, in fact, have been shown to inhibit both TH1 and TH2 cells, and therefore are likely to play a critical role in HPV-related immune responses as well. Few studies have evaluated TH17 or Treg cells. The recent study by Molling et al. (Molling, de Gruijl et al. 2007) is among the few that have measured these cells. Using flow cytometry in HPV16 E7 stimulated PBMCs, they determined that Treg frequencies were significantly greater in women with persistent HPV16 infection and in women with detectable HPV16 E7 specific IL-2 producing T-helper cells, suggesting that HPV infection may affect Treg development. These findings may also be supported by tissue-based studies of MHC class II expression. Although data are limited, one study found evidence of increased MHC class II expression in HPV-positive versus negative patients (Cromme, Meijer et al. 1993), while another found reduced expression of the CD86 MHC class II costimulatory molecule (Ortiz-Sanchez, Chavez-Olmos et al. 2007). It could be hypothesized that HPV upregulates MHC class II expression and down-regulates MHC class II costimulatory molecules in order to increase T-cell anergy through incomplete signaling. Additional studies are needed to better understand these relationships.

For studies of cervical secretions, the collection method can have a large impact on the results. Of the seven cervical secretion studies included in this review, two collected cervical secretions through cervicovaginal lavage (Tjiong, van der Vange et al. 2001; Guha and Chatterjee 2009), four used Weck-cel® (Crowley-Nowick, Ellenberg et al. 2000; Gravitt, Hildesheim et al. 2003) or Merocel® (Lieberman, Moscicki et al. 2008; Marks, Viscidi et al. 2011) ophthalmic sponges, and one used cytobrush sample suspensions (Scott, Stites et al. 1999). Cervicovaginal lavages may not be specific enough to the cervix and may overly dilute the specimen. Even studies that used ophthalmic sponges tended to use Weck-cel® sponges (Gravitt, Hildesheim et al. 2003; Moscicki, Ellenberg et al. 2004), which may not provide adequate cytokine recovery, especially compared to Merocel® sponges (Castle et al.(Castle, Rodriguez et al. 2004).

Studies evaluating tissue have seldom considered both stroma and epithelium. In this chapter, only two studies examined inflammation in both stroma and epithelium (Butsch Kovacic, Katki et al. 2008; Ovestad, Vennestrom et al. 2011). One study found opposite inflammatory patterns by HPV status ((Butsch Kovacic, Katki et al. 2008)). This study also found that neutrophils tended to be found only in the superficial epithelial layers, whereas mononuclear cells were found mainly near the basement membrane, suggesting that inflammatory patterns in the stroma and the epithelium may depend on the specific cell type. The second study only reported differences by CD8 in the stroma (Øvestad 2011).

Tissue-based studies of cytokines are also heterogeneous. Only two studies evaluated cytokine proteins in tissue (Fernandes, Gonçalves et al. 2005; Ortiz-Sanchez, Chavez-Olmos et al. 2007). It is not surprising that few studies have evaluated cytokine proteins in tissue since it can be challenging to find an appropriate antibody and optimize the assay. For example, antibodies that perform well in western blots may not work for staining since staining requires fixation, which can change the confirmation of the cytokine protein, thereby preventing antibody binding (Sachdeva and Asthana 2007). Most tissue-based studies of cytokines in this review measured RNA expression, but accurate measurement of RNA expression requires high quality tissue. If the tissue was not snap frozen immediately after surgery and well maintained, endogenous RNases may have degraded the RNA. RNA quality is rarely addressed. Although the presence of cytokine transcripts in tissue may be meaningful, the absence is not given the short-lived nature of RNA, even for high quality tissues (Sachdeva and Asthana 2007).

To clarify the role of immune response in cervical carcinogenesis, future studies should be conducted in well-characterized epidemiologic studies that can address most or all of the characteristics and considerations described above. Studies should include large numbers of women, evaluate a broader spectrum of cytokines/immune markers and measure and adjust for potential confounders concurrently. Possible usefulness of tissue microarrays and multiplex arrays with well-defined phenotypes should be considered as they are likely to make these studies more feasible. Emerging results must be repeated in different study populations and specimen types, but are encouraging. Accumulating evidence indicates that there is a cell-mediated immune response to HPV. As technologies improve, it should become possible to better characterize these responses to distinguish between women at risk of developing cervical cancer and women who can effectively resolve their HPV infections.

5. Appendix 1. Search strategy for immune function in cervical carcinogenesis

("humans"[MeSH Terms] AND "female"[MeSH Terms] AND English[lang]) AND ("cervix uteri"[MeSH Terms] OR "Uterine Cervical Neoplasms/immunology"[Mesh] OR "Uterine Cervical Neoplasms/pathology"[Mesh] OR "Uterine Cervical Neoplasms/blood" [Mesh] OR "Cervical Intraepithelial Neoplasia/metabolism"[Mesh] OR "Mucus/metabolism" [Mesh]) AND ("Cytokines/blood*"[Mesh] OR "Cytokines/metabolism"[Mesh] OR "Immunity, Innate"[Mesh] OR "Adaptive Immunity"[Mesh] OR "Immunity, Cellular"[Mesh] OR "Immunity, Humoral"[Mesh] OR "Immunity, Mucosal"[Mesh] OR "Immunity, Innate/immunology"[Mesh] OR "immune infiltrates" OR immunity OR "immune response" OR "immune cells" OR "immune cell" OR inflammation OR infiltration OR "Lymphocyte Subsets/immunology"[Mesh] OR "TH1 Cells/ immunology" [Mesh] OR "TH2 Cells/ immunology" [Mesh]) NOT (mice OR mouse OR "cell line" OR "cell lines" OR "mouth" OR "oropharynx" OR "Antiretroviral Therapy, Highly Active"[Mesh] OR "Models, Theoretical"[Mesh] OR "Papillomavirus Vaccines/administration & dosage"[Mesh] OR "Premature Birth/immunology"[Mesh] OR "HIV Infections/immunology"[Mesh] OR "Combined Modality Therapy"[Mesh] OR "Complementary Therapies"[Mesh] OR "Blood Vessels/chemistry"[Mesh] OR "Laser Therapy"[Mesh] OR "Labor Stage, First/physiology"[Mesh] OR "Foreign-Body Reaction/pathology"[Mesh] OR "Postoperative Complications/pathology"[Mesh] OR "Male"[Mesh] OR "Labor, Obstetric/metabolism"[Mesh])

6. References

FUTURE II Study Group (2007). "Quadrivalent vaccine against human papillomavirus to prevent high-grade cervical lesions." *N Engl J Med* 356(19): 1915-1927.

Abike, F., A. B. Engin, et al. (2011). "Human papilloma virus persistence and neopterin, folate and homocysteine levels in cervical dysplasias." *Arch Gynecol Obstet* 284(1): 209-214.

Adam, R. A., I. R. Horowitz, et al. (1999). "Serum levels of macrophage colony-stimulating factor-1 in cervical human papillomavirus infection and intraepithelial neoplasia." *Am J Obstet Gynecol* 180(1): 28-32.

Anderson, B. L. and S. Cu-Uvin (2011). "Clinical parameters essential to methodology and interpretation of mucosal responses." *American journal of reproductive immunology (New York, N Y : 1989)* 65(3): 352-360.

Bais, A. G. (2005). "A shift to a peripheral Th2-type cytokine pattern during the carcinogenesis of cervical cancer becomes manifest in CIN III lesions." *Journal of Clinical Pathology* 58(10): 1096-1100.

Baker, R., J. G. Dauner, et al. (2011). "Increased plasma levels of adipokines and inflammatory markers in older women with persistent HPV infection." *Cytokine* 53(3): 282-285.

Bermudez-Morales, V. H., L. X. Gutierrez, et al. (2008). "Correlation between IL-10 gene expression and HPV infection in cervical cancer: a mechanism for immune response escape." *Cancer investigation* 26(10): 1037-1043.

Bhat, P., S. R. Mattarollo, et al. (2011). "Regulation of immune responses to HPV infection and during HPV-directed immunotherapy." *Immunological reviews* 239(1): 85-98.

Bontkes, H. J., T. D. de Gruijl, et al. (1999). "Human papillomavirus type 16 E2-specific T-helper lymphocyte responses in patients with cervical intraepithelial neoplasia." *J Gen Virol* 80 (Pt 9): 2453-2459.

Bontkes, H. J., T. D. de Gruijl, et al. (2000). "Human Papillomavirus Type 16 E6/E7-Specific Cytotoxic T Lymphocytes In Women With Cervical Neoplasia." *Int. J. Cancer* 88: 92-98.

Bouvard, V., R. Baan, et al. (2009). "A review of human carcinogens--Part B: biological agents." *Lancet Oncol* 10(4): 321-322.

Brismar Wendel, S., T. Kaldensjo, et al. (2010). "Slumbering mucosal immune response in the cervix of human papillomavirus DNA-positive and -negative women." *International journal of oncology* 37(6): 1565-1573.

Butsch Kovacic, M., H. A. Katki, et al. (2008). "Epidemiologic analysis of histologic cervical inflammation: relationship to human papillomavirus infections." *Human Pathology* 39(7): 1088-1095.

Castle, P. E. and A. R. Giuliano (2003). "Chapter 4: Genital tract infections, cervical inflammation, and antioxidant nutrients--assessing their roles as human papillomavirus cofactors." *J Natl Cancer Inst Monogr*(31): 29-34.

Castle, P. E., A. C. Rodriguez, et al. (2004). "Comparison of ophthalmic sponges for measurements of immune markers from cervical secretions." *Clin Diagn Lab Immunol* 11(2): 399-405.

Cromme, F. V., C. J. Meijer, et al. (1993). "Analysis of MHC class I and II expression in relation to presence of HPV genotypes in premalignant and malignant cervical lesions." *Br J Cancer* 67(6): 1372-1380.

Crowley-Nowick, P. A., J. H. Ellenberg, et al. (2000). "Cytokine profile in genital tract secretions from female adolescents: impact of human immunodeficiency virus, human papillomavirus, and other sexually transmitted pathogens." *The Journal of infectious diseases* 181(3): 939-945.

de Gruijl, T. D., H. J. Bontkes, et al. (1999). "Immune responses against human papillomavirus (HPV) type 16 virus-like particles in a cohort study of women with cervical intraepithelial neoplasia. I. Differential T-helper and IgG responses in relation to HPV infection and disease outcome." *J Gen Virol* 80 (Pt 2): 399-408.

de Gruijl, T. D., H. J. Bontkes, et al. (1998). "Differential T helper cell responses to human papillomavirus type 16 E7 related to viral clearance or persistence in patients with cervical neoplasia: a longitudinal study." *Cancer Res* 58(8): 1700-1706.

Dong, D.-d., H. Yang, et al. (2010). "Human leukocyte antigen-G (HLA-G) expression in cervical lesions: association with cancer progression, HPV 16/18 infection, and host immune response." *Reproductive sciences (Thousand Oaks, Calif)* 17(8): 718-723.

Ferlay, J., H. R. Shin, et al. (2010). GLOBOCAN 2008, Cancer Incidence and Mortality Worldwide: IARC CancerBase No. 10 Lyon, France: International Agency for Research on Cancer. Available from: http://globocan.iarc.fr.

Fernandes, A. P. M., M. A. G. Gonçalves, et al. (2005). "HPV16, HPV18, and HIV infection may influence cervical cytokine intralesional levels." *Virology* 334(2): 294-298.

Goncalves, M. A. G., M. Le Discorde, et al. (2008). "Classical and non-classical HLA molecules and p16(INK4a) expression in precursors lesions and invasive cervical cancer." *European journal of obstetrics, gynecology, and reproductive biology* 141(1): 70-74.

Gravitt, P. E., A. Hildesheim, et al. (2003). "Correlates of IL-10 and IL-12 concentrations in cervical secretions." *Journal of Clinical Immunology* 23(3): 175-183.

Gravitt, P. E., A. Hildesheim, et al. (2003). "Correlates of IL-10 and IL-12 concentrations in cervical secretions." *J Clin Immunol* 23(3): 175-183.

Guha, D. and R. Chatterjee (2009). "Cytokine levels in HIV infected and uninfected Indian women: Correlation with other STAs." *Experimental and Molecular Pathology* 86(1): 65-68.

Hildesheim, A., R. Herrero, et al. (2007). "Effect of human papillomavirus 16/18 L1 viruslike particle vaccine among young women with preexisting infection: a randomized trial." *JAMA* 298(7): 743-753.

Hildesheim, A., M. H. Schiffman, et al. (1997). "Immune activation in cervical neoplasia: cross-sectional association between plasma soluble interleukin 2 receptor levels and disease." *Cancer Epidemiol Biomarkers Prev* 6(10): 807-813.

Hong, J. H., M. K. Kim, et al. (2010). "Association Between Serum Cytokine Profiles and Clearance or Persistence of High-Risk Human Papillomavirus Infection." *International Journal of Gynecological Cancer* 20(6): 1011-1016.

Kadish, A. S., G. Y. Ho, et al. (1997). "Lymphoproliferative responses to human papillomavirus (HPV) type 16 proteins E6 and E7: outcome of HPV infection and associated neoplasia." *J Natl Cancer Inst* 89(17): 1285-1293.

Kemp, T. J., A. Hildesheim, et al. (2010). "Elevated Systemic Levels of Inflammatory Cytokines in Older Women with Persistent Cervical Human Papillomavirus Infection." *Cancer Epidemiology Biomarkers & Prevention* 19(8): 1954-1959.

Koshiol, J., L. Lindsay, et al. (2008). "Persistent human papillomavirus infection and cervical neoplasia: a systematic review and meta-analysis." *Am J Epidemiol* 168(2): 123-137.

Lieberman, J. A., A. B. Moscicki, et al. (2008). "Determination of Cytokine Protein Levels in Cervical Mucus Samples from Young Women by a Multiplex Immunoassay Method and Assessment of Correlates." *Clinical and Vaccine Immunology* 15(1): 49-54.

Marks, M. A., R. P. Viscidi, et al. (2011). "Differences in the concentration and correlation of cervical immune markers among HPV positive and negative perimenopausal women." *Cytokine*.

Molling, J. W., T. D. de Gruijl, et al. (2007). "CD4(+)CD25hi regulatory T-cell frequency correlates with persistence of human papillomavirus type 16 and T helper cell responses in patients with cervical intraepithelial neoplasia." *International journal of cancer Journal international du cancer* 121(8): 1749-1755.

Moscicki, A. B., J. H. Ellenberg, et al. (2004). "Risk of high-grade squamous intraepithelial lesion in HIV-infected adolescents." *J Infect Dis* 190(8): 1413-1421.

Munoz, N., X. Castellsague, et al. (2006). "Chapter 1: HPV in the etiology of human cancer." *Vaccine* 24 Suppl 3: S3/1-10.

Murphy, K., P. Travers, et al. (2011). *Janeway's Immunobiology*, Garland Publishing (Taylor & Francis Group).

Ortiz-Sanchez, E., P. Chavez-Olmos, et al. (2007). "Expression of the costimulatory molecule CD86, but not CD80, in keratinocytes of normal cervical epithelium and human papillomavirus-16 positive low squamous intraepithelial lesions." *International journal of gynecological cancer : official journal of the International Gynecological Cancer Society* 17(3): 571-580.

Ovestad, I. T., U. Vennestrom, et al. (2011). "Comparison of different commercial methods for HPV detection in follow-up cytology after ASCUS/LSIL, prediction of CIN2-3 in follow up biopsies and spontaneous regression of CIN2-3." *Gynecol Oncol* 123(2): 278-283.

Sachdeva, N. and D. Asthana (2007). "Cytokine quantitation: technologies and applications." *Front Biosci* 12: 4682-4695.

Schiffman, M., P. E. Castle, et al. (2007). "Human papillomavirus and cervical cancer." *Lancet* 370(9590): 890-907.

Scott, M., D. P. Stites, et al. (1999). "Th1 cytokine patterns in cervical human papillomavirus infection." *Clin Diagn Lab Immunol* 6(5): 751-755.

Seresini, S., M. Origoni, et al. (2007). "IFN-gamma produced by human papilloma virus-18 E6-specific CD4+ T cells predicts the clinical outcome after surgery in patients with high-grade cervical lesions." *Journal of immunology (Baltimore, Md : 1950)* 179(10): 7176-7183.

Sharma, A., M. Rajappa, et al. (2007). "Cytokine profile in Indian women with cervical intraepithelial neoplasia and cancer cervix." *International Journal of Gynecological Cancer* 17(4): 879-885.

Song, S. H., J. K. Lee, et al. 2008. "Interferon-γ (IFN-γ): A possible prognostic marker for clearance of high-risk human papillomavirus (HPV)." *Gynecologic Oncology* 108(3): 543-548.

Song, S., J. Lee, et al. (2007). "The relationship between cytokines and HPV-16, HPV-16 E6, E7, and high-risk HPV viral load in the uterine cervix." *Gynecologic Oncology* 104(3): 732-738.

Stanley, M. (2010). "HPV - immune response to infection and vaccination." *Infect Agent Cancer* 5: 19.

Su, J. H., A. Wu, et al. (2010). "Immunotherapy for cervical cancer: Research status and clinical potential." *BioDrugs* 24(2): 109-129.

Tirone, N. R., B. C. Peghini, et al. (2009). "Local expression of interferon-alpha and interferon receptors in cervical intraepithelial neoplasia." *Cancer Immunology, Immunotherapy* 58(12): 2003-2010.

Tjiong, M. Y., N. van der Vange, et al (2001). "Cytokines in Cervicovaginal Washing Fluid from Patients with Cervical Neoplasia." *Cytokine* 14(6): 357-360.

Trottier, H. and E. L. Franco (2006). "The epidemiology of genital human papillomavirus infection." *Vaccine* 24 Suppl 1: S1-15.

Tsukui, T., A. Hildesheim, et al. (1996). "Interleukin 2 production in vitro by peripheral lymphocytes in response to human papillomavirus-derived peptides: correlation with cervical pathology." *Cancer Res* 56(17): 3967-3974.

2

Viruses Strive to Suppress Host Immune Responses and Prolong Persistence

Curtis J. Pritzl, Young-Jin Seo and Bumsuk Hahm
Departments of Surgery and Molecular Microbiology & Immunology
University of Missouri – Columbia
USA

1. Introduction

Viruses regulate host immune responses to propagate their progeny. Indeed, certain viruses successfully establish viral persistence for long periods of time even in the immunocompetent host. Many viruses seem to have developed clever tactics to elude, utilize, or suppress host innate and adaptive immune systems. Unlike the parental strain, the clone 13 (Cl 13) strain of lymphocytic choriomeningitis virus (LCMV) has been shown to persist in mice for 60 – 100 days by nullifying the function of the host immune system. Multiple findings obtained from this mouse model have held true in humans chronically infected with viruses including human immunodeficiency virus (HIV) and hepatitis viruses. These viruses have evolved a repertoire of mechanisms to suppress and evade the host immune system. By utilizing the model for the LCMV infection of mice, this review will focus on the viral mechanisms for inhibition or escape of host immunity, in particular the host dendritic cell (DC) and T cell responses. Investigating the viral strategies will help us better understand the virus-host interplay and design new immunotherapeutic approaches.

1.1 The lymphocytic choriomeningitis virus model of chronic viral infection

The Cl 13 strain of LCMV is a variant isolated from the spleens of mice infected neonatally with the prototypic LCMV strain, Armstrong 53b (Arm) (Ahmed, Salmi et al. 1984). Mice infected with LCMV Arm develop a robust acute immune response of cytotoxic T lymphocytes (CTLs) that rapidly clears the virus from its host (within 10 days). In contrast, the infection of adult mice with LCMV Cl 13 induces a profound suppression of the host immune system leading to viral persistence (60-100 days following the start of infection) (Figure 1) (Borrow, Evans et al. 1995; Sevilla, Kunz et al. 2003). The clinical importance of virus-induced altered or suppressed immune responses is reflected by several human virus infections that inhibit the immune response such as HIV and hepatitis C virus (HCV) (Steinman, Granelli-Piperno et al. 2003; Liu, Woltman et al. 2009). Thus, the system of LCMV Cl 13 infection of its natural host, the mouse, serves as an excellent model for the mechanistic study of virus-induced immunosuppression and for the development of novel targets controlling viral persistence.

Immunosuppression caused by LCMV Cl 13 is associated with the inhibition of DC function and the reduced frequency and impaired activation (exhaustion) of virus-specific T cells

(Borrow et al. 1995; Sevilla et al. 2003; Barber, Wherry et al. 2006; Trifilo, Hahm et al. 2006). Exhausted T cell responses are characterized by the cells' inability to produce antiviral and immune stimulatory cytokines, destroy virus-infected cells, or proliferate, and have been documented following multiple infections including HIV, HCV, and hepatitis B virus (Yi, Cox et al. 2010).

LCMV Cl 13 differs from Arm by only two amino acids (aa); a Leu in the viral glycoprotein at aa 260 in Cl 13 as compared to Phe in ARM is responsible for DC infection and immunosuppression (Salvato, Borrow et al. 1991). LCMV Cl 13 preferentially replicates in the white pulp of the spleen and infects DCs in spleen and bone marrow (BM) of the mice via the receptor α-dystroglycan (Cao, Henry et al. 1998; Smelt, Borrow et al. 2001; Sevilla et al. 2003). The modulation of immuno-regulatory proteins expressed on DCs was reported to explain the failure of DC function to stimulate or maintain T cell responses upon LCMV Cl 13 infection. Such modulation included the downregulation of MHC molecules and co-stimulatory proteins (Sevilla, McGavern et al. 2004), preferential production of the immunosuppressive cytokine, IL-10 (Brooks, Trifilo et al. 2006; Ejrnaes, Filippi et al. 2006; Brooks, Ha et al. 2008), and increased expression of the negative regulator, programmed death-ligand 1 (PD-L1) on DCs for enhanced PD-L1-PD1 interaction leading to T cell exhaustion (2, 11).

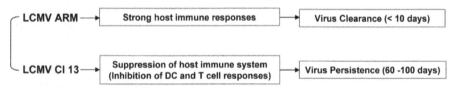

Fig. 1. Characteristics of the different LCMV infection models. LCMV ARM infection of adult mice rapidly generates a strong CD8 T cell response in the host which can clear the virus within 10 days, while an LCMV Cl 13 infection suppresses the host immune responses which leads to a prolonged viral persistence lasting 60 – 100 days.

Furthermore, following LCMV Cl 13 infection, virus-specific CD4+ T cells were functionally dysregulated, which contributes to the inability to sustain CTL function and facilitates viral persistence (Matloubian, Concepcion et al. 1994; Brooks, Teyton et al. 2005). Virus-specific CD4+ T cells were functionally inactivated early during the transition into viral persistence and failed to produce effector cytokines such as IL-2 and TNF-α. Recently, IL-21 was identified as an essential component of CD4+ T cell help to sustain CD8+ T cell effector activity and resolve persistent infection (Elsaesser, Sauer et al. 2009; Frohlich, Kisielow et al. 2009; Yi, Du et al. 2009). The detailed underlying molecular mechanism and intracellular signaling path for the virus-induced immunosuppression and viral persistence, however, are unclear.

2. Chronic viral infections inhibit innate and dendritic cell responses

It is generally thought that a robust CD8+ T cell response is responsible for clearing an acute LCMV infection (Byrne and Oldstone 1984; Fung-Leung, Kundig et al. 1991). However, a strong innate immune response is important for the generation of an effective adaptive response against viral infections (Jung, Kato et al. 2008; Rahman, Cui et al. 2008; Zucchini,

Bessou et al. 2008). Moreover, DCs are indispensible for the generation of the CD8+ effector T cells. The innate immune response provides stimulatory signals, such as type I interferons and IL-12 that promote the priming of CD8+ T cells and favor the T-helper 1 phenotype of CD4+ T cells. DCs are the key intermediate between the innate immune response and the adaptive immune response. DCs are the major professional antigen presenting cell subset that provides the necessary primary and secondary signals to induce the activation and proliferation of virus-specific CTL. A virus that can actively suppress these two responses has a significant advantage over the host immune system and the opportunity to establish a persistent infection.

2.1 Chronic LCMV infections suppress type I interferon expression

Type I interferons (IFN) and inflammatory cytokines are key to the initiation of anti-viral immune responses (Seo and Hahm 2010). Type I IFN is a family of cytokines comprised of IFN-α, IFN-β, IFN-ε, IFN-κ, and IFN-ω. These molecules have been shown to be potent antiviral cytokines by the deletion of the common receptor subunit (IFNAR1). Transgenic mice lacking IFNAR1 have been demonstrated to the lose ability to interfere with the replication of many different viruses (Muller, Steinhoff et al. 1994; Goodman, Zeng et al. 2010; Kolokoltsova, Yun et al. 2010). High levels of type I IFN have been detected at early time points during an acute, LCMV Arm infection (Montoya, Edwards et al. 2005). Zhou et al. have demonstrated that this induction of type I IFN is due at least in part to the recognition of the LCMV RNA genome by retinoic acid-inducible gene I (RIG-I) and melanoma differentiation-associated gene 5 (MDA5) pathway along with toll-like receptor (TLR) 2 and 6 (Zhou, Kurt-Jones et al. 2005; Zhou, Cerny et al. 2010). Similarly, DCs from LCMV Cl 13-infected mice have also been shown to produce type I IFN at early time points of virus infection (Dalod, Salazar-Mather et al. 2002; Diebold, Montoya et al. 2003; Zuniga, Hahm et al. 2007). However, several days later, these cytokines are no longer detectable in the sera of LCMV Cl 13-infected mice (Martinez-Sobrido, Emonet et al. 2009), which suggests that the virus is actively suppressing the host type I IFN response. This observation was confirmed by Zuniga et al. who specifically examined the production of type I IFN by plasmacytoid DCs during an LCMV CL 13 infection (Zuniga, Liou et al. 2008). Plasmacytoid DCs (pDC) are a specialized subset of DCs that rapidly produce large amounts of type I IFN in response to viral infection (Asselin-Paturel and Trinchieri 2005; Delale, Paquin et al. 2005). In response to certain stimulation conditions, these cells have been observed to dedicate 50% of their cellular transcription to the production of type I IFN (Liu 2005; Lee, Lund et al. 2007). Because of this high level of type I IFN, it is suggested that these cells play a key role in the orchestration of antiviral immune responses. In the case of an LCMV Cl 13 infection, the number of pDCs in LCMV Cl 13-infected mice was reduced by 50% compared to mice infected with LCMV Arm at 30 days post-infection (Zuniga et al. 2008). Moreover, the production of type I IFN in response to TLR9 activation was severely impaired in pDCs isolated from LCMV CL 13-infected mice, which suggests that the virus is severely limiting the potential of these cells to respond not only to LCMV, but also additional, unrelated pathogenic stimulation (Zuniga et al. 2008).

Indeed, it has been shown that LCMV Cl 13 utilizes specific molecular mechanisms to inhibit type I IFN production by the host cells. Martinez-Sobrido et al. have shown that the nucleoprotein of LCMV is responsible for the blockade of the host type I IFN response

(Martinez-Sobrido, Zuniga et al. 2006). This inhibition of cytokine production is due to the interaction of the viral protein with the interferon regulatory factor-3 (IRF-3) activation pathway. The data demonstrated that LCMV nucleoprotein (NP) impaired the nuclear translocation of IRF-3, which is involved in the upregulation of type I IFN synthesis. More specifically, amino acid residue 382 of LCMV NP was sufficient to inhibit the host type I IFN response (Martinez-Sobrido et al. 2009).

Additional studies have been carried out to investigate the mechanisms behind the LCMV-mediated blockade of the host type I IFN response. LCMV NP blockade of the IRF-3 pathway also affects the response to RIG-I and MDA5 (Zhou et al. 2010). Moreover, this same study demonstrated that LCMV NP physically interacts with both RIG-I and MDA5. Mutations in LCMV NP that prevented the inhibition of type I IFN however did not affect this interaction, which suggests that there are additional inhibitory mechanisms (Zhou et al. 2010).

This suppression of type I IFN not only affects the host response against LCMV, but it may also reduce the effectiveness of responses against other opportunistic pathogens whose clearance requires type I IFN (Zuniga et al. 2008). The effects of chronic LCMV Cl 13 infections also lead to disruptions in the ability of the host's pDCs to produce type I IFN in response to other unrelated infections such as vesicular stomatitis virus (VSV) or murine cytomegalovirus (MCMV). In addition, LCMV Cl 13 infection had deleterious consequences on the host's natural killer cell population which may be important in the immune response to other viral, bacterial, or parasitic infections such as HIV, influenza virus, *Mycobacterium tuberculosis* (Vankayalapati, Garg et al. 2005), and *Plasmodium falciparum* (Alter, Malenfant et al. 2004; Byrne, McGuirk et al. 2004; Siren, Sareneva et al. 2004; Korbel, Newman et al. 2005; Zuniga et al. 2008). Pre-infection with LCMV Cl 13 was also demonstrated to prevent the host from counteracting the early spread of MCMV and therefore preventing viral clearance (Zuniga et al. 2008).

2.2 Suppression of dendritic cell functions

DCs are key mediators of adaptive immune responses. This group of cells can efficiently present endogenously and exogenously synthesized viral antigens to CD8+ T cells. In addition, these cells provide the necessary co-stimulatory signals to CTL for activation. The effect of chronic LCMV Cl 13 infections on the production of type I IFN by pDCs is only one aspect of the virus-induced restrictions of the host's DC responses. Not only do chronically infecting viruses suppress cytokine production by host DCs, but it has also been shown that they can suppress the development of dendritic cells from hematopoietic precursor cells, inhibit the maturation of DCs following exposure to activation signals, and also lead to the destruction of these cells that are critical for effective anti-viral immune responses.

One major mechanism that LCMV Cl 13 uses to suppress DC responses is to suppress their development from hematopoietic precursor cells (Hahm, Trifilo et al. 2005; Trifilo et al. 2006). The cytokines fms-like tyrosine kinase receptor-3 ligand (Flt3-L) and granulocyte macrophage-colony stimulating factor (GM-CSF) are major signals in the development of DCs from hematopoietic stem cells and can be used to induce the differentiation of DCs both *in vitro* and *in vivo* (Sevilla et al. 2004; Hahm et al. 2005). When Flt3-L is administered to mice, it dramatically increases the number of splenic DCs (Drakes, Lu et al. 1997). When bone marrow is cultured *in vitro* with GM-CSF, the stem cells differentiate into CD11c+

dendritic cells. It has been demonstrated that LCMV Cl 13-infected mice do not respond to Flt3-L treatment, suggesting that the virus induces an Flt3-L-refractory state in the hematopoietic precursor cells (Sevilla et al. 2004; Hahm et al. 2005). Moreover, *in vitro* culture of bone marrow cells infected by LCMV Cl 13 with GM-CSF induced the development of significantly fewer CD11c+ DCs compared to uninfected bone marrow cells (Sevilla et al. 2004; Hahm et al. 2005). Collectively these data indicate that one mechanism that chronic LCMV infection utilizes to evade the immune system is to prevent the development of DCs which are critical to a successful adaptive immune response.

Although LCMV Cl 13 does inhibit the differentiation of DCs from their hematopoietic progenitors, functional DCs do develop. However, the virus employs additional strategies to suppress the responses induced by these cells. Our laboratory and others have demonstrated that LCMV Cl 13 infection of DCs inhibits their ability to upregulate major histocompatibility complex class I (MHC-I) molecules and co-stimulatory molecules such as B7-2 (Figure 2A) (Sevilla et al. 2004). Moreover, the LCMV Cl 13 infection in our studies not only prevented the upregulation of MHC-I and B7-2 but reduced the levels of their expression to below baseline levels. This suppression of MHC-I and co-stimulatory molecule expression renders the DCs unable to efficiently prime CD8+ T cells, which are necessary to clear the infecting virus. Although the inhibition of type I IFN expression may be the cause of this downregulation, there may be additional unknown mechanisms for this phenomenon. Further, the infected DCs were impaired in the ability to synthesize IL-12, a critical cytokine for T cell stimulation, in response to TLR9 ligation (Figure 2B). The results also support the functional abrogation of host immunity in LCMV Cl 13-infected mice upon the invasion of a secondary microbe that contains TLR9 ligand components such as DNA viruses or bacteria.

The final postulated mechanism for LCMV evasion of dendritic cell responses is the targeted killing of these cells. It has been shown that persistently infecting strains of the virus have a mutation in the glycoprotein that affects their tropism and increases the infectivity of DCs (Borrow et al. 1995; Sevilla, Kunz et al. 2000). This dendritic cell-specific infection leads to increased antigen load and therefore makes these cells ideal targets for activated CD8+ T cells. Indeed, a loss of splenic DCs has been observed in the spleens of LCMV Cl 13-infected mice although, the ability of these infected DCs to act as targets has not yet been confirmed. However, DCs are efficient antigen presenting cells and because they are preferentially infected during an LCMV Cl 13 infection, it has been speculated that they are targeted for destruction by activated CD8+ T cells (Odermatt, Eppler et al. 1991; Borrow et al. 1995).

These multiple findings have been recapitulated when DCs were infected with human-tropic viruses. For instance, measles virus (MV) suppressed DC generation from bone marrow progenitor cells under the GM-CSF or Flt3-L-supplemented culture system (Hahm et al. 2005). Further, MV could kill DCs or strongly inhibit the ability of DCs to stimulate anti-viral T cells (Hahm 2009). The decrease in the DC population was also observed in the bloodstream of HCV or HIV-infected patients (Donaghy, Pozniak et al. 2001; Pacanowski, Kahi et al. 2001; Kanto and Hayashi 2004; Kanto, Inoue et al. 2004; Siavoshian, Abraham et al. 2005). Functional abrogation of professional antigen presenting DCs has been reported in multiple cases of patients who were chronically infected with pathogenic viruses.

Like the inhibition of type I IFN, DCs have been shown to play a key role in the host response and elimination of viral infections. Because of this, LCMV and other chronically

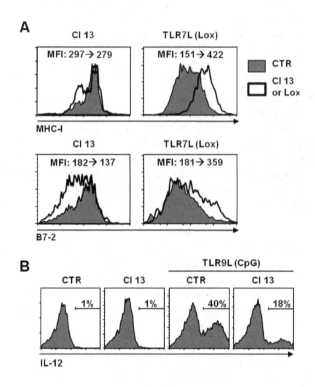

Fig. 2. LCMV Cl 13 suppresses DC responses. (A) Bone marrow-derived DCs were untreated (control, CTR), infected with LCMV Cl 13 (Cl 13), or treated with loxoribine (TLR7 ligand, 0.5mM). DCs were analyzed for the expression levels of MHC-I and B7-2 by flow cytometry on the following day. Mean fluorescent intensities (MFIs) for each molecule are shown. (B) DCs were uninfected (CTR) or infected with LCMV Cl 13. At one day post-infection (dpi), these cells were untreated or treated with CpG (TLR9 ligand, 200 ng/ml) and the synthesis of IL-12 was assessed by flow cytometry.

infecting viruses have developed multiple strategies to counteract and evade the dendritic cell responses. Although a great deal of effort has been focused on these evasion tactics, the underlying mechanisms that the viruses use to suppress these responses are still not yet fully elucidated.

3. Virus-mediated T cell exhaustion

CD8+ Cytotoxic T lymphocytes (CTLs) are a critical line of defense against viral infections. These cells are responsible for the recognition and subsequent killing of virus-infected cells. During an acute virus infection, CTLs recognize antigenic peptides displayed on the surface of professional antigen presenting cells (Carbone, Moore et al. 1988). This recognition, along with co-stimulatory signals activate the CTLs to proliferate and gives them license to kill virus infected cells through their effector functions including the release of the cytotoxic molecules perforin and granzyme B (Lancki, Hsieh et al. 1991). In addition, activated CTLs also upregulate inflammatory cytokines including IFN-γ and TNF-α (Murray, Lee et al. 1990; Martin, Vallbracht et al. 1991; Brehm, Daniels et al. 2005). Following the resolution of the infection this large population of effector CTLs contracts into a small pool of memory cells which are able to quickly respond to subsequent infections by the same pathogen.

Because CTLs are able to eliminate replicative reservoirs, persisting viruses have evolved methods for the evasion of these immune responses. Although the suppression of CTL responses begins with the disruption of dendritic cell responses as described previously, persistently infecting viruses such as LCMV and HIV have developed several mechanisms to specifically perturb CTL responses. The first method involves the exhaustion of CTLs in which the cells lose their ability to kill infected cells, while the other involves the modulation of dominant CTL epitopes, allowing the virus to escape immune recognition. These escape mechanisms give the viruses an additional advantage over the host immune system and allow for chronic viral infections.

3.1 Exhaustion of CD8+ T cells by LCMV Cl 13

3.1.1 Exhaustion of cytotoxic CD8+ T lymphocytes during chronic viral infection

Exhaustion of CTL has been described in multiple viral infections including both LCMV and HIV as the loss of effector functions by antigen-specific CD8+ T cells. The presence of both acutely-infecting and chronically-infecting strains of LCMV have made this virus an outstanding model for determining both the effects of the virus on CTLs as well as the mechanism by which the virus induces T cell exhaustion. During a chronic LCMV infection, the virus-specific CD8+ T cell response is activated and peaks similar to an acute viral infection (Figure 3). However, instead of clearing the virus, the CTLs lose effector functions (Figure 3). The loss of CTL functionality occurs in a stepwise manner. Individual effector functions are lost at distinct time points over the course of the infection (Wherry, Blattman et al. 2003). Initially, the CTLs lose the ability to proliferate and produce IL-2 in the case of most chronic viral infections (Wherry et al. 2003). As the infection continues, the CTLs become dysfunctional in their ability to produce and secrete the inflammatory cytokine TNF-α (Sakuishi, Apetoh et al. 2010). At later time points of the persistent infection, the cells also fail to produce IFN-γ and lose their cytotoxic potential (Wherry et al. 2003; Jin, Anderson et al. 2010). In certain cases, the end result of T cell exhaustion is the death of T cells which leads to the reduction of the total virus-specific T cell population. The culmination of these dysfunctions is the inability of antigen-specific CTLs to kill virus infected cells, thereby allowing the virus to persist. The mechanisms LCMV Cl 13 uses to exhaust CTLs are not yet fully understood. It is known however that the virus activates inhibitory molecules that are involved in the regulation of normal immune responses to exhaust CTLs.

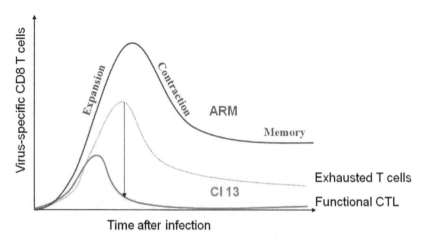

Fig. 3. CD8 T cell response to acute and persistent LCMV infections over time. In response to an acute LCMV infection (ARM, blue line), CD8 T cells rapidly expand until approximately day 7. Following this expansion, the cells contract leaving a small population of memory cells. During a chronic infection (Cl 13, red line), CD8 T cells expand in a similar fashion however quickly lose effector functions (dotted red line) and leave only a small population of functional CTL that are unable to resolve the infection (solid red line).

3.1.2 Inhibitory receptors involved in T cell exhaustion

The inhibitory receptor programmed death – 1 (PD-1) is the most extensively characterized molecule associated with LCMV Cl 13-mediated T cell exhaustion (Wherry, Ha et al. 2007; Blackburn, Shin et al. 2009; Jin et al. 2010; Vezys, Penaloza-MacMaster et al. 2011). PD-1 is a negative immuno-regulatory molecule in the CD28/CTLA-4 family that is expressed on the surface of activated CD8+ T cells. PD-1 has two ligands, PD-L1 and PD-L2 which could be upregulated on the surface of activated DCs and macrophages, although PD-L1 is expressed on multiple cell types (Yamazaki, Akiba et al. 2002; Brown, Dorfman et al. 2003). The expression of this inhibitory receptor has been directly linked to type I IFN production (Terawaki, Chikuma et al. 2011). The role of the PD-1 activation in non-persistent viral infections is the attenuation of T cell responses to prevent unnecessary immunopathology (Freeman, Long et al. 2000). PD-1 is thought to play a critical role in the LCMV-mediated exhaustion of CTLs as virus-specific CD8+ T cells express significantly higher levels of this molecule during chronic LCMV infections. The mechanisms behind the LCMV-mediated upregulation of PD-1 have yet to be fully elucidated. However, the blockade of the PD-1 pathway restores functionality of these cells and leads to clearance of the persistent virus infection (Barber et al. 2006).

Another molecule that has been implicated in the exhaustion of CD8+ T cells during chronic LCMV infections is lymphocyte activated gene – 3 (LAG-3) (Wherry et al. 2007; Grosso, Goldberg et al. 2009). This molecule belongs to the immunoglobulin superfamily and has been shown to be immunomodulatory in the prevention of autoimmune disorders (Workman, Dugger et al. 2002). The expression of LAG-3 does not change on CD8+ T cells during acute infections with LCMV, but is upregulated on CD8+ T cells in LCMV Cl 13-

infected mice (Richter, Agnellini et al. 2010). It has been suggested that LAG-3 functions in a similar fashion to PD-1 during chronic LCMV Cl 13 infections (Blackburn et al. 2009). Although mice deficient in LAG-3 do not demonstrate improved CD8+ T cell responses during persistent LCMV infections (Richter et al. 2010), the simultaneous blockade of both the PD-1 and LAG-3 pathways leads to significant improvements in the CTL responses of LCMV Cl 13-infected mice compared to PD-1 blockade alone (Blackburn et al. 2009).

Multiple other immunomodulatory molecules have been suggested to be involved in the attenuation of virus-specific CD8+ T cell responses. An extensive study by Wherry et al. has shown that the expression of many different genes from multiple cellular processes is affected during CD8+ T cell exhaustion. These markers include natural killer cell marker 2B4 (2B4), which has since been shown to be involved in the regulation of memory CD8+ T cells during chronic LCMV infections (West, Youngblood et al. 2011), T cell Ig- and mucin-domain-containing molecule-3 (Tim-3), CD160, paired Ig-like receptor-B (PIR-B), and GP49B. All of these molecules have been shown to have inhibitory functions during immune responses (Wherry et al. 2007; Jin et al. 2010; Vezys et al. 2011). Although Tim-3 has been shown to act in cooperation with PD-1 in the exhaustion of CD8+ T cells during persistent LCMV infections (Jin et al. 2010), no specific mechanisms in the loss of function of CD8+ T cells have been attributed to these additional markers of T cell exhaustion. Until these markers are investigated individually or in conjunction with the known inhibitory molecules, they are only guilty by association.

The markers and mechanisms that have been described by comparing the persistent and acute LCMV infections are by no means the only ones involved in the suppression of CD8+ T cell responses. Other immunosuppressive molecules have been shown to either be involved in the exhaustion of CD8+ T cell responses or upregulated on exhausted T cells in other persistent viral infections. CTLA-4, among the others discussed above, has been shown to be important in serious human infections such as HIV and HCV (Hryniewicz, Boasso et al. 2006; Kaufmann, Kavanagh et al. 2007; Nakamoto, Cho et al. 2009).

3.1.3 Transcription factors involved in T cell exhaustion

Several transcription factors have also been identified as modulators of the CD8+ T cell response during a persistent LCMV Cl 13 infection (Shaffer, Lin et al. 2002; Agnellini, Wolint et al. 2007). Nuclear factor of activated T cells (NFAT) is a transcription factor that regulates multiple genes involved in the cytotoxicity and inflammatory cytokine production by CD8+ T cells, including IL-2, the loss of which is a hallmark of T cell exhaustion (Wherry et al. 2003). NFAT expression and phosphorylation are unperturbed in the CD8+ T cells from mice persistently infected with LCMV. However, the translocation of NFAT molecules from the cytoplasm to the nucleus is disrupted during chronic LCMV infections which prevents the transcription factor from upregulating genes necessary for complete CTL function (Agnellini et al. 2007). The transcription factor B-lymphocyte-induced maturation protein-1 (Blimp-1) which is known to govern the fate decision of B-cells has also been associated with the exhaustion of CD8+ T cells (Shaffer et al. 2002; Calame 2006). Blimp-1 expression was shown to be dramatically increased in T cells during chronic viral infections (Shin, Blackburn et al. 2009). In this same series of experiments, a conditional knockout of Blimp-1 resulted in significant decreases of the inhibitory receptors PD-1 and LAG-3 in CD8+ T cells during a chronic LCMV Cl 13 infection. Moreover, this conditional knockout resulted in increased cytotoxicity of

LCMV-specific CTL and improved viral control (Shin et al. 2009). Although the research into these transcriptional regulators has revealed another level of immune evasion by LCMV Cl 13, they have not completely elucidated the pathway by which the virus induces T cell exhaustion. Therefore more research is still required to fully understand these mechanisms.

3.1.4 Role of chronic antigen stimulation on T cell exhaustion

One possible mechanism that has been postulated to be involved in the upregulation of these markers and the subsequent exhaustion of virus-specific CD8+ T cells is the prolonged presence of viral antigens. In a study by Bucks et al., repeated exposure to influenza antigen was shown to induce the exhaustion of antigen-specific CTLs. In these experiments, repeated exposure to antigen reduced both the frequency and number of virus specific CD8+ T cells, and significantly impeded the ability of the remaining cells to produce IFN-γ (Bucks, Norton et al. 2009). In support of these findings, a more recent study has investigated the epigenetic regulation CD8+ T cells during a chronic LCMV infection (Youngblood, Oestreich et al. 2011). The results of this study indicate that long-term antigen exposure results in prolonged demethylation of the PD-1 gene locus, leading to extended PD-1 expression which has been observed during chronic LCMV infections. In addition, this demethylation does not resolve rapidly in exhausted T cells due to a downregulation of methyltransferases. Consequently, these exhausted CD8+ T cells have the potential for rapid upregulation of PD-1 upon subsequent antigen encounters (Youngblood et al. 2011).

3.1.5 Cytokines implicated in T cell exhaustion

Another potential inducer of CD8+ T cell exhaustion is the anti-inflammatory cytokine IL-10. IL-10 has been shown to be a potent inhibitor of inflammatory and adaptive immune responses. Two different studies have implicated IL-10 in chronic viral infections (Brooks et al. 2006; Ejrnaes et al. 2006). In these studies it was shown that IL-10-deficient mice chronically infected with LCMV have higher frequencies of virus-specific CTLs and antibody-mediated blockade of the IL-10 receptor can restore the function of exhausted, virus specific CD8+ T cells (Brooks et al. 2006; Ejrnaes et al. 2006). Furthermore, the IL-10 receptor blockade also led to accelerated viral clearance in both studies (Brooks et al. 2006; Ejrnaes et al. 2006). The source of the IL-10 involved in the immune suppression as well as the mechanisms by which IL-10 is induced is still under investigation.

Although the inflammatory cytokine IL-21 has not been shown to be directly involved in the induction of T cell exhaustion, its requirement in the clearance of the virus has been clearly demonstrated. IL-21 is produced primarily by CD4+ T cells and has been shown to induce the proliferation of CD8+ cytotoxic T-lymphocytes in a fashion similar to that of IL-2 (Kasaian, Whitters et al. 2002). Because IL-2 production is lost quickly during a chronic LCMV infection, it is thought that IL-21 may act in a compensatory fashion. The requirement of IL-21 in the clearance of LCMV CL 13 was demonstrated in IL-21 receptor-deficient mice. These mice failed to clear the virus while the wild-type control mice had cleared the infection by day 60 post-infection. (Elsaesser et al. 2009). In the same study by Elsaesser et al., it was shown that IL-21 is produced by CD4+ T cells throughout an LCMV Cl 13 infection (Elsaesser et al. 2009). However, in parallel experiments by Yi et al., it was shown that the number of IL-21-producing CD4+ T cells is 7.8 times lower than in an acute LCMV infection. Therefore, this loss of IL-21-producing, CD4+ T cells may be another critical factor in the rapid exhaustion of CD8+ T cells during a persistent LCMV infection.

The topic of T cell exhaustion is a major focus in the field of viral immunity. It is still not clear if the expression of these markers is due to the presence of a persisting viral infection, or if viruses have evolved specific mechanisms to activate these immunosuppressive pathways. However, multiple studies have demonstrated that the targeting of certain molecules relieves the suppression and allows the host CTL response to reassert control over the infection and accelerate viral clearance. If the mechanisms behind the virus-mediated upregulation of these molecules and CD8+ T cell exhaustion can be determined, the many new targets for immune-based therapies can be designed, giving medicine a much needed advantage in the treatment of chronic viral infections.

3.2 Dysfunction of CD4+ T cells during chronic LCMV infection

CD4+ T cells have been shown to not play a major role in the clearance of an acute, LCMV Arm infection. Experiments conducted with mice deficient in CD4+ T cells demonstrate that they are able to clear the infection as efficiently as their wild-type counterparts (Matloubian et al. 1994). However in the case of a chronic LCMV Cl 13 infection, CD4+ T cells appear to play a more significant role, as depletion of CD4+ T cells prevents mice from clearing the virus (Matloubian et al. 1994). One of the major contributions these cells make is the production of IL-21, which as described above appears to be critical for viral clearance (Elsaesser et al. 2009; West et al. 2011). In addition, there is evidence that CD4+ T cells also become exhausted during an LCMV Cl 13 infection. Brooks et al. have demonstrated that CD4+ T cells begin to lose the ability to make inflammatory cytokines such as IFN-γ and TNF-α as well as IL-2 as early as day 9 post-infection (Brooks et al. 2005). Moreover, an increase in the production of the anti-inflammatory cytokine IL-10 by virus-specific CD4+ T cells was also observed during the chronic LCMV infection (Brooks et al. 2005). There was however no increase in the number of T regulatory CD4+ T cells observed during the course of the viral infection (Brooks et al. 2005). Similar to exhausted CD8+ T cells, exhausted CD4+ T cells have also been shown to upregulate the expression of PD-1 (Day, Kaufmann et al. 2006; Kasprowicz, Schulze Zur Wiesch et al. 2008). In addition, recent evidence suggests that viral persistence actually reprograms the differentiation of CD4+ T cells from the T-helper 1 phenotype to a T-follicular helper cells (Fahey, Wilson et al. 2011).

System Targeted	Disruption of Cellular Function	Phenotype/Mechanism
Type I Interferon	Inhibition of type I IFN production	LCMV NP - Inhibition of IRF3 - Inhibition of MDA5 and RIG-I Inhibition of plasmacytoid DCs
Dendritic Cells	Inhibition of DC development	Decrease in the frequency of CD11c+ cells
	Inhibition of DC maturation	MHC-I and B7-1/B7-2 upregulation impaired following PAMP ligation Loss of IL-12 production Increased IL-10 synthesis
T cells	Suppression of T cell function (exhaustion)	PD-1↑, LAG-3↑, Tim-3↑, Blimp-1↑, NFAT↑ IFN-γ↓, TNF-α↓, IL-2↓, Proliferation↓, Cytotoxic activity ↓

Table 1. Immunological Effects of Persistent LCMV Cl 13 Infections.

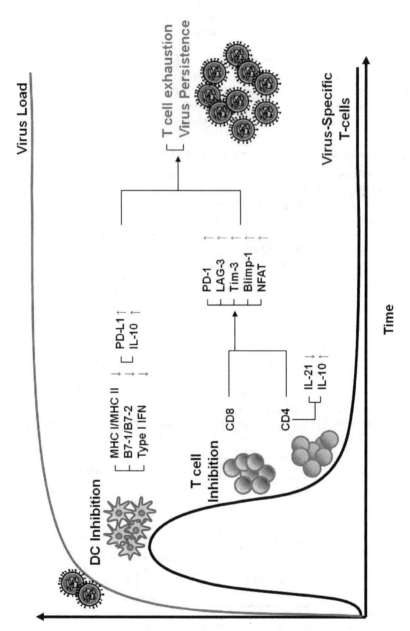

Fig. 4. Schematic representation of the immune cell phenotypes during a chronic LCMV infection. Viral load over time is represented by the red line. The functional T cell response is illustrated using the black line. Alterations in cell surface molecule and cytokine expression is noted with each cell type.

4. Perspectives

Chronic viral infections continue to be a tremendous burden on human health. Many years of research, especially with LCMV Cl 13, has led to a large body of knowledge as to how these viruses subvert and evade both innate and adaptive immune responses (Figure 4 and Table 1). Although there is still a great deal of research needed, several potential molecular immunotherapeutic treatment options have been developed through these studies. First, findings by Brooks *et al.* and Ejarnes *et al.* have clearly demonstrated that the blockade of IL-10 signaling could be used as a potential treatment to restore functionality to exhausted CD8+ T cells. This has been examined recently and it was found that CD8+ T cells from HIV positive patients could be restored using an IL-10-specific antibody (Brockman, Kwon et al. 2009). Similarly, clinical trials are being conducted to evaluate a treatment consisting of inhibition of the PD-1/PD-L1 interaction to recover exhausted CD8+ T cells during HIV infection and certain types of cancer (Sakthivel, Gereke et al. 2011). Other treatment options have been explored including multiple therapeutic vaccination strategies such as DNA vaccines (Martins, Lau et al. 1995), recombinant virus vectors (Wherry, Blattman et al. 2005), and lipo-peptide vaccines (von Herrath, Berger et al. 2000). Finally, the use of IFN-α for the treatment of chronic virus infections was introduced in 1986 for the treatment of hepatitis C virus infections (Hoofnagle, Mullen et al. 1986). However, some evidence suggests that therapeutic vaccination post-infection may not be as effective as hoped because of the immunosuppressed state of the host caused by the infection (Wherry et al. 2005).

In addition to the molecular therapies, immune cell-based therapeutic approaches have been developed. Since CD8+ CTLs are principal players for the eradication of viruses, the CD8+ T cell-based therapy has been implemented (Gottschalk, Bollard et al. 2006; Kapp, Tan et al. 2007). However, the requirement of CD4+ T cells for the maintenance of CTL activity has prompted the use of combined T cell therapies. Further, owing to the extraordinary ability of DCs to serve as natural adjuvants, the potential of antigen-mounted, activated DCs for the treatment of infectious diseases has been confirmed in multiple experimental models (Inaba, Metlay et al. 1990; Fajardo-Moser, Berzel et al. 2008). If DCs are suppressed by chronic viral infections for T cell exhaustion or deletion, provision of active, modulatory DCs presenting viral epitopes could overcome virus-induced suppressive environments and initiate vigorous anti-viral T cell immunity. The proper use of DC subtypes, DC modulation methodology and the way to activate intracellular class I MHC antigen presenting pathways as well as MHC class II pathways need to be considered to maximize the efficacy of DC-based immunocytotherapy.

Collectively, there is a great deal of understanding the mechanisms behind LCMV-induced immunosuppression (Figure 4 and Table 1) that has had practical applications for serious chronic human viral infections and have led to clinical trials for therapeutic interventions. However, many of the underlying causes have yet to be determined and further investigations are needed. In conjunction with molecular mechanistic studies, the approach to subvert the immunosuppressive environment caused by chronic viral infections could aid the development of immune-therapeutic drugs and treatments to combat many viral diseases.

5. Acknowledgements

We thank the editors for invitation of this review. This work was supported by NIH/NIAID grants AI088363 and AI091797 (B.H.).

6. References

Agnellini, P., P. Wolint, et al. (2007). "Impaired NFAT nuclear translocation results in split exhaustion of virus-specific CD8+ T cell functions during chronic viral infection." *Proc Natl Acad Sci U S A* 104(11): 4565-4570.

Ahmed, R., A. Salmi, et al. (1984). "Selection of genetic variants of lymphocytic choriomeningitis virus in spleens of persistently infected mice. Role in suppression of cytotoxic T lymphocyte response and viral persistence." *J Exp Med* 160(2): 521-540.

Alter, G., J. M. Malenfant, et al. (2004). "Increased natural killer cell activity in viremic HIV-1 infection." *J Immunol* 173(8): 5305-5311.

Asselin-Paturel, C. and G. Trinchieri (2005). "Production of type I interferons: plasmacytoid dendritic cells and beyond." *J Exp Med* 202(4): 461-465.

Barber, D. L., E. J. Wherry, et al. (2006). "Restoring function in exhausted CD8 T cells during chronic viral infection." *Nature* 439(7077): 682-687.

Blackburn, S. D., H. Shin, et al. (2009). "Coregulation of CD8+ T cell exhaustion by multiple inhibitory receptors during chronic viral infection." *Nat Immunol* 10(1): 29-37.

Borrow, P., C. F. Evans, et al. (1995). "Virus-induced immunosuppression: immune system-mediated destruction of virus-infected dendritic cells results in generalized immune suppression." *J Virol* 69(2): 1059-1070.

Brehm, M. A., K. A. Daniels, et al. (2005). "Rapid production of TNF-alpha following TCR engagement of naive CD8 T cells." *J Immunol* 175(8): 5043-5049.

Brockman, M. A., D. S. Kwon, et al. (2009). "IL-10 is up-regulated in multiple cell types during viremic HIV infection and reversibly inhibits virus-specific T cells." *Blood* 114(2): 346-356.

Brooks, D. G., S. J. Ha, et al. (2008). "IL-10 and PD-L1 operate through distinct pathways to suppress T-cell activity during persistent viral infection." *Proc Natl Acad Sci U S A* 105(51): 20428-20433.

Brooks, D. G., L. Teyton, et al. (2005). "Intrinsic functional dysregulation of CD4 T cells occurs rapidly following persistent viral infection." *J Virol* 79(16): 10514-10527.

Brooks, D. G., M. J. Trifilo, et al. (2006). "Interleukin-10 determines viral clearance or persistence in vivo." *Nat Med* 12(11): 1301-1309.

Brown, J. A., D. M. Dorfman, et al. (2003). "Blockade of programmed death-1 ligands on dendritic cells enhances T cell activation and cytokine production." *J Immunol* 170(3): 1257-1266.

Bucks, C. M., J. A. Norton, et al. (2009). "Chronic antigen stimulation alone is sufficient to drive CD8+ T cell exhaustion." *J Immunol* 182(11): 6697-6708.

Byrne, J. A. and M. B. Oldstone (1984). "Biology of cloned cytotoxic T lymphocytes specific for lymphocytic choriomeningitis virus: clearance of virus in vivo." *J Virol* 51(3): 682-686.

Byrne, P., P. McGuirk, et al. (2004). "Depletion of NK cells results in disseminating lethal infection with Bordetella pertussis associated with a reduction of antigen-specific Th1 and enhancement of Th2, but not Tr1 cells." *Eur J Immunol* 34(9): 2579-2588.

Calame, K. (2006). "Transcription factors that regulate memory in humoral responses." *Immunol Rev* 211: 269-279.

Cao, W., M. D. Henry, et al. (1998). "Identification of alpha-dystroglycan as a receptor for lymphocytic choriomeningitis virus and Lassa fever virus." *Science* 282(5396): 2079-2081.

Carbone, F. R., M. W. Moore, et al. (1988). "Induction of cytotoxic T lymphocytes by primary in vitro stimulation with peptides." *J Exp Med* 167(6): 1767-1779.

Dalod, M., T. P. Salazar-Mather, et al. (2002). "Interferon alpha/beta and interleukin 12 responses to viral infections: pathways regulating dendritic cell cytokine expression in vivo." *J Exp Med* 195(4): 517-528.

Day, C. L., D. E. Kaufmann, et al. (2006). "PD-1 expression on HIV-specific T cells is associated with T-cell exhaustion and disease progression." *Nature* 443(7109): 350-354.

Delale, T., A. Paquin, et al. (2005). "MyD88-dependent and -independent murine cytomegalovirus sensing for IFN-alpha release and initiation of immune responses in vivo." *J Immunol* 175(10): 6723-6732.

Diebold, S. S., M. Montoya, et al. (2003). "Viral infection switches non-plasmacytoid dendritic cells into high interferon producers." *Nature* 424(6946): 324-328.

Donaghy, H., A. Pozniak, et al. (2001). "Loss of blood CD11c(+) myeloid and CD11c(-) plasmacytoid dendritic cells in patients with HIV-1 infection correlates with HIV-1 RNA virus load." *Blood* 98(8): 2574-2576.

Drakes, M. L., L. Lu, et al. (1997). "In vivo administration of flt3 ligand markedly stimulates generation of dendritic cell progenitors from mouse liver." *J Immunol* 159(9): 4268-4278.

Ejrnaes, M., C. M. Filippi, et al. (2006). "Resolution of a chronic viral infection after interleukin-10 receptor blockade." *J Exp Med* 203(11): 2461-2472.

Elsaesser, H., K. Sauer, et al. (2009). "IL-21 is required to control chronic viral infection." *Science* 324(5934): 1569-1572.

Fahey, L. M., E. B. Wilson, et al. (2011). "Viral persistence redirects CD4 T cell differentiation toward T follicular helper cells." *J Exp Med* 208(5): 987-999.

Fajardo-Moser, M., S. Berzel, et al. (2008). "Mechanisms of dendritic cell-based vaccination against infection." *Int J Med Microbiol* 298(1-2): 11-20.

Freeman, G. J., A. J. Long, et al. (2000). "Engagement of the PD-1 immunoinhibitory receptor by a novel B7 family member leads to negative regulation of lymphocyte activation." *J Exp Med* 192(7): 1027-1034.

Frohlich, A., J. Kisielow, et al. (2009). "IL-21R on T cells is critical for sustained functionality and control of chronic viral infection." *Science* 324(5934): 1576-1580.

Fung-Leung, W. P., T. M. Kundig, et al. (1991). "Immune response against lymphocytic choriomeningitis virus infection in mice without CD8 expression." *J Exp Med* 174(6): 1425-1429.

Goodman, A. G., H. Zeng, et al. (2010). "The alpha/beta interferon receptor provides protection against influenza virus replication but is dispensable for inflammatory response signaling." *J Virol* 84(4): 2027-2037.

Gottschalk, S., C. M. Bollard, et al. (2006). "T cell therapies." *Ernst Schering Found Symp Proc*(4): 69-82.

Grosso, J. F., M. V. Goldberg, et al. (2009). "Functionally distinct LAG-3 and PD-1 subsets on activated and chronically stimulated CD8 T cells." *J Immunol* 182(11): 6659-6669.

Hahm, B. (2009). "Hostile communication of measles virus with host innate immunity and dendritic cells." *Curr Top Microbiol Immunol* 330: 271-287.

Hahm, B., M. J. Trifilo, et al. (2005). "Viruses evade the immune system through type I interferon-mediated STAT2-dependent, but STAT1-independent, signaling." *Immunity* 22(2): 247-257.

Hoofnagle, J. H., K. D. Mullen, et al. (1986). "Treatment of chronic non-A,non-B hepatitis with recombinant human alpha interferon. A preliminary report." *N Engl J Med* 315(25): 1575-1578.

Hryniewicz, A., A. Boasso, et al. (2006). "CTLA-4 blockade decreases TGF-beta, IDO, and viral RNA expression in tissues of SIVmac251-infected macaques." *Blood* 108(12): 3834-3842.

Inaba, K., J. P. Metlay, et al. (1990). "Dendritic cells pulsed with protein antigens in vitro can prime antigen-specific, MHC-restricted T cells in situ." *J Exp Med* 172(2): 631-640.

Jin, H. T., A. C. Anderson, et al. (2010). "Cooperation of Tim-3 and PD-1 in CD8 T-cell exhaustion during chronic viral infection." *Proc Natl Acad Sci U S A* 107(33): 14733-14738.

Jung, A., H. Kato, et al. (2008). "Lymphocytoid choriomeningitis virus activates plasmacytoid dendritic cells and induces a cytotoxic T-cell response via MyD88." *J Virol* 82(1): 196-206.

Kanto, T. and N. Hayashi (2004). "Distinct susceptibility of dendritic cell subsets to hepatitis C virus infection: a plausible mechanism of dendritic cell dysfunction." *J Gastroenterol* 39(8): 811-812.

Kanto, T., M. Inoue, et al. (2004). "Reduced numbers and impaired ability of myeloid and plasmacytoid dendritic cells to polarize T helper cells in chronic hepatitis C virus infection." *J Infect Dis* 190(11): 1919-1926.

Kapp, M., S. M. Tan, et al. (2007). "Adoptive immunotherapy of HCMV infection." *Cytotherapy* 9(8): 699-711.

Kasaian, M. T., M. J. Whitters, et al. (2002). "IL-21 limits NK cell responses and promotes antigen-specific T cell activation: a mediator of the transition from innate to adaptive immunity." *Immunity* 16(4): 559-569.

Kasprowicz, V., J. Schulze Zur Wiesch, et al. (2008). "High level of PD-1 expression on hepatitis C virus (HCV)-specific CD8+ and CD4+ T cells during acute HCV infection, irrespective of clinical outcome." *J Virol* 82(6): 3154-3160.

Kaufmann, D. E., D. G. Kavanagh, et al. (2007). "Upregulation of CTLA-4 by HIV-specific CD4+ T cells correlates with disease progression and defines a reversible immune dysfunction." *Nat Immunol* 8(11): 1246-1254.

Kolokoltsova, O. A., N. E. Yun, et al. (2010). "Mice lacking alpha/beta and gamma interferon receptors are susceptible to junin virus infection." *J Virol* 84(24): 13063-13067.

Korbel, D. S., K. C. Newman, et al. (2005). "Heterogeneous human NK cell responses to Plasmodium falciparum-infected erythrocytes." *J Immunol* 175(11): 7466-7473.

Lancki, D. W., C. S. Hsieh, et al. (1991). "Mechanisms of lysis by cytotoxic T lymphocyte clones. Lytic activity and gene expression in cloned antigen-specific CD4+ and CD8+ T lymphocytes." *J Immunol* 146(9): 3242-3249.

Lee, H. K., J. M. Lund, et al. (2007). "Autophagy-dependent viral recognition by plasmacytoid dendritic cells." *Science* 315(5817): 1398-1401.

Liu, B., A. M. Woltman, et al. (2009). "Modulation of dendritic cell function by persistent viruses." *J Leukoc Biol* 85(2): 205-214.

Liu, Y. J. (2005). "IPC: professional type 1 interferon-producing cells and plasmacytoid dendritic cell precursors." *Annu Rev Immunol* 23: 275-306.

Martin, R., A. Vallbracht, et al. (1991). "Interferon-gamma secretion by in vivo activated cytotoxic T lymphocytes from the blood and cerebrospinal fluid during mumps meningitis." *J Neuroimmunol* 33(3): 191-198.

Martinez-Sobrido, L., S. Emonet, et al. (2009). "Identification of amino acid residues critical for the anti-interferon activity of the nucleoprotein of the prototypic arenavirus lymphocytic choriomeningitis virus." *J Virol* 83(21): 11330-11340.

Martinez-Sobrido, L., E. I. Zuniga, et al. (2006). "Inhibition of the type I interferon response by the nucleoprotein of the prototypic arenavirus lymphocytic choriomeningitis virus." *J Virol* 80(18): 9192-9199.

Martins, L. P., L. L. Lau, et al. (1995). "DNA vaccination against persistent viral infection." *J Virol* 69(4): 2574-2582.

Matloubian, M., R. J. Concepcion, et al. (1994). "CD4+ T cells are required to sustain CD8+ cytotoxic T-cell responses during chronic viral infection." *J Virol* 68(12): 8056-8063.

Montoya, M., M. J. Edwards, et al. (2005). "Rapid activation of spleen dendritic cell subsets following lymphocytic choriomeningitis virus infection of mice: analysis of the involvement of type 1 IFN." *J Immunol* 174(4): 1851-1861.

Muller, U., U. Steinhoff, et al. (1994). "Functional role of type I and type II interferons in antiviral defense." *Science* 264(5167): 1918-1921.

Murray, L. J., R. Lee, et al. (1990). "In vivo cytokine gene expression in T cell subsets of the autoimmune MRL/Mp-lpr/lpr mouse." *Eur J Immunol* 20(1): 163-170.

Nakamoto, N., H. Cho, et al. (2009). "Synergistic reversal of intrahepatic HCV-specific CD8 T cell exhaustion by combined PD-1/CTLA-4 blockade." *PLoS Pathog* 5(2): e1000313.

Odermatt, B., M. Eppler, et al. (1991). "Virus-triggered acquired immunodeficiency by cytotoxic T-cell-dependent destruction of antigen-presenting cells and lymph follicle structure." *Proc Natl Acad Sci U S A* 88(18): 8252-8256.

Pacanowski, J., S. Kahi, et al. (2001). "Reduced blood CD123+ (lymphoid) and CD11c+ (myeloid) dendritic cell numbers in primary HIV-1 infection." *Blood* 98(10): 3016-3021.

Rahman, A. H., W. Cui, et al. (2008). "MyD88 plays a critical T cell-intrinsic role in supporting CD8 T cell expansion during acute lymphocytic choriomeningitis virus infection." *J Immunol* 181(6): 3804-3810.

Richter, K., P. Agnellini, et al. (2010). "On the role of the inhibitory receptor LAG-3 in acute and chronic LCMV infection." *Int Immunol* 22(1): 13-23.

Sakthivel, P., M. Gereke, et al. (2011). "Therapeutic intervention in cancer and chronic viral infections: Antibody mediated manipulation of PD-1/PD-L1 interaction." *Rev Recent Clin Trials*.

Sakuishi, K., L. Apetoh, et al. (2010). "Targeting Tim-3 and PD-1 pathways to reverse T cell exhaustion and restore anti-tumor immunity." *J Exp Med* 207(10): 2187-2194.

Salvato, M., P. Borrow, et al. (1991). "Molecular basis of viral persistence: a single amino acid change in the glycoprotein of lymphocytic choriomeningitis virus is associated with suppression of the antiviral cytotoxic T-lymphocyte response and establishment of persistence." *J Virol* 65(4): 1863-1869.

Seo, Y. J. and B. Hahm (2010). "Type I interferon modulates the battle of host immune system against viruses." *Adv Appl Microbiol* 73: 83-101.

Sevilla, N., S. Kunz, et al. (2000). "Immunosuppression and resultant viral persistence by specific viral targeting of dendritic cells." *J Exp Med* 192(9): 1249-1260.

Sevilla, N., S. Kunz, et al. (2003). "Infection of dendritic cells by lymphocytic choriomeningitis virus." *Curr Top Microbiol Immunol* 276: 125-144.

Sevilla, N., D. B. McGavern, et al. (2004). "Viral targeting of hematopoietic progenitors and inhibition of DC maturation as a dual strategy for immune subversion." *J Clin Invest* 113(5): 737-745.

Shaffer, A. L., K. I. Lin, et al. (2002). "Blimp-1 orchestrates plasma cell differentiation by extinguishing the mature B cell gene expression program." *Immunity* 17(1): 51-62.

Shin, H., S. D. Blackburn, et al. (2009). "A role for the transcriptional repressor Blimp-1 in CD8(+) T cell exhaustion during chronic viral infection." *Immunity* 31(2): 309-320.

Siavoshian, S., J. D. Abraham, et al. (2005). "Hepatitis C virus core, NS3, NS5A, NS5B proteins induce apoptosis in mature dendritic cells." *J Med Virol* 75(3): 402-411.

Siren, J., T. Sareneva, et al. (2004). "Cytokine and contact-dependent activation of natural killer cells by influenza A or Sendai virus-infected macrophages." *J Gen Virol* 85(Pt 8): 2357-2364.

Smelt, S. C., P. Borrow, et al. (2001). "Differences in affinity of binding of lymphocytic choriomeningitis virus strains to the cellular receptor alpha-dystroglycan correlate with viral tropism and disease kinetics." *J Virol* 75(1): 448-457.

Steinman, R. M., A. Granelli-Piperno, et al. (2003). "The interaction of immunodeficiency viruses with dendritic cells." *Curr Top Microbiol Immunol* 276: 1-30.

Terawaki, S., S. Chikuma, et al. (2011). "IFN-alpha directly promotes programmed cell death-1 transcription and limits the duration of T cell-mediated immunity." *J Immunol* 186(5): 2772-2779.

Trifilo, M. J., B. Hahm, et al. (2006). "Dendritic cell inhibition: memoirs from immunosuppressive viruses." *J Infect Dis* 194 Suppl 1: S3-10.

Vankayalapati, R., A. Garg, et al. (2005). "Role of NK cell-activating receptors and their ligands in the lysis of mononuclear phagocytes infected with an intracellular bacterium." *J Immunol* 175(7): 4611-4617.

Vezys, V., P. Penaloza-MacMaster, et al. (2011). "4-1BB signaling synergizes with programmed death ligand 1 blockade to augment CD8 T cell responses during chronic viral infection." *J Immunol* 187(4): 1634-1642.

von Herrath, M. G., D. P. Berger, et al. (2000). "Vaccination to treat persistent viral infection." *Virology* 268(2): 411-419.

West, E. E., B. Youngblood, et al. (2011). "Tight regulation of memory CD8(+) T cells limits their effectiveness during sustained high viral load." *Immunity* 35(2): 285-298.

Wherry, E. J., J. N. Blattman, et al. (2005). "Low CD8 T-cell proliferative potential and high viral load limit the effectiveness of therapeutic vaccination." *J Virol* 79(14): 8960-8968.

Wherry, E. J., J. N. Blattman, et al. (2003). "Viral persistence alters CD8 T-cell immunodominance and tissue distribution and results in distinct stages of functional impairment." *J Virol* 77(8): 4911-4927.

Wherry, E. J., S. J. Ha, et al. (2007). "Molecular signature of CD8+ T cell exhaustion during chronic viral infection." *Immunity* 27(4): 670-684.

Workman, C. J., K. J. Dugger, et al. (2002). "Cutting edge: molecular analysis of the negative regulatory function of lymphocyte activation gene-3." *J Immunol* 169(10): 5392-5395.

Yamazaki, T., H. Akiba, et al. (2002). "Expression of programmed death 1 ligands by murine T cells and APC." *J Immunol* 169(10): 5538-5545.

Yi, J. S., M. A. Cox, et al. (2010). "T-cell exhaustion: characteristics, causes and conversion." *Immunology* 129(4): 474-481.

Yi, J. S., M. Du, et al. (2009). "A vital role for interleukin-21 in the control of a chronic viral infection." *Science* 324(5934): 1572-1576.

Youngblood, B., K. J. Oestreich, et al. (2011). "Chronic Virus Infection Enforces Demethylation of the Locus that Encodes PD-1 in Antigen-Specific CD8(+) T Cells." *Immunity* 35(3): 400-412.

Zhou, S., A. M. Cerny, et al. (2010). "Induction and inhibition of type I interferon responses by distinct components of lymphocytic choriomeningitis virus." *J Virol* 84(18): 9452-9462.

Zhou, S., E. A. Kurt-Jones, et al. (2005). "MyD88 is critical for the development of innate and adaptive immunity during acute lymphocytic choriomeningitis virus infection." *Eur J Immunol* 35(3): 822-830.

Zucchini, N., G. Bessou, et al. (2008). "Cutting edge: Overlapping functions of TLR7 and TLR9 for innate defense against a herpesvirus infection." *J Immunol* 180(9): 5799-5803.

Zuniga, E. I., B. Hahm, et al. (2007). "Type I interferon during viral infections: multiple triggers for a multifunctional mediator." *Curr Top Microbiol Immunol* 316: 337-357.

Zuniga, E. I., L. Y. Liou, et al. (2008). "Persistent virus infection inhibits type I interferon production by plasmacytoid dendritic cells to facilitate opportunistic infections." *Cell Host Microbe* 4(4): 374-386.

Is Chronic Lymphocytic Leukemia a Mistake of Tolerance Mechanisms?

Ricardo García-Muñoz[1], Judit Anton-Remirez[2], Jesus Feliu[3],
María Pilar Rabasa[1], Carlos Panizo[4] and Luis Llorente[5]

[1]*Hematology Service, Hospital San Pedro, Logroño, La Rioja,*
[2]*Rehabilitation Service, Complejo Hospitalario de Navarra, Pamplona, Navarra,*
[3]*Hematology Service, Complejo Hospitalario de Navarra, Pamplona, Navarra,*
[4]*Hematology Service, Clínica Universidad de Navarra, Pamplona, Navarra,*
[5]*Department of Immunology and Rheumatology, Instituto Nacional
de Ciencias Médicas y Nutrición Salvador Zubirán, Mexico City*
[1,2,3,4]*Spain*
[5]*México*

1. Introduction

Chronic Lymphocytic Leukemia (CLL) is a chronic lymphoproliferative disorder of the B lymphocytes. Small lymphocytic lymphoma (SLL) is considered to be the same disease in a non-leukemic form. CLL remains as an incurable tumour and clinical features have very variable presentation, course, and outcome. The progressive accumulation of monoclonal B lymphocytes leads to leukocytosis, lymphadenopathy, hepatosplenomegaly and marrow failure, and is sometimes associated with autoimmune manifestations.

It has been suggested that CLL cells are defective in apoptosis, which leads to the accumulation of malignant B cells. Furthermore, patients with proliferation rates greater than 0.35% per day have been found to have a more aggressive disease[18,19]. Proliferation of CLL cells is most prominent in proliferative centers that include specific areas in lymph nodes and bone marow[20,21]. Numerous CD4 T cells and dendritic cells are in close contact with CLL B cells [22], and micro environmental interactions like BM stromal cells are able to extend the survival of CLL upon direct contact[21]. Thus, the CLL population may originate from a clone with few or no V- domain mutations, or from a more mature clone whose V-domains have undergone the hypermutation process. This creates two separate pools of B cells, both of which originate from antigen-stimulated B lymphocytes. Additionally, IGHV unmutated CLL B cells expressing polyreactive antibodies whereas most IGHV mutated CLL´s did not. However, reversion of the IGHV mutated sequences to germline counterparts restored the polyreactivity (Herve et al 2005). Despite these features, the biological etiology of the divergent natural histories of IgVH unmutated vs mutated CLL and the origin of this type of leukemia/lymphoma remains unknown. For this reason we review the immunologic aspects that can help to understand this complex disease based in the findings that suggest that both unmutated and mutated subgroups of patients originally derive from autoreactive clones.

2. Diagnosis

The diagnosis of CLL requires the presence of at least 5000 B lymphocytes/µL in the peripheral blood (Hallek, et al 2008). CLL/SLL can be identified by the immunophenotype CD5+, CD10-, CD19+, CD20+, dim expression of surface immunoglobulin, CD23+, CD43 +/-, and cyclin D1- (Matutes, et al 2007). The absence of cyclin D1 is critical in distinguishing CLL/SLL from MCL. Bone marrow involvement is characteristically more than 30% of the nucleated cells in the aspirate are lymphoid.

Prognostic Markers and Genomic Aberrations

A favorable prognosis in CLL/SLL is associated with the presence of a mutated immunoglobulin heavy chain variable region, and low CD38 and zeta-chain–associated protein kinase 70 protein expression(Damle et al 1999;Kröber et al 2002;Hamblin et al 1999; Tobbin et al 2002; Crespo et al 2003). Chromosomal aberrations in CLL include del 6q, del 11q, del 13q, trisomy 12, and del 17p (Döhner et al 2000). Importantly, specific genomic aberrations have been associated with disease characteristics such better survival for patients with 12q trisomy and 13q deletion, poor survival and massive lymphadenopathy in 11q deletion and resistance to therapy in the group of patients with 17p deletion and p53 abnormalities (Döhrner et al 2000; Döhrner et al 1995; Döhrner et al 1997;Krober et al 2006). In addition, two miRNA (miR-15a and miR-16-1) were recently identified to be located in the critical region of the 13q14 deletion and their absence in CLL appears to be a major factor in preventing apoptosis and progression through the cell cycle (Aqeilan et al 2010; Cimmino et al 2005; Callin et al 2004; Mertens et al 2006).

Pathophysiology and cell of origin/normal counterpart of CLL

Different from other types of malignancies derived from mature B cells, the pathogenesis of B-CLL/SLL is much less understood. Notwithstanding extensive searching it is not known whether there is an equivalent normal cell in which the CLL arise. However, several cell types have been suggested as giving rise to chronic lymphocytic leukemia included memory, transitional, B1 and marginal zone B cells (Chiorazzi and Ferrarini 2011; Griffin et al 2011). In addition, it is not certain at what stage in lymphocyte maturation the CLL cell arises, since roughly equal numbers seem to come from pre-germinal center B lymphocytes (unmutated group) and post-germinal center B lymphocytes (mutated group). However, the comparison of CLL gene expression profiles with those of purified normal B cell subpopulations indicates that the common CLL gene expression profile is more related to memory B cells than to those derived from naïve B cells, CD5+ B cells, or germinal center centroblasts and centrocytes (Klein et al 2001; Rosenwald et al 2001, Klein and Dalla-Favera 2005). Interestingly, unmutated and mutated chronic lymphocytic leukemias derive from self reactive B cell precursors despite expressing different antibody reactivity (Herve et al 2005). This similar expression profile also suggest that the consequences or even the mechanism of transformation may be similar, irrespective of IGHV mutations status. This too suggests that rather than having a cellular origin or cellular subtype, CLL is originated by a coordinated normal immunologic tolerance mechanism to destroy self-reactive B cells and to avoid autoimmunity during their process of differentiation. This point of view is supported by the fact that some CLL mutated and unmutated cases derive from self-reactive B cells (Herve et al 2005) had evidence of multiple, related rearranged heavy and light chain immunoglobulin genes (Volkheimer et al 2007; Hadzidimitriou et al 2009, Stamatopoulos et al 1996); some express more than one functional Ig heavy chain (Rassenti et al 1997), some had been anergized (Mockridge et al 2007; Muzio et al 2008), edited (Hadzidimitriou et al 2009, Stamatopoulos et al 1996), switched (Cerutti et al 2002) and/or had progressive immunoglobulin gene mutation (Volkheimer et al 2007; Roudier et al 1990; Ruzickova et al 2002).

Hypothesis: Autoimmunity as origin of CLL

The basic hypothesis of the origin of autoimmune disease depends of the emergence of a clone or a small number of clones of T and B lymphocytes capable of damaging interaction with normal cells of organ or tissue involved. Each clone is initiated from a cell which has developed an immune receptor adequately reactive with an accessible self antigen as a result of a V/D/J gene recombination in bone marrow (unmutated) or during somatic mutations in germinal centers (mutated). Importantly, this newly self-reactive cell ("forbidden clone") is anomalously resistant to inactivation by central and peripheral tolerance check points (Burnet 1972). Similar to an autoimmune disease, some lymphoproliferative diseases (marginal zone lymphomas and chronic lymphocytic leukemia) depends of the emergence of a clone capable of interact with an (auto) antigen and with other normal cells and an specific microenvironment to proliferate and survive. In a parallel way, newly malignant B cells are anomalously resistant to apoptosis and proliferate as result of acquisition of genetic damage during V/D/J gene recombination, somatic mutations, class switching and receptor edition/revision. Importantly, with the exception of class switching, the other mechanisms to increase the diversity of B cell receptors might induce both self-reactivity and/or DNA damage.

B cell development and autoimmunity

The current model of the pathogenesis of CLL suggest that stimulation by (self) antigens provides a pro-survival and possibly pro-proliferative advantage for CLL (precursor) cells, most likely leading initially to oligoclonal and subsequently monoclonal selection of malignant cells (Mertens et al 2011)

In humans, B cells develop from progenitors within the bone marrow (Fig1). The stages of B cell ontogeny from pro-B to pre-B to early B to mature B cells are marked by phenotypic changes, the most important of which is expression of the BCR for antigen on the cell surface at the early B cell stage of development (van Lochem et al 2004; Fuda et al 2009) . During the course of ontogenesis, B cells mature in the bone marrow according to the evolution of the Ig chain synthesis. Starting with the rearrangement of the V/D/J genes for the heavy chain at the pre-B stage, the recombination process continues through the VJ gene rearrangements for kappa light chain or for the lambda light chain at the immature stage. Thus, the resulting receptor (BCR) comprised of randomly selected heavy and light chains have an unpredictable specificity that could include ability to bind "self". However, there are tolerance check points at every stage of B cell activation and maturation (table 1 and 2). This tolerance mechanisms in bone marrow include receptor editing, clonal deletion, clonal anergy and differentiation to B1 cells (Goodnow et al 2005; Radic et al 1993; Tiegs et al 1993; Nemazee et al 2000; Luning Prak et al 2011) Notably, current evidence suggest that anergy, receptor edition and differentiation to B1 B cells could be implicated in the generation of CLL B cells (Herve et al 2005; Chu et al 2010; Mockridge et al 2007; Hadzidimitriou et al 2009, Stamatopoulos et al 1996; Ghia et al 2008a; Rassenti & Kipps 1997; Murray et al 2008;

Griffin et al 2011). Additionally , hematopoietic stem cells sorted from a CLL patient´s bone marrow produce CLL like disease when transplanted into immunosuppresed mice (Kikushige et al 2011). Importantly, autoreactive B cells may suffer receptor editing and anergy in bone marrow. At the same, recent evidence shows that L chain receptor editing occurs not only in bone marrow with a pre-B/immature B cell phenotype but also in immature/transitional splenic B cells. Nevertheless, editing at the H chain locus appears to occur exclusively in bone marrow cells with pro-B phenotype (Nakajima et al 2009).

Repertoire analyses of antibodies cloned from B cells derived from bone marrow and peripheral blood of healthy donors provide evidence for both a central tolerance check point in the bone marrow and a second peripheral checkpoint, as evidenced by a decrease in the frequency of autoreactive antibodies from 75% in bone marrow to 20% in the circulating naïve compartment (Yurasov, et al. 2005). Other tolerance mechanisms and peripheral check points include memory development check points (Tsuiji et al 2006) CD5+ expression (Morikawa et al 1993; Gary-Gouy et al 2002; Hillion et al 2005; Hippen et al 2000, Gary-Gouy et al 2002b, Dallou et al 2008), germinal centre exclusion (Cappione et al 2005; Pugh-Bernard et al 2001), receptor edition/revision (Luning Prack et al 2011), antibody feedback (Ravetch & Bolland 2001), anti-idiotypic network (Jerne 1974; Jerne 1984; Forni et al 1980) and all contribute to maintain tolerance and avoid autoimmune diseases.

The contribution of this mechanism in the development of CLL remain unknown, however, Ghia et al describe that CLL expressing IGHV3-21/IGVL3-21 most likely were derived from B cells that had experienced somatic mutation and germinal center maturation in an apparent antigen driven immune response previous to undergoing Ig receptor editing and after germinal-center leukemogenic selection (Ghia et al 2008b). This suggest that peripheral tolerance mechanism also contribute to the shape of self reactive CLL B cells generated and selected after somatic hypermutation. Other mechanisms as germinal centre exclusion, defects in antibody feedback and anti-idiotypic network in lymphoproliferative disorders remain unsolved, however some conjectures about their role have been proposed (García-Muñoz 2009a; García-Muñoz et al 2009b).

The fact that unmutated and mutated chronic lymphocytic leukemias derive from self reactive B cell precursors despite expressing different antibody reactivity (Herve et al 2005) suggest that this B cells escape from tolerance mechanisms. Even more Chiorazzi and Ferrarini suggest that CLL derives from competent B lymphocytes selected for clonal expansion and eventual transformation by multiple encounters and responses to (auto)antigen(s) (Chiorazzi and Ferrarini 2003). This two characteristics of CLL B cells guide us to think that CLL is the product of the selective pressure of tolerance check points in an auto-reactive B cell.

Development of Unmutated CLL B cells

Tumors displaying unmutated V genes have a shorter median survival, in one study of 99 months vs 293 months in the mutated cases (Hamblin et al 1999). Here, a cut-off of $\geq 98\%$ homology to donor germline gene has been used to define unmutated tumor V genes to allow for a low degree of polymorphic allelic variation. There is an association between unfavorable cytogenetic aberrations (del 17p and del 11q) and unmutated CLL, although 13q- is more frequent in mutated CLL. However, there are discrepancies with many cases having some high-risk and other low-risk molecular features and more than 50% of IgVH unmutated cases have no unfavorable cytogenetics (Krober et al 2006). Prominently unmutated CLL B cells are self reactive or polyreactive (Herve et al 2005) and seem that they are resistant to several tolerance mechanism.

Are unmutated CLL B cells invulnerable to anergy?

Low BCR signaling induced by weak reactivity to self antigens induce B cells to enter a tolerized but alive state referred to as anergy (Gauld et al 2006; Getahun et al 2009) . In most cases, anergic B cells are characterized by chronic low level BCR signaling and exhibit reduced surface IgM levels but can express high levels of IgD (Getahun et al 2009; Goodnow et al 1998; Dolmetsh et al 1997). Interestingly, anergy depends on the degree of BCR occupancy and require constant transduction of a BCR signal (Goodnow et al 1989; Benshop et al 2001;Gauld et al 2005). Although it is clear that stimulation through the BCR occurred during the natural history of all types of CLL, it is quite peculiar that unmutated CLL cells retain the capacity to transmit signals through the BCR via surface IgM (Lanham et al 2003). The low expression of the BCR is the hallmark of CLL cells and anergic B cells, and appears to contribute towards producing poorer responses to BCR stimulation. Despite low levels of surface expressed immunoglobulin, signalling through the B cell receptor is possible. ZAP-70 expression has shown to augment signalling via IgM ligation in CLL cells as measured by phosphorylation of downstream mediators such as Syk, BLNK and PLC and calcium influx (Chen et al 2005) This increased signalling might lead to enhanced proliferation or survival of the leukemic cell (Bernal et al 2001). Significantly, a number of studies have shown a strong association between ZAP-70 expression and unmutated IGHV genes. This findings could imply that if an immature self-reactive B cell recognize an auto-antigen and also express ZAP-70 survival and activating signals prevail over anergy. In this case a self reactive CLL B cell selected by a self-antigen during B cell development in bone marrow might mature despite they undergo an anergy process and likely to progress to transitional and mature B cell.

Unmutated CLL cases are more frequently CD38 (66-77%) and ZAP-70 (93%) positive, exhibit IgM+ and IgD+ surface immunoglobulin, express higher amounts of BCR and response better to stimulation compared with mutated CLL´s (Wiestner et al 2003, Hamblin et al 2002; Thumberg et al 2001; Döhner et al 2000; Mockridge et al 2007; Guarini et al 2008). This characteristics suggest that this unmutated CLL B cells where resistant to anergy and progress to mature autoreactive naive B cells.

Receptor editing be unsuccessful to avoid self-reactivity and might induce polyreactive BCR in unmutated CLL B cells

Immature B cells expressing self-reactive IgM antibodies may undergo repeated rounds of light chain rearrangement to lessen the self specificity of the antibody, a process termed receptor editing (Nemazee et al 2000; Luning Prak et al 2011). Evidence of receptor editing in CLL is provided by the fact that a number of CLL´s have multiple light chain rearrangements (Hadzidimitriou et al 2009). B cell receptor of CLL B cells react with recurrent self antigens in vitro including IgG, thyroglobulin, DNA, actin, cardiolipin and others as well as microbial antigens and epitopes exposed on cell surface as a result of apoptosis and also could be stimulated by stroma-derived antigens (Sthoeger et al 1989; Dighiero et al 1991; Chiorazzi et al 2005; Lanemo Myhrinder et al 2008). Sustained or repetitive BCR signaling promotes survival in CLL cells (Petlickovsky et al 2005; Bernal et al

2001). Notably, unmutated CLL B cells are self reactive or polyreactive (Herve et al 2005). Interestingly, 79.3% of unmutated CLL antibodies are polyreactive (Herve et al 2005), and reactivity with a particular form of apoptotic cells is a common feature of this subset (Chu et al 2010). Even more, recently Rozcova et al revealed that Toll like receptor 9 (TLR-9) agonists are a potent stimulus from CLL B cells and induce proliferation, expression of CD38 and secretion of cytokines (Rozcova et al 2010). Outstandingly, TLR-9 recognition of self-molecules (nucleic acids in apoptotic cells) of the host, which are not easily distinguishable from those of no-self (infectious organisms) has the potential to provoke autoimmune diseases. Intriguingly, the unmutated CLL subset expresses antibodies with long heavy and light chain CDR3 (Herve 2005) and some cases of unmutated CLL with 100% of IGHV identity have multiple light chain rearrangements (Hadzidimitriou et al TS25 2009), associated with receptor edition. This suggest that receptor editing mechanisms could be not working well in this subset, even more is possible that increase polyreactivity (Luning Prak et al 2011; Binder et al 2010) and promote survival of self-reactive (Sandel et al 1999) CLL B cells. Consequently, BCRs that react with diverse epitopes may be more prone to sustained signaling. As a result, some unmutated CLL B cells expressing multireactive BCR have a more aggressive course than CLLs expressing less reactive BCRs (Binder et al 2010).

Are unmutated CLL B cells insensitive to CD5 action?

Induction of CD5 by autoantigen might be a mechanism by which the production of autoantibodies is avoided and also maintains tolerance in anergic B cells (Berland et al 2002; Hippen et al 2000). Recently, a very interesting observation was made that many CLL leukemia antibodies recognize non-muscle myosin heavy chain IIA exposed apoptotic cells (MEACs) and that natural antibodies from human serum also react with MEACs. In this study 15 of 16 MEAC-reactive CLL mAbs carried unmutated IGVH genes (Chu et al 2010). Several mechanisms are involved in the tolerance associated with expression of CD5. Likewise, CD5 expression prevents B lymphocytes from uncontrolled self reactivity increasing the BCR signalling threshold[51], and is associated with reexpresion of RAG, receptor edition/revision, and lack of responsiveness to BAFF in some cells outside bone marrow and germinal centres (Lee et al 2009; Hippen et al 2000, Hillion et al 2005). Along this line, the fact that anergic autoreactive B cells may express CD5+ and that immunoglobulin secreted by unmutated B-CLL cells is often autoreactive and react with a variety of autoantigens (including Fc portion of IgG, DNA, histones, cardiolipin, cytoskeletal proteins and insulin) support the notion that unmutated self-reactive B CLL cells are under check to avoid pathogenic autoimmunity (Broker et al 1988; Caligaris-Cappio et al 1996; Morbach et al 2006). We speculate that the expression of ZAP-70 and CD38 could encourage the stimulation of unmutated CLL B cells and overcome the inhibition induced by CD5. In addition, CD5 does not inhibit properly the BCR mediating signalling in leukemic B cells and in some cases provide viability signals or/and promote CLL B cell survival (Perez-Chacon et al 2007; Perez-Chacon 2007b; Gary-Gouy et al 2007; Gary-Gouy et al 2002; Gary-Gouy et al 2002).

Are unmutated CLL B cells transformed human B1 cells?

Similarities between normal human B1 cells and malignant chronic lymphocytic leukemia (CLL) cells, include that both are CD20+CD27+CD43+CD70-; most normal B1 cells express CD5, as do malignant CLL cells; and, both express relatively nonmutated IGHV. In addition, normal human B1 cells are ZAP-70+ like unmutated CLL cells. As a final point, in respect to pathophysiology, Griffin et al propose that the chronically activated phenotype of normal B1 cells may predispose to malignant transformation (Griffin et al 2011).

Are unmutated CLL naïve self-reactive B cells efficiently excluded by germinal centres?

In order to prevent autoimmunity, censoring mechanisms, including anergy and sequestration into the marginal zone, ultimately forbid the participation of mature autoreactive B cells in productive germinal centres reactions, thereby precluding their expansion into the long-lived IgG memory and plasma cell compartments. Importantly, most self reactive and polyreactive IgG antibodies originate from non self-reactive B cells that acquired reactivity by somatic hypermutation (Tiller et al 2007). Significantly, somatic hypermutation does not appear to occur uniformly among CLL IGHV genes(Chiorazzi et al 2005; Fais et al 1998; Tobin et al 2002; Ghia et al 2005) and might suggest the effect of germinal centre exclusion and tolerance mechanisms to maintain the self-reactive BCR in a germ line state and avoid the participation of unmutated CLL cases in germinal centres reactions.

Development of Mutated CLL B cells

Fifty percent of CLL patients have undergone somatic hypermutation in IGHV, and these patients have a more indolent clinical course and longer survival than those without somatic hipermutation (Hamblin et al 1999; Damle et al 1999). The majority of cases of mutated CLL fail to signal via IgM in vitro (Lanham et al 2003; Chen et al 2002). Interestingly, CLL B cells that express only IgD+ are linked to mutated IGHV genes, negative or low CD38 expression, and 50% of mutated CLL cases unable to signal via IgM were able to signal via IgD (Stevenson et al 2004). Muzio et al, showed that CLL B cells (typically IGH-mutated cases) that do not respond to BCR ligation show activation cellular pathways that suggest anergy (Muzio et al 2008). Essentially, mutated CLL cases derive from B cells with self-reactive receptors that were anergized, edited or regulated to avoid autoimmunity. This is supported by the fact that when mutated non autoreactive immunoglobulin sequences of mutated CLL cases were reverted to their germline counterparts, they encoded polyreactive and autoreactive antibodies (Herve 2005). Despite somatic hypermutation had been proposed as a mechanism to change original BCR self reactivity (germ line) towards some non-self BCR (Murray et al 2008), this is an eccentric mode to loss self reactivity because, self reactive naïve B cells are efficiently excluded from germinal centres (Tsuji et al 2006; Cappione A 3rd et al 2005; Pugh-Bernard et al 2001) and if this check point is bypassed B cells progress to plasmatic cells that produce auto-antibodies. Still, a significant fraction of self-reactive BCR fail to be edited or trigger deletion in primary lymphoid tissues, either because the self-antigen are bound with only low avidity or because they are not sufficiently abundant in primary lymphoid organs. For receptors with intermediate avidity for self antigens, the risk they pose for autoimmunity may not overshadow their potential use in fighting infection. B cells with receptors that fall into this zone undergo a conditional type of clonal deletion that is extrinsically regulated through competition with B cells bearing less self reactive BCR (Cyster et al 1994; Lanemo Myhrinder et al 2008). This also can explain that unmutated CLL cases and mutated CLL cases express different antibody repertoires and different VH genes (Fais et al 1988; Johnson et al 1997). Current data support that CLL cells are in active (auto) antigen driven receptor editing, presumably by keeping away from autoreactivity associated with preferential autoimmune linked IGHV gene utilization in CLL patients like IGHV3-21, IGHV4-34, IGKV1-17 (Foreman et al 2007; Hadzidimitruiou et al 2009) and also IGHV5-51 and IGHV1-69 in unmutated IgVH genes (Chapal et al 2000; Vanura et al 2008). Interestingly, highly polyreactive antibodies are expressed frequently by unmutated CLL, but only rarely by mutated cases, supporting the view that the receptor editing mechanism is significantly active to try to elude autoimmunity in CLL.

In mutated CLL cases quite a lot of cellular strategies are used to regulate self-reactive receptors at different points during B cell differentiation.

1. The receptor is edited to one that is less self reactive by V(D)J recombination (Hadzidimitriou et al 2009; Rassenti et al 1997 Ghia et al 2008b; Kalinina et al 2011).
2. Regulation by BCR downregulation and anergy (Muzio et al 2008).
3. Induction of inhibitory receptors as CD5 by self-reactive BCR (Hippen et al 2000; Morikawa et al 1993; Dallou et al 2008; Hillion et al 2005).

Table 1. BCR tolerance mechanisms in central lymphoid organs (bone marrow) include receptor edition, anergy and induction of inhibitory receptors as CD5.

Regulation of self reactive receptor in follicles

Each of the checkpoints described above deal with self-reactive receptor generated by V(D)J recombination in the primary lymphoid organs; however, self-reactive BCRs are also generated in a second wave of receptor-gene-diversification through somatic hypermutation in germinal centre follicles of peripheral lymphoid tissues (Shiono et al 2003; Radic et al 1994; Ray et al 1996). Despite somatic hypermutation could produce modifications in BCR to ablate self-reactivity (Murray et al 2008) also might produce new self-reactive BCR. In addition somatic hypermutation poses a particular severe threat of autoimmunity for the reason that increase the affinity of antibodies for self-antigens, the follicular pathway of B cell differentiation generates long lived plasma and memory cells and numerous apoptotic cells be present in germinal centres with self components that are trapped and displayed as immune complexes on follicular dendritic cells. For these reasons the immune system contain a number of mechanisms to elude the maturation of self-reactive B cells that encourage an autoimmune disease. Self-reactivity of mutated CLL cases may derive from immature self-reactive B cells that suffer somatic hypermutation or by non-self reactive B cells that acquire self-reactive BCR during somatic hypermutation in germinal centres. In humans two types of memory B cells have been described: IgM+ memory B cells and class-switched memory B cells (Agematsu et al 1997; Klein et al 1998; Tangye et al 1998). Transition from naive B cells into circulating IgM+ memory B cells is accompanied by efficient counter selection against self reactive naive B cells before the onset of somatic hypermutation and that self reactive IgM+ memory B cells present in the circulation of healthy humans gain self-reactivity as a result of somatic hypermutation (Tsuji et al 2006).

The increase in self-reactivity during transition between mature naive and IgG+ memory B cells might be due to selective advantage for pre-existing self-reactive cells, or selection for cells with self reactive antibodies produced by somatic hypermutation. (Tiller et al 2007) This mechanisms could contribute to generate the IgG+ CLL cases (Ghiotto F, et al 2004).

1. Germinal centre exclusion (Tsuji et al 2006; Cappione A 3rd et al 2005; Pugh-Bernard et al 2001).
2. The receptor is modified to one that is less self reactive by BCR hypermutation (Murray et al 2008, Tiller et al 2007).
3. Receptor edition/revision (Hadzidimitriou et al 2009; Kalinina et al 2011; Rochas et al 2007)
4. CD5 expression (Hillion et al 2005).
6. Absence of T cell help (Shokat et al 1995)
7. Competition for follicular niches (Cyster et al 1994)

Table 2. Tolerance mechanisms in peripheral lymphoid organs.

Tolerance induced by absence of T-cell help:

A substantial portion of the activated B cells migrate to germinal centers where they undergo the process of somatic hypermutation. These B cells first remove the BCR from their surface, then undergo several rounds of division, and finally re-express mutated immunoglobulin receptors. The cells then undergo a negative selection process similar to that of transitional B cells. The antigen is provided from antigen-antibody complexes on follicular dendritic cells. Survival requires the receptor to be of high enough affinity to out-compete the already circulating antibody and allow B cell uptake and processing of antigen For display peptides to primed helper T cells, which have also moved into the germinal centers (Kearneay et al 1994). If the B cell receives T cell-help it survives and is stimulated to undergo another round of expansion and differentiation. If T cell help is not received, the B cell can become anergized or die by apoptosis (Shokat, et al 1995).

We suggest that in CLL with mutated Ig genes, the proliferating B cells is likely to have traversed a germinal center and acquire "*de novo* self-reactivity" originated in the process of somatic hypermutation mechanism or by receptor editon revision. After this "*de novo* autoreactivity" a normal CD5- B cell can theoretically be transformed into a "*de novo* autoreactive memory B cell" that express CD5+ (increase the threshold for BCR activation), suffer receptor revision (change light chains to evade autoimmunity), down regulate surface Ig (to avoid activation), and remain under check by germinal center exclusion (to diminish the chance to progress in the maturation and become plasma cells that produce autoantibodies). Finally, all this tolerance mechanism converts this B CD5- B cell into an "anergic-edited-CD5+CD27+ memory B cell" excluded from germinal centres. These "*de novo* autoreactive" memory B cells could retain a process of "self-renewal", a specificity that changes (receptor editing-revision) and/or that can not be activated because this "new malignant cell" is an "anergic cell" excluded from germinal centres. This speculation could explain why mutated IGVH CLL susbsets ("anergic cells") have an indolent course related to the absence of BCR signalling activation.

IGVH gene usage in CLL is highly selective, and often associated with autoantibody reactivity (Oscier et al 1987). The fact that almost 30 % of CLL patients share BCRs with restricted, quasi-identical immunoglobulins sequences should aid the understanding of the functional interplay between CLL cells and the microenvironment. On the one hand, unmutated IGVH CLL subsets recognizes apoptotic cells in bone marrow and spleen and express a functionally competent BCR, as shown by the fact that most of it can be stimulated following Ig ligation *in vitro*. On the other hand, CLL mutated that has acquired "*de novo*" autoreactivity induced by somatic hypermutation recognizes apoptotic cells in germinal centres; however they become anergic and are unresponsive throughout BCR stimulation. In a CLL mutated subset the "memory-anergic" B cell returns to bone marrow in the same way that normal memory B cells.

Other immunologic alterations that theoretically might predispose the lost of CLL clone control: Impaired immunologic synapses

CD4 and CD8 T cells of patients with CLL show impaired immunological synapse formation with antigen presenting cells (APC)(Ramsay et al 2008). This dysfunction is in part induced by the CLL B cells. This impaired immunological synapse within T cells and APC could contribute to the failure to mount an effective immune response in patients with CLL. Moreover, it may also add other immunological abnormalities like hipogammaglobulinemia (impaired T cell – B cell interactions), autoimmunity (impaired regulatory T cell control), and second tumours (diminished immunosurveillance mediate by NK and CD8 T cells). Interestingly, lenalidomide, an immunomodulatory drug, could repair this synapses with an enhancement of immune cell function. This effect is clinically observed during treatment of CLL patients with this agent because lenalidomide probably induces a strong activation of the immune system complicated by swelling of involved lymph nodes and fever named tumour flare reaction (Chanan-Khan et al 2006; Aue et al 2009)

Antibody mediated immunoregulation:

The antigen-antibody complexes are also likely to be responsible for the phenomenon known as original antigenic sin, in which memory B cells, generated during a prior exposure to a cross-reacting antigen, present or down-regulate the response to these unique new determinants on the antigen[70]. Memory B cells seem to have an advantage for rapid activation and this produces antibodies that feed back to inhibit the priming of naïve B cells possessing receptors that are specific to unique determinants of the second immunogen. This feedback mechanism is most likely mediated through antigen-antibody complexes that interact with FcγRIIb on the naïve B cells and inhibit signal transduction through their IgM receptors (Ravetch et al 2001). In patients with hipogammaglobulinemia this feedback mechanism is impaired and might contribute to expansion of autoreactive B cells (García-Muñoz 2009b) , and in patients with CLL it may add an additional risk to uncontrolled proliferation of CLL clones.

Anti-idiotypic B cell regulation: In 1974 Jerne proposed that antibody production could be regulated by other antibodies that recognized unique idiotypic determinants in the V regions of the first antibody. He postulated that an increase in the production of the first antibody could negatively regulate the production of anti-idiotypic antibodies, and vice versa. Because of the interconnected pathways in such a network, perturbation of one segment would be dampened by the presence of others segments and thus the original steady state would be buffered (Jerne 1984; Jerne 1970; Forni et al 1980).

Patients with CLL have an increased proportion of autoimmune haemolytic anemia (AIHA) and idiopatic autoimmune thrombocytopenia (ITP) and infections. It is probable that the idiotypic network is disrupted in CLL patients and that this could lead to an increased risk of autoimmunity on one hand and immunodeficiency on the other. Treatment with intravenous immunoglobulins (IVIg) could in theory restore idiotypic network and antigen-antibody-complexes feedback in CLL B cells. Remarkably, patients with AIHA treated with IVIg experiment a reduction of the size of lymph nodes and spleen (Diehl et al 1998). This suggests that immune-complexes feedback and idiotypic network could contribute indirectly in the control of CLL.

MYD88 Mutation

Interestingly, mutations in MYD88 and KLHL6 genes have been reported recently in patients with mutated CLL patients (Puente et al 2011). Significantly, similar to CLL patients, patients with MYD88-deficiency do not secrete autoantibodies (Isnardi et al 2008). We speculate that if mutations in MYD88 gene were acquired during germinal center reaction, is possible that self-reactive B cells cannot progress to plasmatic cells but retain some features or memory B cells. Even more, TLR-9 acts via MYD88 and might induce proliferation of CLL B cells. However, mutations in MYD88 might disturb the function of this TLR-9 and contribute to the biology and better prognosis of mutated CLL cases.

IGHV gene usage in CLL is highly selective, and often associated with autoantibody reactivity. The fact that almost 30 % of CLL patients share BCRs with restricted, quasi-identical immunoglobulins sequences should aid to the understanding of the functional interplay between CLL cells and the microenvironment. On the one hand, unmutated *IGHV* CLL subsets recognizes apoptotic cells in bone marrow and spleen and express a functionally competent BCR, as shown by the fact that most of it can be stimulated following Ig ligation *in vitro*. On the other hand, CLL mutated that has acquired *"de novo"* autoreactivity (¿mutations in MYD88?) induced by somatic hypermutation recognizes apoptotic cells in germinal centres; however they become anergic and are unresponsive throughout BCR stimulation. In a CLL mutated subset the "memory-anergic" B cell returns to bone marrow in the same way that normal memory B cells.

3. Conclusion

Chronic lymphocytic leukemia can be separated into cases that harbour somatic mutation in their IGVH genes, or cases without somatic mutations. IGVH gene usage in CLL is highly selective, and often associated with autoantibody reactivity. Despite the fact that the cell surface markers and gene expression of CLL cells suggest that both subsets originate from a precursor cell of the same developmental stage, these findings could be only the result of several immunologic mechanisms that try to destroy or avoid the persistence of self-reactive CLL B cells. CLL is characterized by multiple immune deficiencies and autoimmune phenomena associated with persistent tolerance mechanism trying to control self-reactive CLL B cells growth.

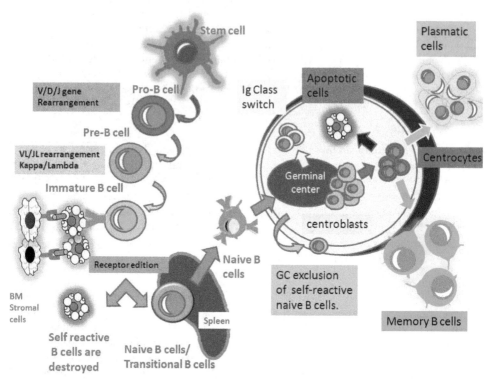

B-cell development occurs initially in the bone marrow and subsequently in lymphoid organs. In bone marrow, hematopoietic progenitor cells (HSC) differentiate into the earliest identifiable cell type committed to the B-cell lineage, the pro-B cell. The pro-B cell undergoes a rearrangement of its immunoglobulin (Ig) heavy chain genes and is called a pre-B cell. Subsequent rearrangement of the light chain enables the cell to express surface IgM and the cell becomes an immature transitional B lymphocyte. These cells leave the bone marrow and are called naïve B cells. They are arrested in the G0 phase of the cell cycle. These naïve B cells enter the lymphoid tissue, where they are exposed to antigen-presenting cells, become activated and differentiate into plasma cells or memory B cells. Through activation by an antigen, B cells differentiate into centroblasts, resulting in Ig isotype switching and somatic mutations in the variable region of the Ig with the generation of high-affinity antibodies. Centroblasts then progress to the centrocyte stage and re-express surface Ig. The centrocytes with high-affinity antibodies differentiate into either memory B cells or plasmablasts, which subsequently move to the bone marrow and terminally differentiate into plasma cells.

Fig. 1. Normal B cell development.

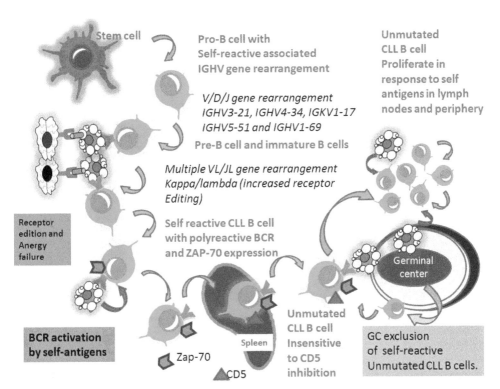

Unmutate CLL B-cell development occurs initially in the bone marrow and subsequently in lymphoid organs. In bone marrow, hematopoietic progenitor cells (HSC) differentiate into the pro-B cell that use IGHV genes related with autoimmunity. The pro-B cell undergoes a rearrangement of its immunoglobulin (Ig) heavy chain genes and is called a pre-B cell. Subsequent rearrangement of the light chain enables the cell to express surface self reactive BCR that fail to be corrected by several rounds of receptor edition. This self-reactive B cells acquire Zap-70 or other alterations that induce increased BCR activation. This is the way in which this self-reactive CLL B cells pass up tolerance mechanisms as anergy and inhibition exerted by CD5. These cells leave the bone marrow as unmutated polyreactive CLL B cells. These unmutated polyreactive CLL B cells enter in the lymphoid tissue, where they are exposed to antigen-presenting cells and self-antigens, however, they cannot be converted into plasma cells or memory B cells with mutations because they are efficiently excluded by germinal centers.

Fig. 2. Hypothesis about generation of unmutated B cells (García-Muñoz et al. Ann Hematol. Accepted).

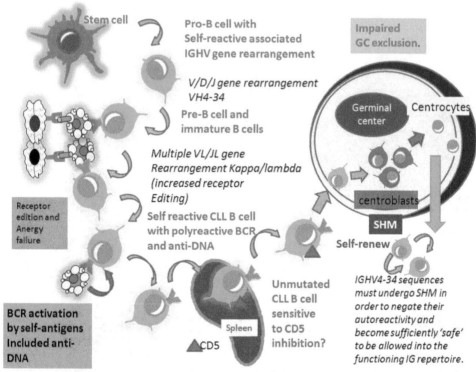

Mutated CLL B-cell development occurs initially in the bone marrow and subsequently in lymphoid organs. In bone marrow, hematopoietic progenitor cells (HSC) differentiate into the pro-B cell that use IGHV genes related with autoimmunity. The pro-B cell undergoes a rearrangement of its immunoglobulin (Ig) heavy chain genes and is called a pre-B cell. Subsequent rearrangement of the light chain enables the cell to express surface self reactive BCR that fail to be corrected by several rounds of receptor edition. This self-reactive B cells enter in germinal centres and undergo somatic hypermutation in order to negate their autoreactivity. This is the way in which this self-reactive CLL B cells pass up tolerance mechanisms as germinal centre exclusion, however, fortunately they suffer some mutations to reverse their self reactivity and avoid autoimmune diseases as SLE. These cells leave the germinal center as mutated CLL B cells memory like cells.

Fig. 3. "Impaired Germinal Centre exclusion model for development of mutated CLL cases wiht VH4-34.

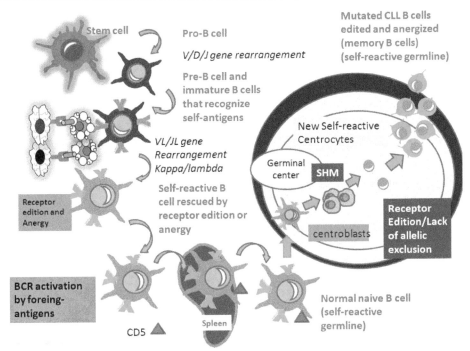

Mutated CLL B-cell development occurs initially in the bone marrow and subsequently in lymphoid organs. In bone marrow, hematopoietic progenitor cells (HSC) differentiate into the pro-B cell that use IGHV genes related with autoimmunity. The pro-B cell undergoes a rearrangement of its immunoglobulin (Ig) heavy chain genes and is called a pre-B cell. Subsequent rearrangement of the light chain enables the cell to express surface self reactive BCR that succeed to be corrected by several rounds of receptor edition. This ex-self-reactive B cells acquire CD5 or other alterations that induce lesser BCR activation. This is the way in which this ex-self-reactive CLL B cells suffer tolerance mechanisms as receptor edition, anergy and inhibition exerted by CD5. These cells leave the bone marrow as unmutated normal naïve B cells. These naïve ex-self reactive B cells enter in germinal centres and suffer somatic hypermutation (SHM) and acquire a new self-reactive BCR, however, again tolerance mechanisms as receptor edition/revision and CD5 expression make this cells in an anergic memory ex-self-reactive B cells. Importantly, reversion of the IGHV mutated sequences to germline counterparts restored the polyreactivity and self-reactivity.

Fig. 4. Mutated CLL B cells generated by somatic hypermutation (García Muñoz et al. Ann Hematol. Accepted).

4. Acknowledgment

The authors declare that a review paper on immunological aspects in CLL is actually accepted in Ann of Hematology.

5. References

Agematsu K, Nagumo H, Yan FC et al. (1997) B cell subpopulations separated by CD27 and crucial collaboration of CD27+ B cells and helper T cells in immunoglobulin production. Eur J Immunol 1997;27:2073-2079

Aqeilan RI, Calin GA, Croce CM, et al. (2010) miR-15 and miR-16-1 in cancer: discovery, function and future perspectives. Cell Death Differ 2010;17:215-20.

Aue G, Njuguna N, Tian X, Soto S, Huges T, Vire B, et al. (2009) Lenalidomide-induced upregulation of CD80 on tumor cells correlates with T cell activation, the rapid onset of a cytokine release syndrome and leukemic cell clearance in chronic lymphcytic leukemia. Haematologica. 2009;94:1266-73.

Bernal A, Pastore RD, Asgary Z, et al.(2001) Survival of leukemic B cells promoted by engagement of the antigen receptor. Blood 2001;98:3050-7

Berland R, Wortis HH.(2002) Origins and functions of B-1 cells with notes on the role of CD5 Annu Rev Immunol 2002;20:253-300

Benschop RJ, Aviszus K, Zhang X et al. (2001) Activation and anergy in bone marrow B cells of a novel immunoglobulin transgenic mouse that is both hapten specific and autorreactive. Immunity 2001;14:33-43.

Binder M, Le'chenne B, Ummanni R, Scharf C, Balabanov S, et al. (2010) Stereotypical Chronic Lymphocytic Leukemia B-Cell Receptors Recognize Survival Promoting Antigens on Stromal Cells. PLoS ONE 2010;5: e15992. doi:10.1371

Binder M, Muller F, Jackst A, Léchenne B, Pantic M, Bacher U, et al. B-cell receptor epitope recognition correlates with the clinical course of chronic lymphocytic leukemia Cancer 2011;117:1891-1900

Broker BM, Klajman A, Youinou P, et al. (1988) Chronic lymphocytic leukemia (CLL) cells secrete multispecific autoantibodies. J Autoinmune 1988;1:469-481Burnet M. (1972) Pathogenesis of auto-immune disease. In Auto-immunity and auto-immune disease (1972). Medical and Technical Publishing CO LTD. 173-290

Caligaris-Cappio F. B chronic lymphocytic leukemia: a malignancy of anti-self B cells. Blood 1996;87:2615-2620

Callin GA,Liu CG, Shimizu M, et al (2004) MicroRNA profiling reveals distinct signatures in B cell chronic lymphocytic leukemia. Proc Natl Acad Sci USA 2004;101:11755-60

Cappione A 3rd, Anolik JH, Pugh-Bernard A, Barnard J, Dutcher P, Silverman G, Sanz I. Germinal center exclusion of autoreactive B cells is defective in human systemic lupus erythematosus. J Clin Invest. 2005;115:3205-3216

Cerutti A, Zan H, Shan S, Schattner E, et al. Ongoing in vivo class switch DNA recombination in chronic lymphocytic leukemia B cells. J Immunol 2002;169:6594-603

Chanan-Khan A, Miller KC, Musial L, Lawrence D, Padmanabhan S, Tajeshita K, et al. (2006) Clinical efficacy of lenalidomide in patients with relapsed or refractory chronic lymphocytic leukemia: results of a phase II stody. J Clin Oncol. 2006;24:5343-9

Chapal N, Peraldi-Roux S, Bresson D, et al. (2000) Human anti-thyroid peroxidase single-chain fragment variable of Ig isolated from a combinatorial library assembled in cell: insights into the In Vivo Situation. J Immunol 2000;114:4162-4169.

Chen L, Apgar J, Huynh L, et al. (2005) Zap-70 directly enhances IgM signaling in chronic lymphocytic leukemia. Blood 2005;105:2036-41.

Chen L, Withopf G, Huynh L, et al. (2002) Expression of ZAP-70 is associated with increased B-cell receptor signaling in chronic lymphocytic leukemia. Blood. 2002;100:4609-46-14

Chiorazzi N, Ferrarini M. (2003) B cell CLL: lessons learned from studies of the B-cell antigen receptor. Ann Rev Immunol. 2003;21:841-94.

Chiorzzi N, Ferrarini M.(2011) Cellular origin(s) of chronic lymphocytic leukemia: cautionary notes and additional considerations and possibilities. Blood.2011;117:1781-1791.

Chiorazzi N, Hatzi K, Albesiano E (2005) B-cell chronic lymphocytic leukemia, a clonal disease of B lymphocytes with receptors that vary in specificity for (auto)antigens. Ann N Y Acad Sci 2005;1062: 1-12.

Chiorazzi N, Rai KR, Ferrarini M. (2005) Chronic lymphocytic leukemia. N Engl J Med 2005;352:804-815

Chu CC, Catera R, Zhang L, Didier S, Agagnina BM, Damle RN, et al. (2010) Many chronic lymphocytic leukemia antibodies recognize apoptotic cells with exposed nonmuscle myosin heavy chain IIA: implications for patient outcome and cell of origin. Blood. 2010;115:3907-3915.

Cimmino A, Callin GA, Fabbri M, et al. (2005) miR-15 and miR-16 induce apoptosis by targeting BCL2. Proc Natl Acad Sci 2005;102:13944-9

Crespo M, Bosch F, Villamor N, et al. (2003) Zap-70 expression as a surrogate for IgV-region mutations in CLL. N Engl J Med 2003;348:1764-1775.

Cyster JG, Hartley SB, Goodnow CC.(1994) Competition for follicular niches excludes self-reactive cells from the recirculating B cell repertoire. Nature 1994;371:389-395.

Dallou A. (2008) CD5: a safeguard against autoimmunity and a shield for cancer cells. Autoimmun Rev 2008;8:349-353

Damle RN, Wasil T, Fais et al,(1999) IGVH gene mutation status and CD38 expression as novel prognostic indicators in CLL. Blood 1999:94:1840-1847.

Diehl LE, Ketchum LH (1998): Autoimmune disease and chronic lymphocytic leukemia: Autoimmune haemolytic anemia, pure red cell aplasia and autoimmune thrombocytopenia. Semin Hematol 25:80-97,1998

Dighiero G, Hart S, Lim A, Borche L, Levy R, et al. (1991) Autoantibody activity of immunoglobulins isolated from B-cell follicular lymphomas. Blood 1991; 78:581-585.

Döhner H, Fischer K, Bentz M, et al.(1995) P53 gene deletion predicts for poor survival and non response to therapy with purine analogs in chronic B-cell leukaemias. Blood 1995;85:1580-9

Döhner H, Stilgenbauer S, Benner A, et al.(2000) Genomic aberrations and survival in CLL. N Engl J Med. 2000:343:1910-1916.

Döhner H, Stilgenbauer S, James MR, et al. (1997) 11q deletions identify a new subset of B-cell chronic lymphocytic leukemia characterized by extensive nodal involvement and inferior prognosis. Blood 1997;89:2516-22.

Dolmetsh RE, Lewis RS, Goodnow CC, et al. (1997) Differential activation of transcription factors induced by Ca2+ response amplitude and duration. Nature 1997;386:855-858

Fais F, et al (1998) Chronic lymphocytic leukemia B cells express restricted sets of mutated and unmutated antigen receptors. J Clin Invest 1998;102:1515-1525.

Forni L, Coutinho A, Köhler G, Jerne NK.(1980) IgM antibodies induce the production of antibodies of the same specificity. Proc Natl Acad Sci USA 1980;77:1125-8

Foreman AL, van de Water J, Gougeon ML, Gershwin ME. (2007) B cells in autoimmune diseases: insights from analyses of immunoglobulin variable (Ig V) gene usage. Autoimmun Rev.2007;6:387-401

Fuda FS, Karandikar NJ, Chen W. (2009) Significant CD5 expression on normal stage 3 hematogones and mature B lymphocytes in bone marrow. Am J Clin Pathol 2009; 132: 733-737

García-Muñoz R. (2009a) Overrall reduction in antibody production could contribute to generate pathogenic autoantibodies and autoimmune manifestations. Clin Rheumatol 2009;28:361-3.

García-Muñoz R, Panizo C, Bendandi M, Llorente L. (2009b). Autoimmunity and lymphoma: is mantle cell lymphoma a mistake of receptor editing mechanism? Leuk Res 2009;11:1437-1439.

García-Muñoz R, Galiacho VR, Llorente L. (2012). Immunological aspects in chronic lymphocytic leukemia (CLL) development. Ann Hematol. (in press)

Gary-Gouy H, Sainz-Perez A, et al. (2007) Natural Phosporylation of CD5 in chronic lymphocytic leukemia B cells and Analysis of CD5 regulated genes in a B cell line suggest a role of CD5 in malignant phenotype. J Immunol 2007;179:4335-4344

Gary-Gouy H, Harriague J, Bismuth G, Platzer C, Schmitt C, Dallou AH. (2002a)Human CD5+ promotes B cell survival through stimulation of autocrine IL-10 production. Blood 2002;100:4537-4543

Gary-Gouy H, Harriague J, Dallou A, Donnadieu E, Bismuth G. (2002b) CD5-negative regulation of B cell receptor signalling pathways originates from tyrosine residue Y429 outside an immunoreceptor tyrosine-based inhibitory motif. J Immunol 2002;168:232-239

Gauld SB, Benschop RJ, Merrel KT, et al. (2005) Maintenance of B cell anergy requires constant antigen receptor occupancy and signaling. Nature Immunol 2005;6:1160-1167).

Gauld SB, Merrell KT, Cambier JC. (2006) Silencing of autoreactive B cells by anergy; a fresh prerspective. Curr Opin Immunol 2006;18:292-297.

Getahun A, O'Neil SK, Cambier JC. (2009) Establishing anergy as a Bona Fide in vivo mechanisms of B cell tolerance. J Immunol 2009;5430-5441

Ghia EM, Jain F, Widhopf II GF, et al.(2008b) Use of IGHV3-21 in chronic lymphocytic leukemia is associated with high risk disease and reflects antigen-driven, post-germinal center leukemogenic selection. Blood 2008;111:5101-5108.

Ghia P, Chiorazzi N, Stomatopoulos K. (2008a) Microenvironmental influences in chronic lymphocytic leukemia: the role of antigen stimulation. J Internal Med. 2008;264:549-62.

Ghia P, Stamatopoulos K, Belessi C, et al. (2005) Geographic patterns and pathogenetic implications of IGHV gene usage in chronic lymphocytic leukemia: the lesson of IGHV3-21 gene. Blood 2005;105:1678-1685.

Ghiotto F, Fais F, Valleto A, et all. (2004) Remarkably similar antigen receptors among a subset of patients with chronic lymphocytic leukemia, J Clin Invest 2004;113:1008-1016.

Goodnow CC. et al. (2005) Self tolerance checkpoints in B cell lymphocyte development. Adv. Immunol 2005;58:279-368.

Goodnow CC, Crosbie J, Adelstein S, et al. (1998) Altered immunoglobulin expression and functional silencing of self reactive B lymphocytes in transgenic mice. Nature 1998;334:676-682.

Goodnow CC, Crosbie J, Jorgensen H, et al. (1989) Induction of self tolerance in mature peripheral B lymphocytes Nature 1989;342:385-391

Griffin DO, Holodick NE, Rothstein TL.(2011) Human B1 cells in umbilical cord and adult peripheral blood express the novel phenotype CD20+CD27+CD43+CD70-. J Exp Med 2011:208:67-80.

Guarini A, Chiaretti S, Tavolaro S, et al. BCR ligation induced by IgM stimulation results in gene expression and functional changes in only in IgVH unmutated chronic lymphocytic leukemia (CLL) cells. Blood 2008;112:782-792.

Hallek M, Cheson D, Catovsky D, Caligaris-Cappio F, Dighiero G, Döner H, Hillmen P, Keating MJ, Montserrat E, Rai KR, Kipps TJ. (2008) Guidelines for the diagnosis and treatment of chronic lymphocytic leukemia: a report from the international Workshop on Chronic Lymphocytic Leukemia updating the National Cancer Institute-Working Group 1996 guidelines. Blood. 2008;111:5446-5456.

Hadzidimitriou A, Darzentas N, Murray F, et al. (2009) Evidence for the significant role of immunoglobulin light chains in antigen recognition and selection in chronic lymphocytic leukemia. Blood 2009;113:403-411.

Hamblin TJ, Davis Z, Gardiner A et al. (1999) Unmutated IGVH genes are associated with a more aggressive form of CLL. Blood 1999;94:1848-1854.

Hamblin TJ, Orchard Ja, Ibbotson RE et al. (2002) CD38 expression and immunoglobulin variable region mutations are independent prognostic variables in chronic lymphocytic leukemias, but CD38 may vary during the course of the disease. Blood 2002;99:1023-1029.

Herve M, Xu K, Ng YS, et al. (2005) Unmutated and mutated chronic lymphocytic leukemias derive from self reactive B cell precursors despite expressing different antibody reactivity. J Clin Invest 2005;115:1636-1643

Hillion S, Saraux A, Youinou P, Jamin C. Expression of RAGs in peripheral B cells outside germinal centers is associated with the expression of CD5. J Immunol 2005;174:5553-61

Hippen KL, Tze LE, Behrens T. (2000) CD5 maintains tolerance in anergic B cells. J Exp Med 2000;191:883-889

Isnardi I, Ng YS, Srdanovic I, Motaghedi R, Rudchenko S, von Bernut H, et al. (2008) IRAK-4/MyD88 dependent pathways are essential for the removal of developing of autoreactive B cells in humans. Immunity 2008;29:746-757

Jerne NK. Idiotipyc networks and other preconceived ideas. (1984) Immunol Rev. 1984:79:5-24

Jerne NK. (1974) Towards a network theory of the immune system. Ann Immunol (Paris) 1974;125C:373-89

Johnson TA, Rassenti LZ, Kipps TJ (1997) Ig VH1 genes expressed in B cell chronic lymphocytic leukemia exhibit distinctive molecular features. J Immunol 1997;158:235-246.

Kalinina O, Doyle-Cooper, Miksanek J et al. Alternative mechanisms of receptor editing in autoreactive B cells. PNAS 2011;108:7125-7130

Kearney ER, Pape KA, Loh DY, et al. Visualization of peptide-specific T cell immunity and peripheral tolerance induction in vivo. Immunity. 1994;1:327-339

Kikushige Y, Ishikawa F, Miyamoto T, et al (2011) Self-renewing hematopoietic stem cell is the primary target in pathogenesis of human chronic lymphocytic leukemia. Cancer Cell. 2011;20:246-59

Klein U, Dalla-Favera R. (2005) New insights into the phenotype cell derivation of B cells in chronic lymphocytic leukemia. Curr Top Microbiol Immunol 2005;294:31-49

Klein U, Rajewsky K, Kuppers R. (1998) Human immunoglobulin (Ig)M+IgD+ peripheral blood expressing CD27 cell surface antigen carry somatically mutated variable region genes: CD27 as a general marker for somatically mutated (memory) B cells. J Exp Med 1998;188:1679-1689

Klein U, Tu Y, Stolovitzky GA, et al. (2001) Gene expression profiling of B cell chronic lymphocytic leukemia reveals a homogeneous phenotype related to memory B cells. J Exp Med 2001;194:1625-1638.

Krober A, Seiler T, Benner A et al. (2002) V(H) mutation status, CD38 expression level, genomic aberrations and prognosis in CLL. Blood 2002;100:1410-1416.

Krober A, Bloehdom J, Hafner S, et al. (2006) Additional genetic high risk features such as 11q deletion, 17p deletion and V3-21 usage characterize discordance of ZAP-70 and VH mutation status in CLL. J Clin Oncol. 2006;24:969-975.

Lanemo Myhrinder A, Hellqvist E, Sidorova E, et al. A new perspective: molecular motifs on oxidized LDL, apoptotic cells, and bacteria are targets for CLL antibodies. Blood. 2008;111:3838-3848

Lanham S, Hamblin T, Oscier D, et al. Differential signaling via surface IgM is associated with VH gene mutational status and CD38 expression in chronic lymphocytic leukemia. Blood 2003;101:1087-1093

Lee J, Kuchen S, Ficher R, et al. (2009) Identification and characterization of circulating human CD5+ pre-naïve B cell population. J Immunol 2009;182:4116-4126.

Luning Prak E, Monestier M, Eisenberg RA. (2011) B cell receptor editing in tolerance and autoimmunity. Ann NY Acad Sci 2011;1217:96-121.

Matutes E, Wrotherspoon A, Catovsky D. (2007) Differential diagnosis in chronic lymphocytic leukemia. Best Pract Res Clin Haematol 2007;20:367-84

Mertens D, Wolf S, Tschuch C et al. (2006) Allelic silencing at the tumor-suppressor locus 13q14.3 suggest an epigenetic tumor-suppressor mechanism. Proc Natl Acad Sci USA 2006;103:7741-6

Mertens D, Bullinger L, Stilgenbauer S. (2011). Chronic lymphocytic leukemia –genomics lead the way. Haematologica 2011;96:1402-1405

Mockridge CI, Potter KN, Wheatley I, Neville LA, Packham G, Stevenson FK. (2007) Reversible anergy of sIgM-mediated signalling in the two subsets of CLL defined by VH-gene mutational status. Blood 2007;109:4424-4431.

Morbach H, Singh S K, Faber C, Lipsky P E, Girschick H J. (2006) Analysis of RAG expression by peripheral blood CD5+ and CD5- B cells in patients with childhood systemic lupus erythematosus Annals of the Rheumatic Diseases 2006;65:482-487

Morikawa K, Oseko F, Morikawa S. (1993) Induction of CD5 antigen on human CD5- B cells by stimulation with staphylococcus Aureus Cowan strain. Int. Immunol 1993;5:809-816.

Murray F, Darzentas N, Hadzidimitriou A, et al.(2008) Stereotyped patterns of somatic hypermutation in subsets of patients with chronic lymphocytic leukemia: implications for the role of antigen selection in leukemogenesis. Blood 2008;111:1524-1533

Muzio M, Apollino B, Scielzo C, et al.(2008) Constitutive activation of distinct BCR-signaling pathways in a subset of CLL patients: a molecular signature of anergy. Blood 2008;112:188-195.

Nakajima PB, Kieffer K, Price A et al. (2009) Two distinct populations of H chain edited B cells show differential surrogate L chain dependence J Immunol. 2009;182:3583-3596.

Nemazee DA, Weigert MG.(2000) Revising B cell receptors. J Exp Med 2000;191:1813-1818.

Oscier DG, Thompsett A, Zhu D, Stevenson FK. (1987) Differential rates of somatic hypermutation in V(H) genes among subsets of chronic lymphocytic leukemia defined by chromosomal abnormalities. Blood 1987;89:4153-4160

Perez-Chacon G, Vargas JA, Jorda J, et al.(2007a) CD5 does not regulate the signalling triggered through BCR in B cells from a subset of B-CLL patients. Leuk Lymphoma 2007;48:147-157.

Perez-Chacon G, Vargas JA, Jorda J, et al.(2007b) CD5 provides viability signals to B cells from a subset of B-CLL patients by a mechanism that involves PKC. Leuk Res 2007;31:183-193

Petlickovski A, Laurenti L, Li X, et al. Sustained signaling through the B-cell receptor induce Mcl-1 and promotes survival of chronic lymphocytic leukemia B cells. Blood. 2005;105:4820-4827.

Puente XS, Pinyol M, Quesada V, Conde L, Ordoñez GR, Villamor N, et al. (2011) Whole genome sequencing identifies recurrent mutations in Chronic lymphocytic leukemia. Nature 2011

Pugh-Bernard, A.E. et al. (2001) Regulation of inherently autoreactive VH4-34 B cells in the maintenance of human B cell tolerance. J Clin Invest. 2001;108:1061-1070.

Rassenti LZ, Kipps TJ. (1997) Lack of allelic exclusion in B cell Chronic lymphocytic leukemia. J Exp Med 1997;185:1435-1445

Radic MZ, Erickson J, Litwin S, et al. (1993) Lymphocytes may scape tolerance by revising their antigen receptor. J Exp Med. 1993;177:1165-1163.

Radic MZ, Wigert M.(1994) Genetic and structural evidence for antigen selection of anti-DNA antibodies. Ann Rev Immunol 1994;12:487-520

Ramsay AG,Johnson AJ, Lee M, Gorgun G, Le Dieur R, Blum W, et al. (2008) Chronic lymphocytic leukemia T cells show impaired immunological synapse formation that can be reversed with an immunomodulating drug. J Clin Invest 2008;118:2427-37

Ravetch JV, Bolland S. IgG Fc Receptors. Annu Rev Immunol. 2001;19:275-290

Ray SK, Putterman C, Diamond B. Pathogenic autoantibodies are routinely generated during response to foreing antigen: a paradigm for autoimmune disease. Proc Natl Acad Sci. USA 1996;93:2019-2024.

Rochas C, Hillion S, Youinou P et al. (2007) RAG mediated secondary rearrangements of B cell antigen receptors in rheumatoid synovial tissue. Autoimmun Rev 2007;7:155-9

Rosenwald A, Alizadeh AA, Widhopf G, et al. (2001) Relation of gene expression phenotype to immunoglobulin mutation genotype in B cell chronic lymphocytic leukemia. J Exp Med 2001;194:1639-1647

Roudier J, Solverman GJ, Chenn PP et al.(1990) Intraclonal diversity in the VH genes expressed by CD5-chronic lymphocytic leukemia producing pathologic IgM rheumatoid factor. J Immunol 1990:144:1526-1530

Rozkova D, Novodna L, Pytlic R, e tal. (2010) Toll like receptors on B cells: Expression and functional consequences of their stimulation. Int J Cancer 2010;126:1132-43

Ruzickova S, Pruss A, Odendahl M, et al. Chronic lymphocytic leukemia preceded by cold agglutinin disease: intraclonal immunoglobulin light chain diversity in VH4-34 expressing single leukemic B cells. Blood 2002;100:3419-3422.

Sandel PC, Monroe JG. (1999) Negative selection of immature B cells by receptor editing or deletion is determined by site of antigen encounter, Immunity. 1999;10:289-299

Shiono H, et al. (2003) Scenarios of autoimmunization of T and B cells in myasthenia gravis. Ann NY Acad Sci 2003;998:237-256.

Shokat KM, Goodnow CC. Antigen induced B cell death and elimination during germinal centre immune responses. Nature 1995;375:334-338.

Stamatopoulos K, Kosmas C, Stavroyianni N, et al (1996) Evidence of immunoglobulin heavy chain variable region gene replacement in a patient with B cell chronic lymphocytic leukemia. Leukemia 1996;10:1551-1556.

Stevenson FK and Caligaris-Cappio F. Chronic lymphocytic leukemia: revelations from the B cell receptor. Blood 2004;103:4389-4395.

Sthoeger ZM, Wakai M, Tse DB, Vinciguerra VP, Allen SL, et al. (1989) Production of autoantibodies by CD5-expressing B lymphocytes from patients with chronic lymphocytic leukemia. J Exp Med 1989;169: 255–268.

Tangye SG, Liu YJ, Aversa G, et al. (1998) Identification of functional human splenic memory B cells by expression of CD148 and CD27. J Exp Med 1998;1691-1703

Thumberg U, Johonson A, Roos G et al.(2001) CD38 is a poor predictor for VH gene mutational status and prognosis in chronic lymphocytic leukemia. Blood 2001;97:1892-1894

Tiegs SL, Russel DM, Nemazee D.(1993) Receptor editing in self-reactive bone marrow B cells. J Exp Med 1993;177:1009-1020.

Tobbin G, Thunberg U, Johnson A, et al. (2002) Somatically mutated Ig V(H)3-21 genes characterize a new subset of chronic lymphocytic leukemia. Blood 2002:99:2262-4.

Tiller T, Tsuiji M, Yurasov S, et al. (2007) Autoreactivity in Human IgG+ Memory B cells. Immunity 2007;26:205-213

Tsuiji M, Yurasov S, Velinzon K, Thomas S, Nussenzweig MC, Wardemann H.(2006) A check point for autoreactivity in human IgM memory B cell development. J Exp Med 2006;203:393-400.

Van Lochem EG, van der Valden VHJ, Wind HK, et al. (2004) Immunophenotypic differentiation patterns of normal hematopoiesis in human bone marrow: Reference patterns for age-related changes and disease induced shifts. Cytometry B Clin Cytom 2004;60:1-13

Vanura K, Le T, Esterbauer H, et al. (2008) Autoimmune conditions and chronic infections in chronic lymphocytic leukemia patients at diagnosis are associated with unmutated IgVH genes. Haematologica 2008;93:1912-16.

Wiestner A, Rosengwald A, Barry TS, et al.(2003) Zap-70 expression identifies a chronic lymphocytic leukemia subtype with unmutated immunoglobulin genes, inferior clinical outcome, and distinct gene expression profile. Blood 2003;101:4944-4951

Yurasov S, Hammersen J, Tiller T, et al. (2005) B cell tolerance check points in healthy humans and patients with systemic lupus erythematosus. Ann N Y Acad Sci. 2005;1062:165-174.

4

T$_H$17 Cells in Cancer Related Inflammation

Rupinder K. Kanwar and Jagat R. Kanwar

Nanomedicine-Laboratory of Immunology and Molecular Biomedical Research (LIMBR),
Centre for Biotechnology and Interdisciplinary Biosciences (BioDeakin),
Institute for Technology & Research Innovation, Deakin University, Geelong,
Technology Precinct, Waurn Ponds, Geelong, Victoria,
Australia

1. Introduction

Until 2005, T helper (CD4+) cells were proposed to be a binary system, consisting of T$_H$1 and T$_H$2 cells (Mosmann TR *et al.*,1986) , when a third T helper -cell subset, known as T$_H$17 (interleukin-17 (IL-17) expressing cells), was identified (Harrington LE *et al.*, 2005, Park H *et al.*, 2005). This was followed up by the another independent discovery in three different laboratories of the differentiation factors cytokines such as interleukin (IL)-6 and transforming growth factor beta (TGF-β), that simplified *in vitro* analysis of this T cell subset to a large extent (Veldhoen M *et al.*, 2006, Bettelli E *et al.*, 2006, Mangan *et al.*, 2006). The discovery of these unique T$_H$17 cells has opened up exciting new avenues for research into the etiology and therapeutics of a broad spectrum of human diseases and data on the biology of these cells have emerged at an astounding pace in just 5 years. The reason for these cells to receive considerable attention in these recent years is their emerging involvement as principal mediators of pathogenesis in several autoimmune and chronic inflammatory disorders. Many reviews of the field have already highlighted the important role of T$_H$17 cells in the diverse group of human autoimmune and inflammatory diseases (Tesmer *et al.*, 2008, Sallusto and Lanzavecchia 2009, Torrado and Cooper 2010, Kimura and Kishimoto 2011, Cosmi *et al.*, 2011).

With regards to cancer, the involvement of T$_H$17 cells in tumour immunology has raised their status as a target for cancer therapy. However based on the reported evidence on the potential anti-tumourigenic and pro-tumourigenic activities of T$_H$17 cells, their role as friends or foes, respectively is still under debate; could be because of a few studies have focused on primary T$_H$17 cells in the human tumour microenvironment (Wilke *et al.*, 2011). The link between cancer development and inflammation is now widely accepted and cancer patients have local and systemic changes in inflammatory parameters (Chechlinska, *et al.*, 2010). Tumours frequently display the characteristics of chronically inflamed tissue, including immune cell infiltration and an activated stroma (Kanwar *et al.*, 2008, Mantovani *et al.*, 2008). Indeed inflammation has been proposed as the seventh trait of cancer by supplementing Hanahan and Weinberg's model that identifies six hallmarks of cancer (Mantovani 2009). This chapter focuses on the role of T$_H$17 cells in cancer by understanding its links with chronic inflammation.

2. Association of cancer with inflammation

Inflammation is the first line of defence against various extracellular stimuli (microbes, trauma, chemicals, heat or any other phenomenon) and can be acute or chronic. Acute or physiological inflammation is when body cells respond to external stimuli for short periods of time. Normal inflammation, for example, inflammation associated with acute infections, injury, wound healing is usually self-limiting; however, dysregulation of any of the involved factors leads to abnormalities. If the stimulus sustains for longer time, it results in a pathological state known as chronic or pathological inflammation as seen in autoimmune and chronic inflammatory diseases such as atherosclerosis, multiple sclerosis, rheumatoid arthritis, allergic inflammation of the lung leading to asthma (Kanwar *et al.*, 2001a, Kanwar 2005, Kanwar *et al.*, 2008, Kanwar *et al.*, 2009, Barreiro *et al.*, 2010). Chronic inflammation is also the case during tumour progression in cancer. The patients with chronic inflammatory conditions have a greatly increased risk of cancer in the affected organs. Also chronic inflammation resulting from viral or bacterial infections can often lead to or hasten the development of malignancy (Coussens and Werb 2002, Kanwar *et al.*, 2011). Table 1 summarizes the chronic inflammatory conditions associated with cancer.

Inflammatory Condition	Associated Cancer(s)
AIDS	Non-Hodgkin's lymphoma, squamous cellcarcinomas, Kaposi's sarcoma
Asbestosis, silicosis	Mesothelioma, lung carcinoma
Barrett's oesophagus	Oesophageal carcinoma
Bronchitis	Lung carcinoma
Chronic cholecystitis	Gall bladder cancer
Chronic pancreatitis, hereditary pancreatitis	Pancreatic carcinoma
Coeliac disease	Lymphoma
Gingivitis	Oral squamous cell carcinoma
Helicobacter pylori infection	Gastric cancer
Hepatitis B or C	Hepatocellular carcinoma
Inflammatory bowel disease, Crohn's disease, chronic ulcerative colitis	Colorectal carcinoma
Lichen sclerosus	Vulvar squamous cell carcinoma
Mononucleosis	B-cell non-Hodgkin's lymphoma, Burkitts lymphoma,
Obesity related inflammation	Liver cancer
Opisthorchis, Cholangitis	Cholangiosarcoma, colon carcinoma
Osteomyelitis	Sarcoma
Pelvic inflammatory disease, chronic cervicitis	Ovarian carcinoma, cervical/anal carcinoma
Prostate inflammatory atrophy	Prostate cancer
Rheumatoid arthritis	Lymphoma
Shistosomiasis, bladder inflammation	Bladder carcinoma
Sialadenitis	Salivary gland carcinoma
Sjögren syndrome, Hashimoto's thyroiditis	MALT lymphoma
Skin inflammation	Melanoma

Modified from Coussens and Werb, 2002, Conro y *et al.*, 2010

Table 1. Chronic inflammatory conditions and infections associated with cancer.

When the control of cell proliferation, growth and cell death (apoptosis) is lost, we obtain a clone of cells known as benign tumour. By growing its own blood supply (angiogenesis), the tumour feeds itself, grows indefinitely and spreads (metastasizes) in the body thereby leads to malignant cancer. Tumour cells are known to produce various pro inflammatory cytokines such as IL-1β, IL-6, IL-23 and tumour necrosis factor (TNF)-αand chemokines that attract inflammatory leukocytes which include neutrophils, dendritic cells, macrophages, eosinophils, mast cells and lymphocytes (Coussens and Werb 2002, Kanwar *et al.*, 2008,). These cells further produce growth factors, various cytokines, chemokines, cytotoxic mediators like reactive oxygen species, matrix metalloproteinases (MMPs), membrane-perforating agents and soluble mediators of cell killing such as TNF-α, interleukins and interferons (Wahl *et al.*, 1998, Kuper *et al.*, 2000, Coussens and Werb 2002, Kanwar *et al.*, 2008). The recruitment of dendritic cells capture antigen and stimulate anti-tumour immunity by T lymphocyte activation which kill cancer cells via cell mediated cytotoxicity (Kanwar *et al.*, 1999). According to the immune surveillance theory, tumours arise only if cancer cells are able to escape immune surveillance, yet sometimes a robust immune response might result in a favourable effect that might be due to CD8+ cytotoxic T cells which have the capacity to kill tumour cells (Kanwar *et al.*, 2001b) CD4+ T cell responses are also important as they help recruiting CD8+ cytotoxic T cell and generate an inflammatory response that chains the function of CTLs activity (Kanwar *et al.*, 2003). The growth factors asnd cytokines released by inflammatory cells can also have pro-tumour actions. They can lead to proliferation, survival and migration of the tumour by promoting angiogenesis and lymphanogenesis, remodelling extracellular matrix to facilitate invasion, coating tumour cells to make available receptors for spreading cells via lymphatics and capillaries, and evading host mechanisms (Coussens and Werb 2002, Rigo *et al.*, 2010). In this context tumour-associated macrophages (TAMs) have a significant role. After migration the monocytes, recruited largely by monocyte chemotactic protein (MCP) chemokine become the significant component of inflammatory infiltrates as TAMs in neoplastic tissues, and has a dual role in neoplasms. TAMs may kill neoplastic cells following activation by IL-2, interferon and IL-12 or potentiate neoplastic progression through the production of a number of potent angiogenic and lymphangiogenic growth factors, cytokines and proteases, all of which are mediators for tumour growth (Brigati *et al.*, 2002, Tsung *et al.*, 2002). Further TAMs and tumour cells also produce IL-10, which effectively blunts the anti-tumour response by cytotoxic T cells, and prevent maturation of anti-tumour dendritic cells *in situ* leading to immunosuppression and immune evasion (Coffelt *et al.*, 2009). Increasing evidences have suggested that many types of cancer are closely associated with inflammation (Table 1). Thus, inflammation is a process used by immune cells to eliminate cancer and by cancer cells to promote tumour progression and metastasis.

3. CD4+ T cell subsets as essential regulators of immune responses and inflammatory diseases

Immune system consists of innate and adaptive immunity. Adaptive immunity is mediated by T and B cells. T helper cells/CD4+ cells are the key actors in establishing an immune response. Naive CD4+ T cells differentiate into different types of effector cells depending upon the combination of cytokines in milieu, antigen and the antigen presenting cell (APC). There are four types known so far (Figure 1) and include T$_H$1, T$_H$2, T- regulatory (Treg) and T$_H$17. T$_H$1 cells, induced by IL-12, express T$_H$1 specific Transcription factors (T-bet) and produce IFN-γ as their signature cytokine and evoke cell-mediated immunity and phagocyte-dependent inflammation. Vigorous pro-inflammatory activities of T$_H$1 cells has been seen to cause tissue damage and elicit unwanted T$_H$1-dominated responses in the pathogenesis of organ-specific autoimmune/inflammatory disorders, Crohn's disease, sarcoidosis, acute kidney allograft rejection, and some unexplained recurrent abortions (Romagnani, 2000).

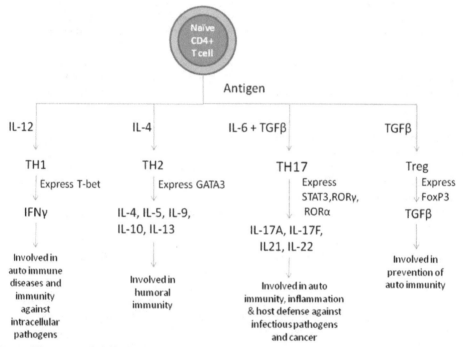

Fig. 1. CD4+ T- Cell differentiation: Naive CD4+ T cells differentiate into different effector cells under the influence of the pool of cytokines present in the surroundings. There are four known types of effector T$_H$ cells which have different functions based on the expression of unique transcription factors and characteristic cytokines.

T$_H$2 cells are induced by IL-4, express GATA 3 and produce IL-4, IL-5, IL-9, IL-10 and IL-13. These are associated with the humoral immunity and resistance against extracellular forms of pathogens. T-regulatory (Treg) cells, characterized by expression of FoxP3 (forkhead/winged helix transcription factor), produce TGF-β (transforming growth factor-β1). These distinct regulatory T cell subsets suppress adaptive T cell responses, have anti-inflammatory role and are involved in maintaining tolerance to self components (prevent autoimmunity).

T$_H$17 cells, a newly defined lineage of CD4+ cells, are not only distinct from other T$_H$ cells in their gene expression and regulation, but also in terms of their biological function (Dong 2008) T$_H$17 cells are characterized in particular through the production of IL-17 and IL-17F, and have functions in autoimmune diseases, inflammation and host defence against infectious pathogens. Recently accumulating evidence suggests that T$_H$ cells possess functional 'plasticity' (Bettelli *et al.*, 2006, Yang *et al.*, 2008a, Crome *et al.*, 2010a) i.e. they can be converted into other types of T_H cells under *in vitro* as well as *in vivo* conditions. This property seems to be certainly beneficial to mount different and varied responses for combating immunological insults given at short notices.

T_H17 cells: a new lineage of effector T_H cells Discovery: The presence of T_H17 cells as a specific lineage was recognized when it was demonstrated that lipopeptides from the spirochete *Borrelia burgdorferi* triggered the increased levels of IL-17A mRNA in T cells to produce IL-17 (member of IL-17 family composed of 6 cytokines, IL-17A-F), TNF-α and GM-CSF while these cells were negative for IFN-γ or IL-4, revealing a novel cytokine phenotype distinct from T_H1 or T_H2. (Infante-Duarte *et al.*, 2002). This was the first report to establish the link between bacterial infection and a new effector T cell phenotype later to become T_H17 while foretelling the description of a factor later identified as critical to T_H17 development: IL-6 (Weaver *et al.*, 2007) . Further hint came when, Aggarwal *et al.* 2003, who demonstrated that IL-23 stimulates murine CD4+ T cells to secrete IL-17 following stimulation of the T- cell receptor (TCR). These crucial findings that IL-23 but not IL-12, stimulated memory, but not naive, CD4 T cells to produce IL-17A and IL-17F, were consistent with a unique effector CD4 T cell population similar to that previously reported by Infante-Duarte and colleagues in 2002. Then the findings that IL-17 secreting CD4+ T cells arise in the absence of T_H1 and T_H2 induced transcription factors and cytokines solidified the lineage separation between T_H1/T_H2 and T_H 17 cells (Harrington *et al.*, 2005; Park *et al.*, 2005).

Differentiation and transcriptional regulation: Although early studies by Aggarwal and colleagues in 2003 implicated IL-23 in driving T_H17 expression and generation , it was later on demonstrated that IL-23 receptor (IL-23R) is not expressed on naïve T cells. Instead, IL-23, as well as TNF-α, acts as survival signals for T_H17 cells. It is apparent now as reviewed recently (Weaver *et al.*, 2007, Torchinsky and Blander 2010, Kimura and Kishimoto 2011) that IL-23 is important only for T_H17 cells' expansion, survival and pathogenicity. The key cytokines required for T_H17 differentiation, surprisingly, are a combination of pro-inflammatory and anti-inflammatory cytokines; i.e. IL-6 and TGF-β respectively (Veldhoen M *et al.*, 2006, Mangan *et al.*, 2006, Betteli *et al.*, 2006). The studies by Betteli and colleagues identified TGF-β as a critical factor for T_H17 commitment while IL-6 acted to deviate TGF-β-driven development of Foxp3-expressing Tregs toward T_H17 (Betteli *et al.*, 2006).

Further attempts were made to delineate the precise signalling mechanisms through which IL-6 and TGF-β cooperate to induce T_H17 differentiation. Studies have shown that the key transcription factors in determining the differentiation of the T_H17 lineage are retinoid-related orphan receptor γt (RORγt) and RORα which can be induced by the combination of IL-6 and TGF-β (Ivanov *et al.*, 2006, Yang *et al.*, 2008b). RORγt was shown to be specifically expressed by mouse and human T_H17 cells (Ivanov *et al.*, 2006, Wilson *et al.*, 2007). Further a central role for IL-6-induced STAT3 activation was made evident. Although IL-6 activates both STAT3 and STAT1, it has been demonstrated that STAT3 activation is maintained while STAT1 activation is suppressed in T_H17 cells (Kimura *et al.*, 2007). Interferon regulatory factor (IRF) 4 and T-bet are other players in the scene of transcriptional regulation, which act as positive and negative regulators of $T_H17$commitment, respectively (Brüstle *et al.*, 2007, Rangachari *et al.*, 2006). Further Aryl hydrocarbon receptor (Ahr) was shown to be induced under T_H17-polarizing conditions such as in the presence of TGF-β plus IL-6, and promotes T$_H$17 cell development through inhibiting STAT1 and STAT5 activation. More recently, an AP-1 transcription factor, BATF was shown to also play a role in T$_H$17 differentiation. BATF-/- mice had a defect specifically in differentiation of T$_H$17 cells, and were resistant to autoimmune encephalomyelitis (Schraml *et al.,* 2009). IL-1 (Chung *et al.,* 2009) and IL-21 (Korn *et al.,* 2007) have also been shown to be required for their differentiation. And certain studies have shown that IL-10 released by Treg cells and IL-2 inhibit T$_H$17 cell development (Weaver et al., 2007). - Apart from IL-17 as its major cytokine, T$_H$17 cells also release IL-21 and IL-22 (Wei *et al.,* 2007, Dong 2008). As IL-21 is required for T$_H$17 cells' differentiation as well as is produced by them, it may be acting as a positive feedback loop to amplify the production of these cells (Torchinsky and Blander 2010). T$_H$17 cells also express CCR6, CXCR4, CD49 integrins and CD161 (Kryczek, *et al.,* 2009). Crome *et al.,* 2010b established a novel method to isolate *in vivo* differentiated T$_H$17 cells from peripheral blood by sorting CD161+CCR4+CCR6+CXCR3-CD4+T cells. These authors also suggested low expression of granzyme A and B as another distinguishing feature of T$_H$17 cells. T$_H$17 cells also express IL-23R at high levels. There exists also a negative regulatory system for T$_H$17 cell differentiation and IL-27 was shown to important role in curbing T$_H$17 responses by limiting development of T$_H$17 effectors (Batten *et al.,*2006, Stumhofer *et al.,* 2006). Thus, various cytokines and transcription factors can either enhance or inhibit T$_H$17 differentiation (Figure 2). Very recently, Martinez *et al.* in 2010 suggested that Smad2 positively regulates the generation of T$_H$17 cells *in vivo* and *in vitro* (Figure 3).

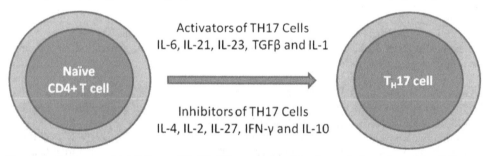

Fig. 2. Activators and inhibitors of T$_H$17 differentiation: The figure below shows the different activators and inhibitors which promote or inhibit the differentiation of T$_H$17 cells.

Cytokine production: The T$_H$17 lineage was originally defined by the production of hallmark cytokines interleukin-17 (also known as IL-17A) and IL-17F, members of IL-17 family (Aggarwal *et al.,* in 2003) as homodimers or heterdimers (Liang *et al.,* 2007). Later on studies have shown that T$_H$17cells are also characterized by the production of IL-10 family cytokine, IL-22 (Liang *et al.,* 2006). IL-21, besides acting in concert with TGF-β to promote T$_H$17 differentiation, is also produced by T$_H$17 cells (Korn *et al.* ,2007). T$_H$17 cells are also known to produce certain cytokines that are expressed by other T helper cell lineages, including TNF-α and lymphotoxin-β, and the T$_H$17 subset can be characterized by expression of chemokine receptor CCR6 and the CCR6 ligand, CCL20 (Hirota *et al.,* 2007, Torchinsky and Blander 2010). A subset of T$_H$17 cells is reported to co-expresses IFN-γ in humans where as many as half of all the IL-17+ cells also express IFN-γ. It is not yet clear if these cells represent a stable phenotype or a transitional phase, undergoing a switch from T$_H$17 to T$_H$17 or vice versa (reviewed by Tesmer *et al.,* 2008) (Figure 3).

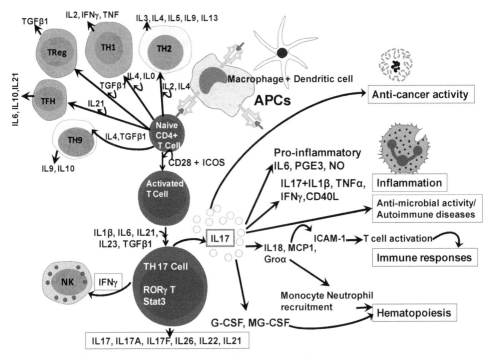

Fig. 3. T_H17 differentiation and activation of immune cells for immune responses, inflammation, anti-cancer activity and hematopoiesis.

Biological activities/functions: The important roles of IL-17 in host defence against many extracellular and intracellular pathogens have already been established (reviewed by Torchinsky and Blander 2010). IL-17A, F released by T_H17 cells, is involved in the recruitment, activation and migration of neutrophils which help the body to fight against infection with various bacterial and fungal species (Yang *et al.*, 2008c). Non-immune cells are major targets for the effector functions of T_H17 cells. Specifically, cytokines produced by T_H17 cells act on cells such as fibroblasts and keratinocytes (Chrome *et al.*, 2010) and thereby contribute to immunity in barrier tissues such as the skin and gut. T_H17 cells have also been involved with tissue repair functions through their production of the cytokine IL-22 along with IL-10 (Dong C 2008). Further the anti-infective and anti-inflammatory roles of IL-22 are associated with its functions in maintaining the integrity of epithelial barriers (Torchinsky and Blander 2010). More interestingly, it was shown that TGF-β and IL-6 from antigen presenting dendritic cells, that recognized apoptotic cells carrying TLR ligands, were able to drive differentiation of naïve CD4+ T cells to the T_H17 lineage (Torchinsky *et al.*, 2009). Thus T_H17 cells may be uniquely suited to serve in host response against pathogens causing significant apoptosis and tissue damage (Figure 3).

There are effector molecules as discussed above (cytokines, chemokines and integrin α3) associated with T_H 17 cells that act as pro-inflammatory mediators of inflammation and upregulate the expression of adhesion molecules thereby mediating the migration of circulating mixed leukocytes, such as monocytes, neutrophils, T cells and natural killer (NK) cells. The infiltrated leukocytes further augment the ongoing inflammation, indirectly by secreting an elaborated number of chemokines and cytokines, including IL-1, IL-6, TNF-α, monocyte chemoattractant protein-1(MCP-1), keratinocyte-derived chemokine (KC), IFN-γ, IL-17, and IL-23 (Coussens and Werb 2002, Kryczek et al, 2009a, Barreiro et al., 2010),. When these inflammatory signals are altered or misprocessed, the inflammation can become chronic, causing extensive tissue damage. To combat chronic inflammation in autoimmune diseases, novel therapeutic strategies targeting T$_H$17 cells and their effector molecules thus represent opportunities for therapeutic intervention.

4. Association of T$_H$17 cells with chronic inflammation

Earlier, T$_H$1 phenotype was associated with inflammation and autoimmunity and now the T$_H$17 subset has also been described as pro-inflammatory to play a role in autoimunity and chronic inflammation. The findings that IFN-γ and IFN-γ receptor-deficient mice and mice lacking IL-12p35 and other molecules involved in T$_H$1 differentiation were not protected from experimental autoimmune encephalomyelitis (EAE), but rather developed more severe disease have challenged the concept that autoimmunity is a T$_H$1 driven disease process (Gran B et al., 2002, Torchinsky and Blander 2010). The suggestion about another subset of T cells, distinct from the T$_H$1 lineage that might be required for the induction of EAE and other organ-specific autoimmune diseases has recently established role and importance of T$_H$17 cells in the pathogenesis of organ-specific autoimmune inflammation based on animal studies and clinical findings. The topic on the broad implications of T$_H$17 cells in the pathogenesis of number of immune-mediated diseases such as psoriasis, rheumatoid arthritis, multiple sclerosis, inflammatory bowel disease, and asthma is beyond the scope of this chapter, but readers are referred to excellent recent reviews (Tesmer et al., 2008, Dong C 2008, Torchinsky and Blander 2010, Cosmi et al., 2011) (Figure 1).

Inflammation and pathogenesis induced by T$_H$17 cells is a result of the pro-inflammatory cytokines, chemokines and chemokine receptors these cells produce and express, respectively. Recently, T$_H$17 polarized cells have been shown to be associated with cancers. Cancer and inflammation are now considered to be inextricably linked. Inflammatory mediators and cellular effectors are important constituents of the local environment of tumours. Many cancers arise from the sites of infection, chronic irritation and inflammation as shown in Table 1, the inflammatory conditions are present before a malignant change occurs. To understand the kinetics and targets of inflammation in a discussion of T$_H$17 cells and cancer, the relationship between T$_H$1-derived IFNγ, T$_H$17 cells and antigen-presenting cells (APCs) in humans was recently studied (Kryczek et al., 2008a). These authors demonstrated in a cutting edge study that IFNγ could rapidly induce elevated B7-H1 expression on APCs and stimulate their production of IL-1 and IL-23. B7-H1 signaling resulted in abrogation of the T$_H$1-polarizing capacity of APC, whereas IL-1 and IL-23 directed them toward a memory T$_H$17-expanding phenotype. These findings thus suggest that in the course of inflammation, that the acute T$_H$1-mediated response is attenuated by IFNγ-induced B7-H1 on APCs and is subsequently evolved toward T$_H$17-mediated chronic inflammation by APC derived IL-1 and IL-23. This study in addition to challenging the dogma that IFNγ suppresses T$_H$17 and enhances T$_H$1 development, also strengthens the notion that T$_H$17 kinetics depends strongly on the context of the ongoing immune reactions and the constituents of the cytokine milieu, both of which are influenced by disease progression (Figure 3).

5. T$_H$ 17 cells in cancer

Various studies have been carried out in the recent years with rapid progress on different cancer types to investigate the association of cancer and T$_H$17 cells. It has been seen that, T$_H$17 cells, might either promote tumour growth or regulate antitumour responses. This may be due to the irregular conflicting data based on the studies in humans versus those in mice and contradictory data from experiments in immunocompetent versus immunodeficient mice (Wilke *et al.*, 2011). There is, however, a strikingly high frequency of tumour-infiltrating T$_H$17 cells in patients with diverse cancer types. These cells when examined in cancer patients, the findings reveal that human tumour-associated T$_H$17 cells express minimal levels of human leukocyte antigen (HLA)-DR, CD25 and granzyme B, suggesting that they are not a 'conventional' effector cell population (Wilke *et al.*, 2011). On examining the associated mechanisms and clinical significance of T$_H$17 cells in 201 ovarian cancer patients, it was found that T$_H$17 exhibited a polyfunctional effector T-cell phenotype, were positively associated with effector cells, and were negatively associated with tumour-infiltrating Treg cells (Kryczek *et al.*, 2009a). The study authors further reveal that for homing molecules, tumour-associated T$_H$17 highly express chemokine receptors CXCR4 and CCR6, c-type lectin receptor CD161 and the CD49 integrin isoforms c, d and e, while CCR2, CCR5 and CCR7 are not present on these cells (Figure 3).

Several biological activities of T$_H$17 cells are directly or indirectly linked to human tumour pathogenesis. Tumour-associated T$_H$17 cells have the ability to influence the tumour immune response through the action of their cytokines products in cancer patients which reportedly include high levels of pro inflammatory granulocyte-macrophage colony stimulating factor (GM-CSF), TNF-α, IL-2 and IFNγ, but negligible levels of anti-inflammatory IL-10 . This phenotype was observed in six types of human cancers which include ovarian, colon, liver, skin, pancreatic and renal (Kryczek *et al.*, 2009a). 50% of T$_H$17 cells, in patients with hepatocellular carcinoma (HCC) produced IFNγ-IFNγ, a typical T$_H$1-type cytokine (Zhang *et al.*, 2009, Kryczek *et al.*, 2009, Wilke *et al.*, 2011). Further, on *in vitro* expansion, the T$_H$17cells from tumour-infiltrating lymphocyte populations in melanoma, breast and colon cancers secrete elevated amounts of IL-8 and TNF-α, but no IL-2 (Su *et al.*, 2010). Since this profile has been seen previously in T$_H$17 cells isolated from healthy donors (Liu and Rohowsky-Kochan 2008) and patients with autoimmune diseases (Kryczek *et al.*, 2008b), it may indicate a possible difference in the phenotypes of freshly isolated T$_H$17cells and those expanded or induced *in vitro* from tumour-associated populations (Figure 3). Earlier information reviewed from both experimental animal systems and human cancer patients suggested that IL-17 and IL-23 are generally favourable to the growth of tumours thus overshadowing their roles in the generation of T-cell anti-tumour immunity (Tesmer *et al.*, 2008).

Still the role of IL-17 producing T$_H$17 cells in cancer is elusive as different immunopathological implications of these cells have been observed in different malignancies. Analysis of tumour-derived naive and memory CD4$^+$ T cells revealed that IL-17 producing T cells are in memory phase as they are positive for CD45RO, but negative for CD45RA, CD62L, and CCR7 (Miyahara *et al.*, 2008). These authors also indicated that tumour cells may secrete key cytokines required for the expansion of T_H17 cells. Further Su et al., 2010 demonstrated elevated CD4+ T_H17 cell populations in the tumour-infiltrating lymphocytes (TILs) and suggested development of tumour-infiltrating T_H17 cells may be a general feature in cancer patients, when they extended their studies from ovarian cancers to melanoma, breast and colon cancers. Their study further demonstrated that tumour cells and tumour-derived fibroblasts, mediate the recruitment of T_H17 cells by secreting chemokines RANTES (regulated upon activation, normal T cell expressed and secreted) and MCP-1 in the tumour microenvironment. The tumour microenvironments produce a pro-inflammatory cytokine milieu and provide cell–cell contact engagement that facilitates the generation and expansion of T_H17 cells. They also showed that inflammatory TLR and nucleotide oligomerization binding domain (Nod2) 2 signalling promote the attraction and generation of T_H17 cells and that this was induced by tumour cells and tumour-derived fibroblasts.

6. Dynamic interaction between T_{reg} and T_H17 cells

Levels of both T_{reg} and T_H17 cells increase synchronically following tumour development and are inversely associated. TGF-β promotes T_{reg} development and both TGF-β plus IL-6 are required for T_H17 differentiation (Veldhoen M et al., 2006, Mangan et al., 2006, Betteli et al., 2006). Although, both the cytokines needed for T_H17 cell development have been seen to be present in high levels in tumours (Zhou 2005), yet the levels of T_{reg} cells and other T subsets are more than T_H17 cells in both mouse and human tumours (Kryczek et al., 2007). So there must be something that prevents differentiation of T_H17 cells. An interesting study by Kryczek and colleagues in 2009 from ovarian cancer patients, raised concerns on the roles of IL-6 an TGF-β, where it has been reported that inhibition of IL-1β, but not IL-6 or TGF-β, decreased T_H17 cell induction by myeloid APCs isolated from patients, and the levels of IL-17 and numbers of T_H17 cells did not correlate with the levels of IL-6 and TGF-β in these patients' samples. These observations hinted a crucial role of only IL-1β, but not of IL-6 or TGF-β, for T_H17 cell development in the ovarian cancer microenvironment. Similar support for a crucial role of IL-1β in promoting T_H17 cell development has been reported in mouse studies (Chung et al., 2009, Gullen et al., 2010).

According to few studies, IL-10 released by T_{reg} cells negatively regulates differentiation of T_H17 cells and IL-2, a growth factor for most T cells promote FoxP3 expression in T_H17 cells and inhibit cellular differentiation to T_H17 cells (Wilson et al., 2007). Retinoic acid has been found to enhance TGF-β signalling and decrease IL-6 signalling, thus, it might also be affecting the balance between T_H17 and T_{reg} cells. Apart from this, it has also been seen that mouse peripheral mature T_{reg} can be converted to T_H17 cells favoured by inflammation and IL-6 ('plasticity') (Yang et al., 2008a). The role of TGF-β in the differentiation of both induced T_{reg} cells as well as T_H17 cells, along with the documented interactions between RORα and FoxP3 that influence the two subsets, suggest a system that balances inflammation with tolerance (Figure 3).

7. Evidences for the negative and positive roles of T_H17 in anti-tumour Immunity

Though reports have addressed the presence of T_H17 cells in experimental and human tumours but they lack regarding the clear indication about either a pro-tumoural or antitumoural activity of these cells (Bronte 2008).There are various biological functions of T$_H$17 cells and their effector molecules as mentioned earlier in the chapter that could be on the basis of experimental and clinical data, suggest T$_H$17 cells might either be positively or negatively co-related with cancer.

Negative role of T$_H$17 cells in anti-cancer

IL-17 produced by T$_H$17 cells is an angiogenic factor (Numasaki *et al.*, 2003) which stimulates the migration and cord formation of vascular endothelial cells *in vitro* and elicits vessel formation *in vivo* which in turn promotes tumour growth and metastasis through *de novo* carcinogenesis and neovascularisation via STAT3 signalling. Another cytokine, IL-23 required for T$_H$17 activity has been identified as a cancer-associated cytokine because it promotes tumour incidence and growth (Langowski *et al.*, 2006). It has been seen that T$_H$17 cells produce negligible levels of HLA- DR, CD 25, granzyme B, PD1 and FoxP3, all of which are involved in effector functions suggesting that they do not contribute to immune suppression in the tumour environment. Thus, as T$_H$17 cells produce pro-inflammatory cytokines and have been found to accumulate in tumour microenvironment and as inflammation is linked to cancer development and progression, it is reasonable to predict a positive relation between these cells and cancer progression. Also, the data from experiments on ovarian cancer suggest that T$_H$17 cells through TNF-α are involved in the development or progression of cancer in mice and humans(Charles *et al.*, 2009).

Further T$_H$17 cells might increase their own frequency in the tumour by both direct and indirect mechanisms (Zou and Restifo 2010). The induction of T$_H$17 cells in the human tumour microenvironment through IL-1β production by the myeloid APCs may in turn promote dendritic cell trafficking into tumour-draining lymph nodes and the tumour environment by producing CCL20 (Kryczek *et al.*, 2009a). Further as CCR6+ T$_H$17 cells are known to efficiently migrate towards CCL20 (Kryczek *et al.*, 2008b, Kryczek *et al.*, 2009a), and CCL20 can then lead to the recruitment of dendritic cells to the tumour-draining lymph nodes and tumour itself in a CCR6-dependent manner (Martin-Orozco *et al.*, 2009). Compared with corresponding non-tumour regions, the levels of T$_H$17 cells were found to be significantly increased in tumours of HCC patients. Most of these intratumoural T$_H$17 cells exhibited an effector memory phenotype with increased expression of CCR4 and CCR6. Furthermore, the intratumoural cell density of T$_H$17 correlated with poor survival in HCC patients (Zhang *et al.*, 2009). A study from Kuang and colleagues in 2010, has demonstrated predominantly enriched levels of IL-17-producing cells in peritumoural stroma of murine HCC tissues, where their levels correlated with monocyte/macrophage density. The level of murine hepatoma-infiltrating CD4+ IL- 17+ cells as well as the tumour growth was reduced significantly when monocyte/macrophage inflammation in liver was inhibited via treatment with a Kupffer cell toxicant (gadolinium chloride).

Similar to humans, healthy mice has limited populations of T$_H$17 cells but these cells expanded in the blood, bone marrow and spleens but not in the tumour draining lymph nodes and largest populations were seen in tumour itself of mice with the aggressive B16 melanoma, fibrosarcoma and advanced head and neck cancers, The number of CD4+IL-17+ T cells gradually increased in the tumour microenvironment during tumour development but interestingly, the number of these cells remained limited during tumour development in the tumour draining lymph nodes, including advanced tumour stages. (Kryczek *et al.*, 2007).On the other hand in nasopharyngeal carcinoma, data from human samples demonstrated no correlation of T_H17 cells with patient clinicopathological characteristics or survival outcomes (Zhang *et al.*, 2010). Studies with patient samples from lung adenocarcinoma or squamous cell carcinoma revealed that malignant pleural effusion from these patients was chemotactic for T_H17 cells, and this activity was partially abrogated by CCL20 and/or CCL22 blockade (Ye *et al.*, 2010). Interestingly, higher infiltration of T_H17 cells in malignant pleural effusion predicted improved patient survival.

Positive role of T_H17 cells in anti-tumour immunity

Both human and mouse tumours study data suggest several lines of evidence about the protective role of T_H17 cells with the induction of protective anti-tumour immune response.T_H17 cells have been seen to positively co-relate with effector immune cells like IFNγ[+] effector T cells, cytotoxic CD8[+] T cells and natural killer (NK) cells in the tumour microenvironment which might be to produce an anti- tumour response against cancer cells to kill them by promoting cell mediated cytotoxicity (Kryczek *et al.*, 2009a). Various experimental studies have shown that IL-17 overexpression or exogenous T_H17 cell induction lead to decreased tumour growth, for example; Muranski and colleagues in 2008, through a first functional study showed that T_H17-polarized CD4+ T cells (following treatment with TGF-β and IL-6), induced potent tumour eradication of large established melanoma in mice. The study provides a support for a clinical trial involving the adoptive transfer of T_H17-polarized, tumour-specific CD4+ T cells to patients with cancer. A year later, another interesting functional study, revealed for the first time that T_H17-polarized CD8+ T cells induce potent tumour eradication in mice, and provided again support for a clinical trial involving the adoptive transfer of T_H17-polarized, tumour-specific CD8+ T cells to cancer patients (Hinrichs *et al.*, 2009). Once *in vivo*, T_H17-polarized CD8+ T cells might be converted to an IFNγ-producing phenotype, induced tumour regression and persisted in the host longer than non-polarized cells. tumourIL-17 deficient mice (IL-17A knockout (IL-17A -/-) have accelerated tumour growth and more lung metastasis than wild-type mice (Kryczek *et al.*, 2009b, Martin-Orozco *et al.*, 2009, Wei *et al.*, 2010). Transgenic expression of human or murine IL-17 in tumour cells suppresses or slows tumour growth and increases tumour-specific cytotoxic responses (Hirahara *et al.*, 2001, Benchetrit *et al.*, 2002). However, contrasting results were shown by Wang *et al.*, 2009 who have reported that transferred tumours of B16 and bladder carcinoma MC49 grew more slowly in IL-17-/- mice.

In prostate cancer patients, a significant inverse correlation was seen between T_H17 cell differentiation and tumour progression (Sfanos *et al.*, 2008). In addition to these evidences, it is known that IL-17 released by T_H17 cells promote dendritic cell maturation which might allow for better tumour antigen presentation and thereby leading to a stronger T cell response. Furthermore, direct mechanistic and functional evidence that T_H17 cells mediate antitumour immunity by promoting dendritic cell trafficking to tumour-draining lymph nodes, and to the tumour itself has also been provided (Martin-Orozco *et al.*, 2009). tumourtumourMore recently, CTLA4 (cytotoxic T lymphocyte antigen 4) blockade was shown to increase T_H17 cells in patients with metastatic melanoma and IL-17 levels in tumour-associated ascites positively predicted patient survival (von Euw *et al.*, 2009). To summarize the above data, there is strong evidence that T_H17 cells can have protective roles in tumour immunity but the exact nature of T_H17 cells in anti-tumour immunity remains to be explored.

8. Conclusions

Rapid and large advances in understanding the development, regulation and function of these cells have been made since T$_H$17 cells are originally identified as a third lineage of effector T helper cells in 2005. The study of T$_H$17 cells has been one of the fast-moving and exciting subject areas in immunology. This has been particularly true in the context of a diverse group of immune-mediated chronic inflammatory diseases and autoimmunity, where the pathogenic role of T$_H$17 cells has been well documented. With regards to cancer, T$_H$17 cells are found to be present in the tumour microenvironment though not as a predominant T cell subset within the tumour. Based on the evidence provided by both human and clinical studies data, T$_H$17 cells and T$_H$17-associated cytokines/effector molecules have been shown to have both pro-tumorigenic and anti-tumorigenic functions. On one hand it seems that the pro-inflammatory T$_H$17 cells might engineer the microenvironment around tumours, and contribute to the proliferation, migration and survival of cancer cells. On the other hand, it is possible that inflammatory cells and molecules play roles to initiate and maintain protective anti-tumour immunity as seen in the case of infectious diseases (Punj et al., 2003). The IL-17 dependent pro-tumorigenic or anti-tumorigenic activity might be due to inherent technical limitations for example source and dose of exogenous versus endogenous IL-17, in each of the studies (Zou and Restifo 2010). Further, based on the results from recent murine model studies, employing T$_H$17-polarized T cells for cancer therapy may appear to be to be a promising approach for translational research. It is also important to study futher the specific nature of inflammatory response and the tissue context, so that the positive or negative effects of T$_H$17 cells on tumour immunopathology can be determined. Equally important to understand is i) how the effector functions of T$_H$17cells are regulated?, ii) how do the regulators of T$_H$17-cell differentiation work? iii), do T$_H$17 play same role in different types and stages of cancer?, and iv) how T$_{reg}$ cells can be suppressed in chronic inflammatory or large tumour burdens to increase the T$_H$17 cells and later activation and proliferation of cytotoxic T cells to clear tumour cells? The answers will, help in designing future novel therapeutic vaccine approaches; specifically targeting inflammatory T$_H$17 cells for cancer therapy.

9. Abbreviations

CD	Cluster of Differentiation
IL	Interleukin
IFN	Interferon
TNF	Tumour Necrosis Factor
TGF	Tumour Growth Factor
MMP	Matrix Metalloproteinase
APC	Antigen Presenting Cells
FoxP3	Forkhead Box P3
MAPK	Mitogen-Activated Protein Kinases
TRAF6	Tumour Necrosis Factor Receptor-Associated Factor-6
TLR	Toll-like Receptors

10. References

[1] Aggarwal S, Ghilardi N, Xie MH, de Sauvage FJ, Gurney AL (2003). Interleukin-23 promotes a distinct CD4 T cell activation state characterized by the production of interleukin-17. J. Biol. Chem. 278:1910-1914.

[2] Barreiro O, Martín P, González-Amaro R, Sánchez-Madrid F (2010). Molecular cues guiding inflammatory responses. Cardiovasc Res 86:174-182.

[3] Batten M, Li J, Yi S, Kljavin NM, Danilenko DM, Lucas S et al. (2006). Interleukin 27 limits autoimmune encephalomyelitis by suppressing the development of interleukin 17-producing T cells. Nat Immunol 7: 929-936.

[4] Benchetrit F, Ciree A, Vives V, Warnier G, Gey A, Sautes-Fridman C et al. (2002). Interleukin-17 inhibits tumor cell growth by means of a T-cell-dependent mechanism. Blood 99: 2114-2121.

[5] Bettelli E, Carrier Y, Gao W, Korn T, Strom TB, Oukka M et al. (2006). Reciprocal developmental pathways for the generation of pathogenic effector T_H17 and regulatory T cells. Nature 441:235-238.

[6] Brigati C, Noonan DM, Albini A, Benelli R. (2002). Tumors and inflammatory infiltrates: friends or foes? Clin Exp Metastasis 19:247-258.

[7] Bronte V. Th17 and cancer: friends or foes?. Blood 112: 214.

[8] Brüstle A, Heink S, Huber M, Rosenplänter C, Stadelmann C, Yu P, et al. (2007). The development of inflammatory T(H)-17 cells requires interferon-regulatory factor. Nat Immunol 8:958-966.

[9] Charles KA, Kulbe H, Soper R, Escorcio-Correia M, Lawrence T, Schultheis A et al. (2009). The tumor-promoting actions of TNF-alpha involve TNFR1 and IL-17 in ovarian cancer in mice and humans. J Clin Invest 119: 3011-3023.

[10] Chechlinska M, Kowalewska M, Nowak, R. (2010). Systemic inflammation as a confounding factor in cancer biomarker discovery and validation. Nat Rev Cancer 10: 2-3

[11] Chung Y, Chang SH, Martinez GJ, Yang XO, Nurieva R, Kang HS et al. (2009). Critical regulation of early Th17 cells differentiation by interleukin-1 signaling. Immunity 30(4):576-587.

[12] Coffelt SB, Hughes R, Lewis CE. (2009). Tumor-associated macrophages: Effectors of angiogenesis and tumor progression. Biochim et Biophys Acta 1796:11-18.

[13] Crome SQ, Wang AY, Levings MK. (2010a). Translational mini-review series on Th17 cells: function and regulation of human T helper 17 cells in health and disease. Clin Exp Immunol 159: 109-119.

[14] Crome S Q, Clive B, Wang AY, Kang CY, Chow V, Yu J et al. (2010b). Inflammatory effects of *ex vivo* human Th17 cells are suppressed by regulatory T cells. J Immunol 185:3199-3208.

[15] Cosmi L, Liotta F, Maggi E, Romagnani S, Annunziato F. (2011). Th17 cells: new players in asthma pathogenesis. Allergy 66:989-998.

[16] Coussens LM and Werb Z. (2002). Inflammation and cancer. Nature 420(6917):860-867.

[17] Dong C. (2008). T_H17 cells in development: An updated view of their molecular identity and genetic programming. Nat Rev Immunol 8:337-348.

[18] Gran B, Zhang GX, Yu S, Li J, Chen XH, Ventura ES et al. (2002). IL-12p35-deficient mice are susceptible to experimental autoimmune encephalomyelitis: evidence for redundancy in the IL-12 system in the induction of central nervous system autoimmune demyelination. J Immunol. 169:7104-7110.

[19] Gulen MF, Kang Z, Bulek K, Youzhong W, Kim TW, Chen Y, et al. (2010). The receptor SIGIRR suppresses Th17 cell proliferation via inhibition of the interleukin-1 receptor pathway and mTOR kinase activation. Immunity 32, 54–66.

[20] Harrington LE, Hatton RD, Mangan PR, Turner H, Murphy TL, Murphy KM, Weaver CT. (2005). Interleukin 17-producing CD4+ effector T cells develop via a lineage distinct from the T-helper type 1 and 2 lineages. Nat Immunol 6:1123-1132.

[21] Hinrichs CS, Kaiser A, Paulos CM, Cassard L, Sanchez-Perez L, Heemskerk B, Wrzesinski C, Borman ZA, Muranski P, Restifo NP. (2009). Type 17 CD8+ T cells display enhanced anti-tumour immunity. Blood 114: 596–599.

[22] Hirahara N, Nio Y, Sasaki S, Minari Y, Takamura M, Iguchi C, Dong M, Yamasawa K, Tamura K.. (2001). Inoculation of human interleukin-17 gene transfected Meth-A fibrosarcoma cells induces T cell-dependent tumor specific immunity in mice. Oncology 61: 79–89.

[23] Hirota K, Yoshitomi H, Hashimoto M, Maeda S, Teradaira S, Sugimoto N, et al. (2007) Preferential recruitment of CCR6-expressing Th17 cells to inflamed joints via CCL20 in rheumatoid arthritis and its animal model. J Exp Med 204:2803–2812.

[24] Infante-Duarte C, Horton HF, Byrne MC, Kamradt T (2000). Microbial lipopeptides induce the production of IL-17 in Th cells. J. Immunol. 165:6107–6115.

[25] Ivanov II, McKenzie BS, Zhou L, Tadokoro CE, Lepelley A, Lafaille JJ, et al.(2006). The orphan nuclear receptor RORγt directs the differentiation program of proinflammatory IL-17+ T helper cells. Cell 126:1121–1133.

[26] Kanwar JR. (2005). Anti-inflammatory immunotherapy for multiple sclerosis/experimental autoimmune encephalomyelitis (EAE) disease. Curr Med Chem. 12(25):2947-2962.

[27] Kanwar JR, Berg RW, Lehnert K, Krissansen GW. (1999). Taking lessons from dendritic cells: multiple xenogeneic ligands for leukocyte integrins have the potential to stimulate anti-tumor immunity. Gene Ther 6:1835–1844.

[28] Kanwar JR, Berg RW, Yang Y, Kanwar RK, Ching LM, Sun X, Krissansen GW. (2003). Requirements for ICAM-1 immunogene therapy of lymphoma. Cancer Gene Ther 10 :468-476.

[29] Kanwar RK, Kanwar JR, Wang D, Ormrod D and Krissansen GW (2001a).Temporal expression of heat shock proteins 60 and 70 at lesion prone sites during atherogenesis in the apolipoprotein E-deficient mouse. Arterioscler Thromb and Vas Biol 21: 1991-1997.

[30] Kanwar JR, Kanwar RK, Burrow H, Baratchi S. (2009). Recent advances on the roles of NO in cancer and chronic inflammatory disorders. Curr Med Chem 16(19):2373-2394.

[31] Kanwar RK, Macgibbon AK, Black PN, Kanwar JR, Rowan A, Vale M et al. (2008). Bovine milk fat enriched in conjugated linoleic and vaccenic acids attenuates allergic airway disease in mice. Clin Exp Allergy 38: 208-218.

[32] Kanwar JR, Palmano KP, Sun X, Kanwar RK, Gupta R, Haggarty N et al. (2008). 'Iron-saturated' lactoferrin is a potent natural adjuvant for augmenting cancer chemotherapy. Immunol Cell Biol 86: 277-288.

[33] Kanwar JR, Shen WP, Kanwar RK, Berg RW, Krissansen GW. (2001b). Effects of survivin antagonists on growth of established tumors and B7-1 immunogene therapy. J Natl Cancer Inst 93:1541-1552.

[34] Kanwar RK, Singh N, Gurudevan S, Kanwar JR (2011). Targeting Hepatitis B Virus and Human Papillomavirus Induced Human Viral Carcinogenesis: Novel Patented Therapeutics. Recent Patents on Anti-Infective Drug Discovery, May 6(2):158-74.

[35] Kimura A and Kishimoto T (2011). Th17 cells in inflammation. Internat Immunopharmacol 11:319-322.

[36] Kimura A, Naka T, Kishimoto T (2007). IL-6-dependent and -independent pathways in the development of interleukin 17-producing T helper cells. Proc Natl Acad Sci USA 104:12099-12104.

[37] Korn T, Bettelli E, Gao W, Awasthi A, Jager A, Strom TB, et al. (2007). IL-21 initiates an alternative pathway to induce proinflammatory TH17 cells. Nature 448:484-487.

[38] Kryczek I, Wei S, Zou L, Altuwaijri S, Szeliga W, Kolls J, Chang A et al. (2007). Cutting Edge: T$_H$17 and regulatory T cell dynamics and the regulation by IL-2 in the tumor microenvironment. J Immunol 178: 6730-6733.

[39] Kryczek, I. Wei S, Gong W, Shu X, Szeliga W, Vatan L, Chen L, Wang G, and Zou W (2008a) Cutting edge: IFN-gamma enables APC to promote memory Th17 and abate Th1 cell development. J. Immunol., 181,5842-5846.

[40] Kryczek I Banerjee M, Cheng, P, Vatan L, Szeliga W, Wei S et al. (2009). Phenotype, distribution, generation, and functional and clinical relevance of Th17 cells in the human tumour environments. Blood 114: 1141-1149.

[41] Kryczek I. Bruce AT, Gudjonsson JE, Johnston A, Aphale A, Vatan L, Szeliga W, Wang Y, Liu Y, Welling TH, Elder JT, Zou W. (2008b) Induction of IL-17+ T cell trafficking and development by IFN-gamma: mechanism and pathological relevance in psoriasis. J. Immunol 181:4733-4741.

[42] Kryczek I. Wei S, Szeliga W. Vatan L. Zou W. (2009b). Endogenous IL-17 contributes to reduced tumor growth and metastasis. Blood 114: 357-359.

[43] Kuang DM, Kuang DM, Peng C, Zhao Q, Wu Y, Chen MS, Zheng L(2010) Activated monocytes in peritumoral stroma of hepatocellular carcinoma promote expansion of memory T helper 17 cells..Hepatology, 51:154-164.

[44] Kuper H, Adami HO, Trichopoulos D. (2000). Infections as a major preventable cause of human cancer. J Intern Med 248:171-183.

[45] Langowski JL, Zhang X, Wu L, et al. (2006). IL-23 promotes tumour incidence and growth. Nature 442: 461 - 465.

[46] Liang SC, Long AJ, Bennett F, Whitters MJ, Karim R, Collins M et al. (2007). An IL-17F/A heterodimer protein is produced by mouse Th17 cells and induces airway neutrophil recruitment. J Immunol 179:7791-7799.

[47] Liang SC, Tan XY, Luxenberg DP, Karim R, Dunussi-Joannopoulos K, Collins M et al. (2006). Interleukin (IL)-22 and IL-17 are coexpressed by Th17 cells and cooperatively enhance expression of antimicrobial peptides. J Exp Med 203:2271-2279.

[48] Liu H, Rohowsky-Kochan C. (2008) Regulation of IL-17 in human CCR6+ effector memory T cells. J. Immunol 180: 7948-7957.

[49] Mangan PR, Harrington LE, O'Quinn DB, Helms WS, Bullard DC, Elson CO et al. (2006). Transforming growth factor-beta induces development of the T(H)17 lineage. Nature 441:231-234.

[50] Mantovani, A. (2009). Inflaming metastasis. Nature 457:36-37.

[51] Mantovani A, Allavena P, Sica, A, Balkwill F. (2008). Cancer-related inflammation. Nature 454:436-444.

[52] Martinez GJ, Zhang Z, Reynolds JM, Tanaka S, Chung Y, Liu T et al. (2010). Smad2 positively regulates the generation of th17 cells. J Biol Chem. 285(38): 29039-29043.

[53] Martin-Orozco N, Muranski P, Chung Y, Yang XO, Yamazaki T, Lu S, Hwu P, Restifo NP, Overwijk WW, Dong C. (2009). T helper 17 cells promote cytotoxic T cell activation in tumour immunity. Immunity 31, 787–798.

[54] Miyahara Y, Odunsi K, Chen W, Peng G, Matsuzaki J, Wang. (2008). Generation and regulation of human CD4+ IL-17-producing T-cells in ovarian cancer. Proc Natl Acad Sci USA 105(40):15505-15510.

[55] Mosmann TR, Cherwinski H, Bond MW, Giedlin MA, Coffman RL. (1986). Two types of murine helper T cell clone. I. Definition according to profiles of lymphokine activities and secreted proteins. J Immunol 136:2348–2257.

[56] Muranski P, Boni A, Antony PA, Cassard L, Irvine KR, Kaiser A, Paulos CM, Palmer DC, Touloukian CE, Ptak K, Gattinoni L, Wrzesinski C, Hinrichs CS, Kerstann KW, Feigenbaum L, Chan CC, Restifo NP. (2008) Tumor specific Th17-polarized cells eradicate large established melanoma. Blood 112: 362 –373.

[57] Numasaki M, Fukushi J, Ono M, Narula SK, Zavodny PJ, Kudo T et al. (2003). Interleukin-17 promotes angiogenesis and tumor growth. Blood 101: 2620–2627.

[58] Park H, Li Z, Yang XO, Chang SH, Nurieva R, Wang YH, et al. (2005). A distinct lineage of CD4 T cells regulates tissue inflammation by producing interleukin 17. Nat Immunol 6(11):1133-1141.

[59] Punj V, Saint-Dic D, Daghfal S, Kanwar JR. (2004). Microbial-based therapy of cancer: a new twist to age old practice. Cancer Biol Ther 3-:708-714.

[60] Rangachari M, Mauermann N, Marty RR, Dirnhofer S, Kurrer MO, Komnenovic V et al. (2006). T-bet negatively regulates autoimmune myocarditis by suppressing local production of interleukin 17. J Exp Med 203:2009–2019.

[61] Rigo, A., Gottardi, M., Zamo, A., Mauri, P., Bonifacio, M, Kramper M et al. (2010). Macrophages may promote cancer growth via a GM-CSF/HB-EGF paracrine loop that is enhanced by CXCL12. Mol Cancer 9: 273.

[62] Romagnani S (2000). T-cell subsets (Th1 versus Th2). Ann Allerg, Asthma Immunol 85: 9-18.

[63] Sallusto F, Lanzavecchia A. (2009). Human Th17 cells in infection and autoimmunity. Microb Infect / Institut Pasteur 11: 620-624.

[64] Schraml BU, Hildner K, Ise W, Lee WL, Smith WA, Solomon B (2009). The AP-1 transcription factor Batf controls T(H)17 differentiation. Nature 460:405–409.

[65] Sfanos KS, Bruno TC, Maris CH, Xu L, Thoburn CJ, DeMarzo AM et al. (2008). Phenotypic analysis of prostate-infiltrating lymphocytes reveals TH17 and Treg skewing. Clin Cancer Res 14:3254-3261.

[66] Stumhofer JS, Laurence A, Wilson EH, Huang E, Tato CM, Johnson LM et al. (2006). Interleukin 27 negatively regulates the development of interleukin 17-producing T helper cells during chronic inflammation of the central nervous system. Nat Immunol 7:937–945.

[67] Su X, Ye J, Hsueh EC, Zhang Y, Hoft DF, Peng G. (2010). Tumor microenvironments direct the recruitment and expansion of human Th17 cells. J Immunol 184: 1630-1641.

[68] Torrado E and Cooper AM. (2010). IL-17 and Th17 cells in tuberculosis. Cytokine Growth Factor Rev 21:455-62.

[69] Torchinsky MB and Blander JM. (2010). T helper 17 cells: discovery, function, andphysiological trigger. Cell. Mol. Life Sci 67:1407–1421.

[70] Torchinsky MB, Garaude J, Martin AP, Blander JM (2009). Innate immune recognition of infected apoptotic cells directs T(H)17 cell differentiation. Nature 458:78–82.

[71] Tsung K, Dolan JP, Tsung YL, Norton JA. (2002). Macrophages as effector cells in interleukin 12-induced T cell-dependent tumor rejection. Cancer Res 62:5069–5075.

[72] Veldhoen M, Hocking RJ, Atkins CJ, Locksley RM, Stockinger B. (2006). TGF beta in the context of an inflammatory cytokine milieu supports de novo differentiation of IL- 17 producing T cells. Immunity 24: 179-89.

[73] Euw, E. et al. (2009). CTLA4 blockade increases Th17 cells in patients with metastatic melanoma. J. Transl. Med. 7: 35.

[74] Wahl LM, Kleinman HK. (1998). Tumor-associated macrophages as targets for cancer therapy. J Natl Cancer Inst 90: 1583–1584.

[75] Wang L, Yi T, Kortylewski M, Pardoll DM, Zeng D, Yu H. (2009). IL-17 can promote tumor growth through an IL-6- Stat3 signaling pathway. J Exp Med 206:1457–1464.

[76] Weaver CT, Hatton RD, Mangan PR, Harrington LE. (2007). IL-17 family cytokines and the expanding diversity of effector T cell lineages. Annu Rev Immunol 25:821-852.

[77] Weaver CT, Murphy KM. (2007). T-cell subsets: the more the merrier. Curr Biol 17:61-63.

[78] Wei L, Laurence A, Elias KM, O'Shea JJ (2007). IL-21 is produced by Th17 cells and drives IL-17 production in a STAT3- dependent manner. J Biol Chem 282:34605–34610.

[79] Wei S. Kryczek I, Namm J, Szeliga W, Vatan L, Chang A. et al. (2010) Endogenous IL-17, tumor growth, and metastasis. Blood 115: 2256–2257.

[80] Wilke CM, Kryczek I, Wei S, Zhao E, Wu K, Wang G, Zou W. (2011). Th17 cells in cancer: help or hindrance? Carcinogenesis 32: 643-649.

[81] Wilson NJ, Boniface K, Chan JR, McKenzie BS, Blumenschein WM, Mattson JD et al. (2007). Development, cytokine profile and function of human interleukin 17-producing helper T cells. Nat Immunol 8:950-957.

[82] Yang XO, Nurieva R, Martinez GJ Kang HS, Chung Y, Pappu BP. et al. (2008a). Molecular antagonism and plasticity of regulatory and inflammatory T cell programs. Immunity 29:44-56.

[83] Yang XO, Pappu BP, Nurieva R, Akimzhanov A, Kang HS, Chung Y et al. (2008b). T helper 17 lineage differentiation is programmed by orphan nuclear receptors RORα and ROR γ. Immunity 28:29-39.

[84] Yang XO, Chang SH, Park H, Nurieva R, Shah B, Acero L, et al. (2008c). Regulation of inflammatory responses by IL-17F. J Exp Med 205: 1063–1075.

[85] Ye ZJ, Zhou Q, Gu YY, Qin SM, Ma WL, Xin JB, Tao XN, Shi HZ. (2010) Generation and differentiation of interleukin-17-producing CD4+ T cells in malignant pleural effusion. J. Immunol, 185: 6348–6354.

[86] Zou, W (2005). Immunosuppressive networks in the tumour environment and their therapeutic relevance. Nature Rev. Cancer 5:263–274.

[87] Zou W, Restifo NP. (2010). T_H17 cells in tumor immunity and immunotherapy; Nat Rev Immunol 10: 246-256.

[88] Zhang JP Yan J, Xu J, Pang XH, Chen MS, et al. (2009) Increased intratumoral IL-17-producing cells correlate with poor survival in hepatocellular carcinoma patients. J. Hepatol 50:980-989.

[89] Zhang YL. Li J, Mo HY, Qiu F, Zheng LM, Qian CN. et al. (2010) Different subsets of tumor infiltrating lymphocytes correlate with NPC progression in different ways. Mol. Cancer 9: 4.

5

Pattern Recognition Receptors and Cancer: Is There Any Role of Inherited Variation?

Anton G. Kutikhin
Kemerovo State Medical Academy
Russian Federation

1. Introduction

1.1 What are pattern recognition receptors?

The group of the pattern recognition receptors (PRRs) includes families of Toll-like receptors (TLRs), NOD-like receptors (NLRs), C-type lectin receptors (CLRs) and RIG-I-like receptors (RLRs). The summary of the most modern conceptual data about members of these families and about their structure and functions can be obtained from the recent comprehensive reviews (Elinav et al., 2011; Kawai and Akira, 2011; Osorio and Reis E Sousa, 2011; Loo and Gale, 2011), and the schemes of their signaling are presented in Figures 1-2.

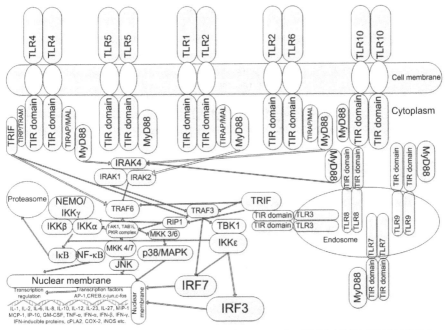

Fig. 1. The signaling of the Toll-like receptor pathway. TLR1, TLR2, TLR4, TLR5, TLR6, and TLR10 are usually located on the cell surface whilst TLR3, TLR7, TLR8 and TLR9 are settled

on the ER membrane (in the resting state) or on the endosomal/lysosomal membrane (after ligand stimulation and trafficking). According to the known data about their structure (Hashimoto et al., 1988), TLRs belong to type I transmembrane glycoproteins and contain three major domains (Matsushima et al., 2007). The ectodomain is oriented towards the extracellular space or cytoplasm (depending on receptor localization) and contains multiple (16-28) leucine-rich repeats (LRRs) that harbor 24–29 amino acids and may contain two types of motifs: typical (T) motifs (LxxLxLxxNxLxxLxxxxF/LxxLxx) and bacterial (S) motifs (LxxLxLxxNxLxxLPx(x)LPxx) (Bell et al., 2003; Matsushima et al., 2007). LRR modules fold into the parallel β-sheets that bend into a concave surface, forming one or two distinct horseshoe structures determining the unique horseshoe shape of TLRs (Matsushima et al., 2007). LRR hydrophobic residues are packed within the interior of ectodomain structure, forming a ligand-binding hydrophobic pocket (Bell et al., 2003, 2006; Kim et al., 2007; Liu et al., 2008). In addition, C-terminal LRRs may control the receptor dimerization and the signal transmission (Takada et al., 2008). The single-spanning transmembrane domain is homologous to IL-1R analog and anchors the receptor in the correct orientation on cell membrane (Huyton et al., 2007; Medzhitov et al., 1997). Third, the cytoplasmic TLR domain (toll/interleukin-1 receptor domain, TIR domain) is usually composed of approximately 150 amino acid residues (Jin and Lee, 2008) and dimerizes after the ligand-ectodomain interaction (TLR ligands are presented in Table 1) and respective alterations in the receptor conformation, triggering the recruitment of the adaptor proteins (MyD88, TIRAP/MAL, TRIF, TRAM, SARM) to initiate the specific signaling pathway of the immune response stimulation (Jin and Lee, 2008; O'Neill and Bowie, 2007). It is important that all TLRs form hetero- or homodimers, and this feature may facilitate the dimerization of the cytoplasmic domain. All adaptors indicated above contain TIR domains, and interactions between such domains of receptor and adaptor are key for the successful signaling (Palsson-McDermott and O'Neill, 2007). The process of TLR signaling is mediated by a number of other adaptor proteins and, finally, leads to activation of NF-κB (Yamamoto et al., 2004), MAPK (Yamamoto et al., 2004), JNK (Takeuchi and Akira, 2001), IRF1, IRF3, IRF5, IRF7 and IRF8 (Honda and Taniguchi, 2006) that move into the nucleus and directly or indirectly control the transcriptional activity of the genes encoding various proinflammatory cytokines (IL-1, IL-2, IL-6, IL-8, IL-10, IL-12, IL-13, IL-23, IL-27, MIP-1, MCP-1, RANTES, SOCS, IP-10, GM-CSF, TNF-α, IFN-α, IFN-β, IFN-γ and IFN-inducible proteins (Chang, 2010; Wong et al., 2011; Zhu and Mohan, 2010).

Member of TLR family	Exogenous ligand	Endogenous ligand
TLR1 (form heterodimers with TLR2)	Triacylated lipopeptides	β-defensin 3
	Lipoarabinomannan	
	Soluble factors of *Neisseria meningitidis* cell wall	
	OspA protein of *Borrelia burgdorferi*	
TLR2	Lipoprotein	HSP22
	Peptidoglycan	HSP60
	Di- and triacylated lipopeptides	HSP70
	Lipoteichoic acid	HSP72
	Zymosan	gp96
	Lipoarabinomannan	HMGB1
	Outer-membrane porins of N.gonorrhoeae and S.dysenteriae	β-defensin 3

		OspA protein of *Borrelia burgdorferi*	Surfactant proteins A and D
		Phenol-soluble modulin of Staphylococcus epidermidis	Eosinophil-derived neurotoxin
		Cell membrane glycolipids of *Trypanosoma cruzi*	Antiphospholipid antibodies
		Hemagglutinin protein of wild-type measles virus	Serum amyloid A
		Envelope proteins of HSV-1 and CMV	Biglycan
		Atypical LPS of *L.interrogans* and *P.gingivalis*	Versican
			Hyaluronic acid fragments
TLR3		dsRNA	mRNA
		Polyinosine-polycytidylic acid	
TLR4		Lipopolysaccharide	HMGB1
		Glucuronoxylomannan	Tenascin-C
		RSV fusion protein	HSP60
		MMTV and MMLV	HSP70
		Taxol	gp96
			Mrp8 and Mrp14
			Neutrophil elastase
			Antiphospholipid antibodies
			Lactoferrin
			Surfactant proteins A and D
			β-defensin-2
			Biglycan
			Low-molecular-weight oligosaccharide fragments of hyaluronan
			Fibrinogen
			Fibronectin
			Heparansulfate
			Oxidized LDL
			Saturated fatty acids
TLR5		Flagellin	
TLR6 (form heterodimers with TLR2)		Diacylated lipoprotein	
		Peptidoglycan	
		Zymosan	
TLR7		Imidazoquinolines	Antiphospholipid antibodies
		ssRNA	ssRNA
TLR8		ssRNA	ssRNA
			Antiphospholipid antibodies
TLR9		Bacterial and viral CpG DNA	IgG-chromatin complexes
		Hemozoin	
TLR10 (may form heterodimers with TLR1 and TLR2)		Unknown	Unknown

Table 1. Ligands of TLRs. Abbreviations: TLR – Toll-like receptor, HSP – heat shock protein, gp – glycoprotein, HSV – herpes simplex virus, CMV – cytomegalovirus, LPS – lipopolysaccharide, dsRNA – double-stranded RNA, HMGB1 - high mobility group box 1, RSV – respiratory syncytial virus, MMTV – mouse mammary tumor virus, MMLV – Moloney murine leukemia virus, Mrp – myeloid related protein.

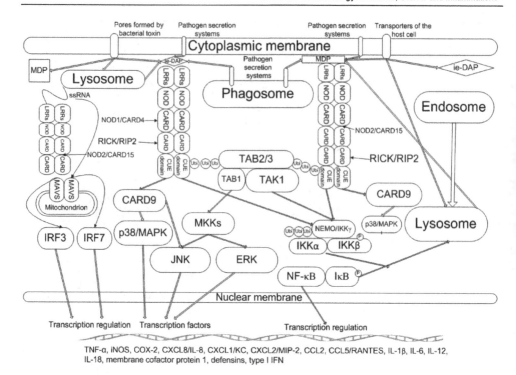

Fig. 2. The signaling of the NOD-like receptor pathway. NLRs usually have three-domain structure (Chen et al., 2009). First, the C-terminal domain, contains multiple leucine-rich repeats (LRRs), directly recognizing exogenous and endogenous ligands (Kumar et al., 2009). The second, central, nucleotide-binding oligomerization domain (NOD) has intrinsic ATPase activity and is responsible for the self-oligomerization and the formation of a complex after the ligand binding for the activation and recruitment of downstream signaling proteins (Kumar et al., 2009). These two domains are common for all known NLRs (Chen et al., 2009). Third, variable, the N-terminal protein-protein interaction domain, may represent a caspase recruitment domain (CARD), death effector domain (DED), pyrin domain (PYD), acidic transactivating domain, or baculovirus inhibitor of apoptosis protein repeat domain (BIR domain) (Kanneganti et al., 2007). The most investigated of NLRs are NOD1/CARD4 and NOD2/CARD15. Both NOD1/CARD4 and NOD2/CARD15 recognize the components of bacteria cell wall: ligands of NOD1/CARD4 are γ-D-glutamyl-m-diaminopimelic acid (iE-DAP) and its synthetic derivatives (particularly having hydrophobic acyl residues) (Chamaillard et al., 2003; Girardin et al., 2003), and the ligand of NOD2/CARD15 is muramyl dipeptide (MDP) (Girardin et al., 2003). These compounds are the components of peptidoglycan (PGN). They can enter the cytosol through the pores formed as a result of bacterial toxin exposure (Ratner et al., 2007), via action of the pathogen secretion systems (Ratner et al., 2007), by endocytosis (Marina-Garcia et al., 2008) or by work of transporters (Ismair et al., 2006), and they can be released in the cytosol of infected cells during a bacterial cell division or from lysosomes where PGN of phagocytosed bacteria is degraded (Shaw et al., 2010). Until the ligand binding, LRR-containing C-terminal domain of NOD1/CARD4 and NOD2/CARD15 prevents the activation of the central domain (NOD)

and its further oligomerization (Faustin et al., 2007); ligand binding causes the conformational alterations in the C-terminal region that, in turn, lead to self-oligomerization of the central domain and to the further activation of N-terminal domain (CARD) that recruits and activates specific adaptor proteins, initiating NOD signaling pathways. Such initiation results in the activation of various transcription factors and, consequently, in the production of proinflammatory mediators (Inohara et al., 1999; Ogura et al., 2001).

Although CLRs and RLRs are investigated relatively less than TLRs and NLRs, it is known that they recognize bacterial, viral, fungal, protozoan, and helminth PAMPs as TLRs and NLRs (Table 2), initiating an immune response against them through their specific signaling pathways (as their structure is not so clear as in the case with signaling pathways of TLRs and NLRs, it will be precisely depicted only in the following years). It is crucially important to note that in many steps signaling pathways of all classes of PRRs may intersect, making possible the crosstalk between them.

Receptor	Ligand
MRC1 (CD206, CLEC13D, mannose receptor)	High mannose, fucose
CD207 (CLEC4K, langerin)	Mannose, fucose, N-acetyl-glucosamine, β-glucan
CD209 (CLEC4L, DC-SIGN)	High mannose, fucose
CLEC7A (Dectin-1)	β-1, 3 glucans
CLEC6A (CLEC4N, Dectin-2)	High mannose, α-mannans
CLEC4E (Mincle)	α-mannose, glycolipids, SAP130
CLEC4A (DCIR)	Mannose, fucose
CLEC4C (BDCA-2, CD303)	Mannose, fucose
RIG-I	Nucleic acids of many viruses
MDA5	Nucleic acids of many viruses

Table 2. The ligands of CLRs and RLRs.

The receptors constituting families of PRRs are united by two general features. Firstly, they directly recognize common antigen determinants of virtually all classes of pathogens (so-called pathogen-associated molecular patterns, or simply PAMPs) and initiate immune response against them via specific intracellular signaling pathways. Secondly, they recognize endogenous ligands (since they are usually released during cell stress, they are called damage-associated molecular patterns, DAMPs), and, consequently, PRR-mediated immune response can be activated without influence of infectious agents. Therefore, PRRs may also initiate the development of aseptic inflammation caused by physical factors such as mechanical pressure, thermal damage, ionizing and non-ionizing radiation, or chemical factors (for instance, acidic damage, alkaline damage, exposure to chemical war gases, croton oil or turpentine, exposure to allergens, liberation of toxic substances during tumor disintegration, aseptic necrosis, internal bleeding, haemolysis, autoimmune processes etc.). It may promote the further progression of inflammation or, on the contrary, prevent the hazardous infectious complications (the combination of these two effects may also be true). The final outcome of PRR working is an enhanced production of the many proinflammatory cytokines participating in a plenty of immune system processes. Expression of PRRs on different levels (transcriptomic or proteomic) was detected in a lot of cells and organs, so it gave an evidence that these receptors control many elements of the complex machinery of human immune system: they allow epithelium and endothelium to defend against infectious agents on their own, they mediate the activation of adaptive immune response by antigen-presenting cells and T-helpers, they stimulate expression of cell adhesion molecules for leukocyte rolling and for other processes of inflammation development, and, finally, they contribute to phagocytosis efficacy (Chang, 2010). As a consequence of all written above, pattern recognition receptors play the key role in realization of innate and adaptive immune response. In addition, many PRRs have a number of other vital functions apart from participation in the immune response realization: they may regulate various aspects of cell proliferation, survival, apoptosis, autophagy, reactive oxygen species generation, pyroptosis, angiogenesis and, consequently, of tissue remodeling and repair (Brown et al., 2007; Fukata et al., 2006; Kim et al., 2007; Rakoff-Nahoum and Medzhitov, 2008).

The fundamental character and diversity of PRR functions have led to amazingly rapid research in this field, and such investigations are very perspective for medicine as immune system plays a key role in vast majority if not all human diseases, and the process of discovering new aspects of the immune system functioning is rapidly ongoing. There is a plethora of papers analyzing the significance of PRRs in various diseases. One of the most actively exploring fields in PRR biology is their role in cancer aetiopathogenesis. Not surprisingly, it is (as well as tumor immunology in general) a hot spot in cancer biology as well.

1.2 The position of pattern recognition receptors in cancer biology

Since PRRs mediate immune response inducing by many immunoadjuvants (Okamoto and Sato, 2003; Seya, 2003), and many of them regulate immune response against potentially carcinogenic infectious agents (*Helicobacter pylori*, EBV, HPV, HHV-8/KSHV, CMV, *Mycobacterium tuberculosis*, *Streptococcus pneumoniae*, enteropathogenic *Escherichia coli*, *Shigella flexneri*, *Salmonella typhimurium*, *Borrelia burgdorferi*, *Chlamydia pneumoniae*, *Chlamydia trachomatis*, *Chlamydia psittaci*, *Campylobacter jejuni*, *Candida spp.*, *Schistosoma mansoni*, *Paracoccidioides brasiliensis*, *Histoplasma capsulatum* etc.), it seems to be possible to stimulate anti-tumor immunity through their enhanced activation. This hypothesis, originally developed for the TLRs, should be also true for the all PRRs as well (Killeen and Wang, 2006; Tsan, 2006). According to this suggestion, a reinforced PRR activation may protect from infectious agents and prevent, inhibit, or block carcinogenesis whilst disrupted functioning of these PRRs may allow infectious agents or tumor cells to avoid recognition by immune system and, consequently, not to be eliminated. At the same time, such PRR activation may promote carcinogenesis, creating a proinflammatory microenvironment (via action of respective cytokines) that is favorable for the tumor progression and chemoresistance development (Chen, 2007). It may also result in immunosuppression caused by chronic inflammation (Tsan, 2006). Chronic inflammation may promote the development of cervical, endometrial, ovarian, breast, prostate, testicular, nasopharyngeal, lung, esophageal, gastric, colorectal, liver, pancreatic, gallbladder, kidney, bladder, lymphatic malignancies, and feasibly several other cancer types (Kinlen, 2004; Okamoto and Sato, 2003). In this case, on the contrary, lower PRR activity should minimize the effects of chronic inflammation such as enhancement of cancer initiation and promotion/progression and, consequently, decrease the probability of tumor development. So, the situation resembles a double-edged sword. The ideal variant, possibly, is the «golden mean» - the balance between low and high PRR activity. This hypothesis, developed for PRRs, may also be successfully projected on PRR intracellular signaling pathways – if their elements are overexpressed/constantly activated, it may lead to similar consequences as enhanced PRR activation. On the other hand, if the members of PRR pathways are underexpressed/inactivated/unable to do their work at the right time in the right place, it may result in the same effects that arise after decreased PRR activity, and the analogical «golden mean» in functioning of all genes encoding proteins constituting PRR signaling pathways will be the optimal variant.

1.3 Structural genomic variation and its relevance to cancer

The novel approaches in healthcare move towards the model of "personalized medicine". Advances in the healthcare service grow annually as well as their social relevance. Diagnostic tests and target therapy have become a part of our life. However, in spite of the neoteric improvements of the screening and treatment modalities, the prognosis of patients with many diseases including cancer remains poor. Thus, modern molecular biology and medicine are concerned on the developing of more and more new genomic markers that possess predictive, therapeutic, or prognostic significance. Several markers may evaluate predisposition of any person to one or another disease with a certain degree of accuracy based on the results of a simple blood test. The widespread application of these tests can reveal the risk groups in populations, and thereafter, the complex of preventive measures among the risk group subjects may be conducted. Moreover, above-mentioned genomic markers can be identified in the perinatal period, so the choice between "include" or "not to include" in the risk group on their basis can be made maximally early, and, consequently, the preventive measures can have the greatest efficacy. As a result, the integrative systems of predictive genomic markers, defined once, will allow to create the programs of cancer prevention based on them and will permit next generations to be informed and forewarned about their risks and predispositions to certain diseases.

Thereby, the discovery and development of predictive, therapeutic, or prognostic markers is the primary problem of biomedicine at the present time. However, the critical barrier for progress in this field is that it is not always easy to find an effective genomic marker that is exactly associated with a particular disease. One of the most widespread and important markers is the type of genomic markers called single nucleotide polymorphisms (SNPs). They represent a variation in the DNA sequence, when a single nucleotide differs between members of a biological species or paired chromosomes in an individual. The finishing of Human Genome Project and the widespread distribution of genotyping technologies have led to the enormous number of studies devoted to the association of the inherited gene polymorphisms with various diseases. The SNPs may result in amino acid substitutions altering protein function or splicing, and they can also change structure of enhancer sequences during splicing (Lamba et al., 2003) or affect mRNA stability (Tierney and Medcalf, 2001). SNPs may also alter transcription factor binding motifs, changing the efficacy of enhancer or repressor elements (Thomas et al., 2006), and they can alter the structure of translation initiation codons that may lead to the downregulation of wild-type transcript (Zysow et al., 1995). Gene polymorphisms located in the leucine-rich repeats constituting ectodomain of PRRs may affect the ability of receptor to bind pathogens they normally recognize (Bell et al., 2003), SNPs in the transmembrane domain can lead to the defects of the intracellular receptor transport that do not allow to locate a receptor on the membrane (Johnson et al., 2007), and, finally, the polymorphisms in the internal domain may result in the altered interaction with the adaptor proteins or in the disrupted dimerization. So, inherited SNPs of the genes encoding PRRs may alter PRR expression and activity, modulating cancer risk and, possibly, influencing on various features of the cancer progression. The same statement should be true for the genes encoding proteins of PRR signaling pathways.

On the basis of the fundamental and epidemiological studies, it is possible to specify the two fundamental mechanisms for the modulation of cancer risk by the polymorphisms of the genes encoding PRRs and proteins of PRR pathways. The first of them is the impairment of the immune response to the certain pathogens (it can be bacteria, viruses, fungi, protozoan, and helminths) that increase the risk of the potentially carcinogenic infection and promote its development along with further chronic persistence. The second mechanism is an increase of production of proinflammatory cytokines after the binding of the ligand (exogenous or endogenous) that create a condition of carcinogenic chronic inflammation.

2. How to connect structural genomic variation in pattern recognition receptors and cancer?

2.1 Relevant malignancies: the first dimension of investigation

There is a variety of cancer types that can be associated with the inherited alterations in the genes encoding PRRs and proteins of PRR signaling pathways:

- Oral cancer (the alteration of the immune response to *Candida spp.* and other infectious agents colonizing oral cavity);
- Esophageal cancer (the variation of immune response to pathogens infecting esophagus);
- Gastric cancer (on the basis of modulation of the immune response to *Helicobacter pylori*, EBV and other infectious agents potentially causing this disease);
- Cancer of the small bowel (the modulation of the immune response to *Campylobacter jejuni*);
- Colorectal cancer (the alteration of the immune response to many infectious agents inhabiting colon and rectum);
- Liver cancer (the variation of the immune response to HBV, HCV, *Helicobacter hepaticus*, or liver flukes);
- Gallbladder cancer (the modulation of the immune response to infectious agents finding in bile);
- Pancreatic cancer (the alteration of the immune response to the pathogens inhabiting the pancreas);
- Endometrial cancer (the modification of the immune response to several kinds of infectious agents colonizing endometrium);

- Cervical cancer (the alteration of the immune response to HPV and some infectious agents colonizing cervix);
- Ovarian cancer (the variation of immune response to *Chlamydia trachomatis*);
- breast cancer (the modulation of the immune response to some viruses infecting breast including HPV and EBV)
- Prostate cancer (the variation of the immune response to *Propionibacterium acnes* and other uncertain pathogens finding in prostate tissue);
- Testicular cancer (the modification of the immune response to EBV);
- Kidney cancer (the variation of the immune response to bacteria and viruses infecting kidneys);
- Bladder cancer (the modulation of the immune response to certain viruses or *Schistosoma spp.*);
- Nasopharyngeal carcinoma (the alteration of the immune response to EBV);
- Lung cancer (the variation of the immune response to *Mycobacterium tuberculosis, Streptococcus pneumoniae, Chlamydia pneumoniae*, and, possibly, to other infectious agents causing chronic inflammatory lung diseases);
- Lymphoma (the modification of the immune response to EBV and many other infectious agents such as *Borrelia burgdorferi* or *Helicobacter pylori*);
- Kaposi sarcoma (the variation of the immune response to HHV-8/KSHV-infection);
- Brain tumors (the alteration of the immune response to CMV and other viruses).

2.2 Selection of valuable polymorphisms: the second dimension of investigation

It is important to remember that there are two main components determining the importance of the SNP in the programs of cancer prevention based on genomic risk markers: the value of odds ratio (OR) between cases and controls (as in the whole population as in subgroups) and the prevalence of the polymorphism in population, and they both may vary in different geographic regions. It is desirable to develop not the one general program, but a number of the individual programs for the different countries/populations/environmental conditions. At the moment, it is possible only to recommend a list of polymorphisms for the further investigation since only small number of studies with perfect design was carried out. The list of relevant polymorphisms that can be admitted as the most perspective for the further oncogenomic investigations may be created according to the following rules:

Gene polymorphism may be included into the short list for the further oncogenomic studies if:

- The SNP leads to the substantial functional consequences on the molecular level (for instance, it strongly affects transcription, splicing, translation, stability and transport of pre-mRNA, mRNA, non-coding RNA or protein encoding by the gene, or it noticeably influences signaling of synthesized protein);
- It is associated with risk of cancer in the population studies;
- It has any functional consequences on the molecular level and it is strongly (threshold OR value may be individual for each cancer type) associated with condition that significantly increases risk of cancer.
- The gene polymorphism can be also included into the extended list if:
- It is characterized by more subtle functional alterations in the gene that, however, still result in qualitative or quantitative alterations of the encoding protein (or non-coding RNA);

- It is associated only with condition that substantially increases risk of cancer but not with risk of cancer.

One question may immediately arise: how to distinguish «substantial» and «more subtle» functional changes on the molecular level? It seems to be difficult to answer only on the basis of general principles of molecular biology since for one gene even the smallest alteration in its structure may lead to critical consequences, for another one converse statement can be true, and the effect also greatly depends on the position of the polymorphism. Therefore, an assessment of power of functional alteration should be individual for each gene, and although conclusions obtained in various investigations may differ, these discrepancies would not distort the general picture: if the polymorphism has «serious» functional consequences according to the results of one research, it definitely should be added into the short list until these conclusions will not be subverted. In any case, the general value of creation of such short and extended lists of the prescriptive polymorphisms seems to overcome difficulties related to these complications. It is important that many polymorphisms can be simply in the linkage disequilibrium with truly functional variants, and fundamental investigations are needed to determine are they only markers of association or indeed causal variants. All polymorphisms that are only in the linkage disequilibrium with functional ones should be excluded from both lists.

In concordance with this conception, the following SNPs of the genes encoding PRRs and proteins of PRR signaling pathways may be accepted as the most valuable for the further oncogenomic investigations on the basis of the analysis of relevant published literature (Table 3):

Gene	Polymorphism
TLR1-TLR6-TLR10 gene cluster:	rs10008492, rs4833103, rs5743815, rs11466657
TLR2	rs3804100, rs4696480, -196 - -174 del (Delta22), GT-microsatellite polymorphism
TLR4	rs4986790, rs4986791, rs16906079, rs11536891, rs7873784, rs1927911, rs10759932, rs10116253, rs11536889, rs11536858
TLR9	rs5743836, rs352140
TIRAP/MAL	rs8177400, rs8177399, rs8177374, rs7932766
MyD88	rs1319438, rs199396
IRAK1	rs1059703, rs3027898, rs10127175
TRAF3	rs7143468, rs12147254, rs11160707
TRAF6	rs331455, rs331457
TOLLIP	rs5743867
IRF3	rs7251
IRF5	rs2004640, rs2280714, rs10954213, 5 bp indel (CGGGG) polymorphism
NOD1	rs2075820, ND(1)+32656
NOD2	rs2066842, rs2066844, rs2066845, rs2006847
MRC1	rs1926736, rs2478577, rs2437257, rs691005
CD209	rs2287886, rs735239, rs735240, rs4804803
CLEC7A	rs16910526
RIG-I	rs36055726, rs11795404, rs10813831

Table 3. The short list of polymorphisms of the genes encoding PRRs and proteins of their signaling pathways promising for the further oncogenomic studies.

The following polymorphisms of the genes encoding PRRs and proteins of PRR signaling pathways may be added into the extended list for the further oncogenomic investigations (Table 4):

Gene	Polymorphism
TLR1-TLR6-TLR10 gene cluster:	rs4833095, rs5743551, rs5743618, rs4129009
TLR2	rs5743704, rs62323857, rs1219178642
TLR3	rs5743305, rs3775291, rs121434431, rs5743316
TLR4	rs1927914, rs2149356
TLR5	rs5744168
TLR7	rs179008
TLR8	rs3764880, rs2407992
TLR9	rs352139, rs187084, rs41308230, rs5743844
TIRAP/MAL	rs7932976, rs595209, rs8177375
MyD88	rs156265, rs7744
IRAK1	rs1059702, rs7061789, rs2239673, rs763737, rs3027907, rs5945174
IRAK3	rs1732886, rs1732888, rs10506481, rs1624395, rs1370128
IRAK4	rs1461567, rs4251513, rs425155
TRAF1	rs6920220, rs10818488, rs3761847, rs7021206
TRAF2	rs7852970
TRAF6	rs540386
TOLLIP	rs5743854
IRF1	rs11242115, rs839, rs9282763
IRF3	rs2304204, rs2304206
IRF5	rs4728142, rs41298401, rs13242262, rs10488631, rs729302, rs3807306
IRF7	rs1131665
IRF8	rs17824933
NOD1	rs72551113, rs72551107, rs6958571, rs2907749, rs2907748, rs2075822, rs2075819, rs2075818
NOD2	rs104895493, rs104895476, rs104895475, rs104895474, rs104895473, rs104895472, rs104895462, rs104895461, rs104895460, rs104895438, rs5743291, rs5743260, rs2076756, rs2066843, Pro371Thr, Ala794Pro, Gln908His
MRC1	rs692527, rs2477664, rs691005, rs2253120, rs2477637
CD209	rs735240
RIG-I	rs3824456, rs669260
MAVS/VISA/IPS-1	rs11905552, rs17857295, rs2326369, rs7269320

Table 4. The extended list of the polymorphisms of the genes encoding PRRs and proteins of their signaling pathways promising for the further oncogenomic studies.

2.3 How to organize the study: the third dimension of investigation

The drawing-up of a rigorous study protocol is the crucial moment in the molecular epidemiology, and in some cases the complexity of the research is considerable. Even if the investigation has a valuable aim, sufficient funding and is carried out in an excellent laboratory, errors in the study design may lead to the misrepresentation of the research results and, hence, to the reduction of their usefulness. All moments that can distort the study accuracy should be taken into account, and certain, the most relevant of them, are discussed below. Obviously, the methods of the sample collection, DNA extraction, and PCR conduction should be reliable enough. Modern methods such as automated DNA extraction, real-time PCR, and pyrosequencing should be used, although traditional methods such as allele-specific PCR with visualization in the agarose gel can be exploited as well, and their application definitely will be continued for the next decade. Anyway, automated methods should be of choice compared to methods where a subjective factor is substantial and can influence the results. The improvement of existing technologies and the development of new ones may elevate the accuracy of DNA extraction and PCR, leading to increase of validity of the results and, consequently, to the further progress in the field.

Other important aspects of the study design also should be considered. To differentiate the impact of the chronic inflammatory conditions from the contribution of the other mechanisms in the association of the polymorphisms of the genes encoding PRRs and proteins of PRR signaling pathways with cancer risk, the stratification of cases and controls by infectious agent status and chronic inflammation status should be mandatory in the further studies devoted to this problem. The sample size should be sufficient, and it depends on the frequency of target polymorphism – if it is high, sample size can be less than in the studies where target SNP frequency is low. There is also a lack of studies investigating functional consequences of the polymorphisms of the genes encoding PRRs and proteins of PRR pathways on molecular level (for instance, alterations in the promoter activity, in the gene expression on the transcriptomic and proteomic levels, in stability or/and localization of the non-coding RNA, pre-mRNA, mRNA and protein inside the cell, in protein structure and functions, etc.). It is important since many polymorphisms can be simply in linkage disequilibrium with the other, truly functional variants, and thus such fundamental studies are necessary to clarify their role (are they only markers of association or indeed causal variants?). In addition, in certain populations replication studies should be conducted to prove results that were obtained in prime investigations, particularly if the sample size was not large.

There are certain disparities in different population studies investigating the association of the polymorphisms of the genes encoding PRRs and proteins of their signaling pathways with various aspects of cancer development. General reasons for these discrepancies may include confounding host, bacterial, or environmental factors in different ethnicities modulating the penetrance of the variant allele and affecting risk of condition increasing cancer risk (such as autoimmune diseases, precancerous gastric lesions, tuberculosis, recurrent pneumonia etc.), different bacterial impact in aetiology of such conditions in different populations (that will be reflected in different features of PRR-mediated immune response because of specific PRR-ligand interaction), differences in the sample size, in age/gender/BMI/ethnicity/TNM stage/other clinicopathological characteristics between the study samples, in the prevalence of infectious agent (e.g. HP or EBV) in case and control groups, differences in diagnostics, stratification, genotyping methods, and chance. In addition, certain studies in which negative results were obtained could never been published (so-called file drawer effect) that may create a significant bias and distort a picture that we can observe at the moment. Unfortunately, although some genome-wide association studies (GWAS) relevant to the discussing problem were performed, it is usually not possible to compare them with the non-GWAS on the same cancer type since there are no non-GWAS investigating association of the same SNPs with similar malignancies. It may be feasible in future when the number of studies devoted to this issue will be enough for correct comparative analysis.

3. Hot spots in the field

The most intriguing moments in the problem of the association of inherited structural variation in the genes encoding PRRs and proteins of PRR signaling pathways with features of cancer development are:

- Are SNPs in the genes encoding PRRs or proteins of PRR signaling pathways associated with the features of cancer progression or only with cancer risk? Existing studies have shown controversial results, and the results of most of them allow to suggest that there is no or weak correlation between such polymorphisms and peculiarities of cancer progression.

- Are the polymorphisms of the genes encoding CLRs, RLRs, or specific proteins of their signaling pathways associated with risk or progression of cancer? If yes, would be appropriate to include them in the list of polymorphisms using in programs of cancer risk determination and further cancer prevention? As it was shown above, there are some premises to think that these SNPs may be associated with cancer risk. Further fundamental and population studies are necessary to answer this question.

- Do the polymorphisms of genes encoding PRRs or proteins of PRR signaling pathways (particularly TLRs and TLR pathway) correlate with altered prostate cancer risk or progression? Despite there are some fundamental mechanisms allowing to hypothesize that *TLR* gene polymorphisms may play a role in prostate cancer aetiology, and a number of comprehensive projects on large samples in various countries was conducted, the reliable associations of these SNPs with prostate cancer risk or with features of prostate cancer progression were not detected, and results vary in different populations.

- Are the polymorphisms of the genes of PRR signaling pathways associated with cancer risk or progression to the same extent as polymorphisms of the genes encoding PRRs? It is logical that if SNP of gene encoding specific PRR is associated with risk or progression features of certain malignancies, polymorphisms in the genes encoding specific signaling molecules constituting pathways of this receptor should correlate with similar neoplasms, if they have substantial functional consequences on the molecular level. In contrast to the polymorphisms of the genes encoding TLRs, whose association with solid tumors is a subject of investigation in a lot of genetic association studies, the polymorphisms of the genes encoding proteins of TLR pathway are investigated mostly in relation to leukemia and lymphoma, and their association with epithelial tumors is discovered very poorly. SNPs affecting functional parts of TLR pathway central elements (MyD88, TRIF/TICAM1, TIRP/TRAM/TICAM2, TIRAP/MAL, IRAKs, TRAF3, TRAF6, TAK1, TAB1, TAB2, PKR, IRF3, IRF7) should be the most significant for the oncogenomic studies analyzing this problem.

- How the polymorphisms of the genes encoding PRRs and proteins of PRR signaling pathways interact with each other in relation to determination of cancer risk and progression? Particularly, how SNPs of positive and negative regulators of PRR activity (especially, miRNA) influence on cancer risk or progression if they are inherited together? Answers to these questions remain elusive at present time, and should be obtained from the fundamental and population studies in the future.

- Which the SNPs of the genes encoding PRRs and proteins of PRR pathways have independent significance, and which are just in the linkage disequilibrium? Knowledge of it may help in listing of the polymorphisms useful in the programs of cancer risk determination and further prevention.

- Which SNPs of the genes encoding PRRs and proteins of PRR pathways should be included in such list? Which of them have universal effect for each cancer type, and which influence on risk or/and progression of one cancer type but have no effect in relation to another malignancy? Differences in the association of the same SNP with different malignancies should be explained by features of specific PAMP-PRR interaction (probably, certain characteristics of ligand binding), or, possibly, on peculiarities of DAMP-PRR interaction. List of SNPs prescriptive for the further oncogenomic investigations may be created according to the conception suggested above.

- How SNPs of the genes encoding PRRs and proteins of PRR pathways affect cancer risk or progression in different populations and their subgroups? How this information may be adjusted for application in the creation of the programs of cancer risk determination and further prevention? Only large, comprehensive, well-designed population studies may give answer to these questions.

- Do the polymorphisms of the genes encoding PRRs and proteins of PRR pathways influence on cancer risk only through increase of risk of chronic inflammatory conditions, or they can affect it also through other mechanisms? How this information may be used in the programs of cancer risk determination and further prevention? To answer these questions, control group in population studies should include not only healthy controls, but also controls with the chronic inflammatory conditions predisposing to investigating cancer type.

- Which infectious agents recognizing by various PRRs are carcinogenic, and which are not? It may help to define the cancer types associated with the SNPs of the genes encoding specific PRRs and proteins constituting PRR signaling pathways. Fundamental studies devoted to the investigation of infectious agent-PRR interactions, to the investigation of carcinogenicity of known infectious agents and to the discovery of new, possibly carcinogenic, infectious agents, should answer this question.

No doubt, the determination of the role of SNPs in genes encoding PRRs and proteins of PRR signaling pathways in fields of tumor immunology and molecular epidemiology of cancer may open new pages in the cancer biology and cancer prevention.

4. Acknowledgements

I would like to thank Prof. Elena B. Brusina and Arseniy Yuzhalin for their support during the writing of this chapter.

5. References

Bell, J.K.; Mullen, G.E.; Leifer, C.A.; Mazzoni, A.; Davies, D.R. & Segal, D.M. (2003). Leucine-rich repeats and pathogen recognition in toll-like receptors. *Trends in Immunology*, Vol.24, No.10, (October 2003), pp. 528–533, ISSN 1471-4906

Bell, J.K.; Botos, I.; Hall, P.R.; Askins, J.; Shiloach, J.; Davies, D.R. & Segal, D.M. (2006). The molecular structure of the TLR3 extracellular domain. *Journal of Endotoxin Research*, Vol.12, No.6, (December 2006), pp. 375-378, ISSN 0968-0519

Brown, S.L.; Riehl, T.E.; Walker, M.R.; Geske, M.J.; Doherty, J.M.; Stenson, W.F.; Stappenbeck, T.S. (2007). Myd88-dependent positioning of Ptgs2-expressing stromal cells maintains colonic epithelial proliferation during injury. *The Journal of Clinical Investigation*, Vol.117, No.1, (January 2007), pp. 258–269, ISSN 0021-9738

Chamaillard, M.; Hashimoto, M.; Horie, Y.; Masumoto, J.; Qiu, S.; Saab, L.; Ogura, Y.; Kawasaki, A.; Fukase, K.; Kusumoto, S.; Valvano, M.A.; Foster, S.J.; Mak, T.W.; Nuñez, G. & Inohara, N. (2003). An essential role for NOD1 in host recognition of bacterial peptidoglycan containing diaminopimelic acid. *Nature Immunology*, Vol.4, No.7, (July 2003), pp. 702-707, ISSN 1529-2908

Chang, Z.L. (2010). Important aspects of Toll-like receptors, ligands and their signaling pathways. *Inflammation Research*, Vol.59, No.10, (October 2010), pp. 791-808, ISSN 1023-3830

Chen, G.; Shaw, M.H.; Kim, Y.G. & Nuñez, G. (2009). NOD-like receptors: role in innate immunity and inflammatory disease. *Annual Review of Pathology*, Vol.4, pp. 365-398, ISSN 1553-4006

Chen, R.; Alvero, A.B.; Silasi, D.A. & Mor, G. (2007). Inflammation, cancer and chemoresistance: taking advantage of the toll-like receptor signaling pathway. *Americam Journal of Reproductive Immunology*, Vol.57, No.2, (February 2007), pp. 93–107, ISSN 1046-7408

Elinav, E.; Strowig, T.; Henao-Mejia, J. & Flavell, R.A. (2011). Regulation of the antimicrobial response by NLR proteins. *Immunity*, Vol.34, No.5, (May 2011), pp.665–679, ISSN 1074-7613

Faustin, B.; Lartigue, L.; Bruey, J.M.; Luciano, F.; Sergienko, E.; Bailly-Maitre, B.; Volkmann, N.; Hanein, D.; Rouiller, I. & Reed, J.C. (2007). Reconstituted NALP1 inflammasome reveals two-step mechanism of caspase-1 activation. *Molecular Cell*, Vol.25, No.5, (March 2007), pp. 713-724, ISSN 1097-2765

Fukata, M.; Chen, A.; Klepper, A.; Krishnareddy, S.; Vamadevan, A.S.; Thomas, L.S.; Xu, R.; Inoue, H.; Arditi, M.; Dannenberg, A.J. & Abreu, M.T. (2006). Cox-2 is regulated by Toll-like receptor-4 (TLR4) signaling: role in proliferation and apoptosis in the intestine. *Gastroenterology*, Vol.131, No.3, (September 2006), pp. 862–877, ISSN 0016-5085

Girardin, S.E.; Boneca, I.G.; Viala, J.; Chamaillard, M.; Labigne, A.; Thomas, G.; Philpott, D.J. & Sansonetti, P.J. (2003). Nod2 is a general sensor of peptidoglycan through muramyl dipeptide (MDP) detection. *Journal of Biological Chemistry*, Vol.278, No.11, (March 2003), pp. 8869-8872, ISSN 0021-9258

Girardin, S.E.; Travassos, L.H.; Hervé, M.; Blanot, D.; Boneca, I.G.; Philpott, D.J.; Sansonetti, P.J. & Mengin-Lecreulx, D. (2003). Nod1 detects a unique muropeptide from gram-negative bacterial peptidoglycan. *Science*, Vol.300, No.5625, (June 2003), pp. 1584-1587, ISSN 0036-8075

Hashimoto, C.; Hudson, K.L. & Anderson, K.V. (1988). The Toll gene of Drosophila, required for dorsal-ventral embryonic polarity, appears to encode a transmembrane protein. *Cell*, Vol.52, No.2, (January 1988), pp. 269-279, ISSN 0092-8674

Honda, K. & Taniguchi, T. (2006). IRFs: master regulators of signalling by Toll-like receptors and cytosolic pattern-recognition receptors. *Nature Reviews. Immunology*, Vol.6, No.9, (September 2006), pp. 644-658, ISSN 1474-1733

Huyton, T.; Rossjohn, J. & Wilce, M. (2007). Toll-like receptors: structural pieces of a curve-shaped puzzle. *Immunology and Cell Biology*, Vol.85, No.6, (August-September 2007), pp. 406–410, ISSN 0818-9641

Inohara, N.; Koseki, T.; del Peso, L.; Hu, Y.; Yee, C.; Chen, S.; Carrio, R.; Merino, J.; Liu, D.; Ni, J. & Núñez, G. (1999). Nod1, an Apaf-1-like activator of caspase-9 and nuclear factor-kappaB. *Journal of Biological Chemistry*, Vol.274, No.21, (May 1999), pp. 14560-14567, ISSN 0021-9258

Ismair, M.G.; Vavricka, S.R.; Kullak-Ublick, G.A.; Fried, M.; Mengin-Lecreulx, D. & Girardin, S.E. (2006). hPepT1 selectively transports muramyl dipeptide but not Nod1-activating muramyl peptides. *Canadian Journal of Physiology and Pharmacology*, Vol.84, No.12, (December 2006), pp. 1313–1319, ISSN 0008-4212

Jin, M.S. & Lee, J.O. (2008). Structures of the toll-like receptor family and its ligand complexes. *Immunity*, Vol.29, No.2, (August 2008), pp. 182-191, ISSN 1074-7613

Johnson, C.M.; Lyle, E.A.; Omueti, K.O.; Stepensky, V.A.; Yegin, O.; Alpsoy, E.; Hamann, L.; Schumann, R.R. & Tapping, R.I. (2007). Cutting edge: a common polymorphism impairs cell surface trafficking and functional responses of TLR1 but protects against leprosy. *Journal of Immunology*, Vol.178, No.12, (June 2007), pp. 7520–7524, ISSN 0022-1767

Kanneganti, T.D.; Lamkanfi, M. & Núñez, G. (2007). Intracellular NOD-like receptors in host defense and disease. *Immunity*, Vol.27, No.4, (October 2007), pp. 549-559, ISSN 1074-7613

Kawai, T. & Akira, S. (2011). Toll-like receptors and their crosstalk with other innate receptors in infection and immunity. *Immunity*, Vol.34, No.5, (May 2011), pp. 637–650, ISSN 1074-7613

Killeen, S.D.; Wang, J.H.; Andrews, E.J. & Redmond, H.P. (2006). Exploitation of the toll-like receptor system in cancer: a doubled-edged sword? *British Journal of Cancer*, Vol.95, No.3, (August 2006), pp. 247–252, ISSN 0007-0920

Kim, D.; Kim, M.A.; Cho, I.H.; Kim, M.S.; Lee, S.; Jo, E.K.; Choi, S.Y.; Park, K.; Kim, J.S.; Akira, S.; Na, H.S.; Oh, S.B. & Lee, S.J. (2007). A critical role of toll-like receptor 2 in nerve injury-induced spinal cord glial cell activation and pain hypersensitivity. *Journal of Biological Chemistry*, Vol.282, No.20, (May 2007), pp. 14975–14983, ISSN 0021-9258

Kim, H.M.; Park, B.S.; Kim, J.I.; Kim, S.E.; Lee, J.; Oh, S.C.; Enkhbayar, P.; Matsushima, N.; Lee, H.; Yoo, O.J. & Lee JO. (2007). Crystal structure of the TLR4-MD-2 complex with bound endotoxin antagonist eritoran. *Cell*, Vol.130, No.5, (September 2007), pp. 906–917, ISSN 0092-8674

Kinlen, L. (2004). Infections and immune factors in cancer: the role of epidemiology. *Oncogene*, Vol.23, No.38, (August 2004), pp. 6341–6348, ISSN 0950-9232

Kumar, H.; Kawai, T. & Akira, S. (2009). Pathogen recognition in the innate immune response. *The Biochemical Journal*, Vol.420, No.1, (April 2009), pp. 1-16, ISSN 0264-6021

Lamba, V.; Lamba, J.; Yasuda, K.; Strom, S.; Davila, J.; Hancock, M.L.; Fackenthal, J.D.; Rogan, P.K.; Ring, B.; Wrighton, S.A. & Schuetz, E.G. (2003). Hepatic CYP2B6 expression: gender and ethnic differences and relationship to CYP2B6 genotype and CAR (constitutive androstane receptor) expression. *The Journal of Pharmacology and Experimental Therapeutics*, Vol.307, No.3, (December 2003), pp. 906–922, ISSN 0022-3565

Liu, L.; Botos, I.; Wang, Y.; Leonard, J.N.; Shiloach, J.; Segal, D.M. & Davies, D.R. (2008). Structural basis of toll-like receptor 3 signaling with double-stranded RNA. *Science*, Vol.320, No.5874, (April 2008), pp. 379–381, ISSN 0036-8075

Loo, Y.M. & Gale, M. Jr. (2011). Immune signaling by RIG-I-like receptors. *Immunity*, Vol.34, No.5, (May 2011), pp. 680-692, ISSN 1074-7613

Marina-García, N.; Franchi, L.; Kim, Y.G.; Miller, D.; McDonald, C.; Boons, G.J. & Núñez, G. (2008). Pannexin-1-mediated intracellular delivery of muramyl dipeptide induces caspase-1 activation via cryopyrin/NLRP3 independently of Nod2. *Journal of Immunology*, Vol.180, No.6, (March 2008), pp. 4050-4057, ISSN 0022-1767

Matsushima, N.; Tanaka, T.; Enkhbayar, P.; Mikami, T.; Taga, M.; Yamada, K. & Kuroki, Y. (2007). Comparative sequence analysis of leucine-rich repeats (LRRs) within vertebrate toll-like receptors. *BMC Genomics*, Vol.8, (May 2007), p. 124, ISSN 1471-2164

Medzhitov, R.; Preston-Hurlburt, P. & Janeway, C.A. Jr. (1997). A human homologue of the Drosophila Toll protein signals activation of adaptive immunity. *Nature*, Vol. 388, No. 6640, (July 1997), pp. 394-397, ISSN 0028-0836

Ogura, Y.; Inohara, N.; Benito, A.; Chen, F.F.; Yamaoka, S. & Nunez, G. (2001). Nod2, a Nod1/Apaf-1 family member that is restricted to monocytes and activates NF-kappaB. J *Journal of Biological Chemistry*, Vol. 276, No.7, (February 2001), pp. 4812-4818, ISSN 0021-9258

O'Neill, L.A. & Bowie, A.G. (2007). The family of five: TIR-domain-containing adaptors in Toll-like receptor signalling. *Nature Reviews. Immunology*, Vol. 7, No.5, (May 2007), pp. 353-364, ISSN 1474-1733

Okamoto, M. & Sato, M. (2003). Toll-like receptor signaling in anti-cancer immunity. *The Journal of Medical Investigation*, Vol. 50, No.1-2, (February 2003), pp. 9–24, ISSN 1343-1420

Osorio, F. & Reis E Sousa, C. (2011). Myeloid C-type lectin receptors in pathogen recognition and host defense. *Immunity*, Vol. 34, No.5, (May 2011), pp. 651–664, ISSN 1074-7613

Pålsson-McDermott, E.M. & O'Neill, L.A. (2007). Building an immune system from nine domains. *Biochemical Society Transactions*, Vol. 35, No.6, (December 2007), pp. 1437-1444, ISSN 0300-5127

Rakoff-Nahoum, S. & Medzhitov, R. (2008). Role of toll-like receptors in tissue repair and tumorigenesis. *Biochemistry (Moscow)*, Vol.73, No.5, (May 2008), pp. 555–561, ISSN 0006-2979

Ratner, A.J.; Aguilar, J.L.; Shchepetov, M.; Lysenko, E.S. & Weiser, J.N. (2007). Nod1 mediates cytoplasmic sensing of combinations of extracellular bacteria. *Cellular Microbiology*, Vol. 9, No.5, (May 2007), pp. 1343-1351, ISSN 1462-5814

Seya, T.; Akazawa, T.; Uehori, J.; Matsumoto, M.; Azuma, I. & Toyoshima, K. (2003). Role of toll-like receptor and their adaptors in adjuvant immunotherapy for cancer. *Anticancer Research*, Vol.23, No.6a, (November-December 2003), pp. 4369–4376, ISSN 0250-7005

Shaw, P.J.; Lamkanfi, M. & Kanneganti, T.D. (2010). NOD-like receptor (NLR) signaling beyond the inflammasome. *European Journal of Immunology*, Vol.40, No.3, (March 2010), pp. 624-627, ISSN 0014-2980

Takada, E.; Okahira, S.; Sasai, M.; Funami, K.;, Seya, T. & Matsumoto, M. (2007). C-terminal LRRs of human Toll-like receptor 3 control receptor dimerization and signal transmission. *Molecular Immunology*, Vol. 44, No.15, (July 2007), pp. 3633-3640, ISSN 0161-5890

Takeuchi, O. & Akira, S. (2001). Toll-like receptors; their physiological role and signal transduction system. *International Immunopharmacology*, Vol.1, No.4, (April 2001), pp. 625-635, ISSN 1567-5769

Thomas, K.H.; Meyn, P. & Suttorp, N. (2006). Single nucleotide polymorphism in 5'-flanking region reduces transcription of surfactant protein B gene in H441 cells. *American Journal of Physiology. Lung Cellular and Molecular Physiology*, Vol.291, No.3, (September 2006), pp. 386–390, ISSN 1040-0605

Tierney, M.J. & Medcalf, R.L. (2001). Plasminogen activator inhibitor type 2 contains mRNA instability elements within exon 4 of the coding region. Sequence homology to coding region instability determinants in other mRNAs. *Journal of Biological Chemistry*, Vol.276, No.17, (April 2001), pp. 13675–13684, ISSN 0021-9258

Tsan, M.F. (2006). Toll-like receptors, inflammation, and cancer. *Seminars in Cancer Biology*, Vol.16, No.1, (February 2006), pp. 32-37, ISSN 1044579X

Wong, Y.; Sethu, C.; Louafi, F. & Hossain, P. (2011). Lipopolysaccharide Regulation of Toll-Like Receptor-4 and Matrix Metalloprotease-9 in Human Primary Corneal Fibroblast Cells. *Investigative Ophthalmology and Visual Science*, Vol.52, No.5, (April 2011), pp. 2796-2803, ISSN 0146-0404

Yamamoto, M.; Takeda, K. & Akira, S. (2004). TIR domain-containing adaptors define the specificity of TLR signaling. *Molecular Immunology*, Vol.40, No.12, (February 2004), pp. 861–868, ISSN 0161-5890

Zhu, J. & Mohan, C. (2010). Toll-like receptor signaling pathways--therapeutic opportunities. *Mediators of Inflammation*, Vol.2010, p. 781235, ISSN 0962-9351

Zysow, B.R.; Lindahl, G.E.; Wade, D.P.; Knight, B.L. & Lawn, R.M. (1995). C/T polymorphism in the 5'untranslated region of the apolipoprotein(a) gene introduces an upstream ATG and reduces in vitro translation. *Arteriosclerosis, Thrombosis and Vascular Biology*, Vol.15, No.1, (January 1995), pp. 58–64, ISSN 1049-8834

Section 2

Basics of Autoimmunity and Multiple Sclerosis

6

Adaptive Immune Response in Epilepsy

Sandra Orozco-Suárez[1,*], Iris Feria-Romero[1], Dario Rayo[2],
Jaime Diegopérez[2], Ma.Ines Fraire[2], Justina Sosa[3], Lourdes Arriaga[4],
Mario Alonso Vanegas[5], Luisa Rocha[6], Pietro Fagiolino[7] and Israel Grijalva[1]
[1]Unidad de Investigación Médica en Enfermedades Neurológicas,
[2]Hospital de Pediatria, CMN Siglo XXI,
[3]Hospital de Especialidades, CM "La Raza",IMSS.México D.F.,
[4]Unidad de Investigación en Inmunoquímica,Hospital de Especialidades,
CMN Siglo XXI, IMSS México D.F.,
[5]Instituto Nacional de Neurología y Neurocirugía,"Manuel Velasco Suárez", México D.F.,
[6]Departamento de Farmacobiología,
Centro de Investigacion y de Estudios Avanzados, Sede Sur,
[7]Centro de Monitoreo de Fármacos, Universidad de la República, Montevideo,
[1,2,3,4,5,6]México
[7]Uruguay

1. Introduction

Various brain injuries in humans such as neurotrauma,stroke, infection, febrile convulsions and status epilepticus are associated with the acute occurrence of seizures and an increased risk of developing epilepsy, Experimental studies in rodents have shown that these events induce a chronic decreased seizure threshold or the development of spontaneous seizures, supporting the notion, that central nervous system (CNS) injury can lead to lasting hyperexcitability. These injuries trigger inflammatory processes in the brain, which are rapidly ensuing and long-lasting, raising the possibility that inflammatory mediators may contribute to the development of epileptogenesis, and the consequent precipitation of spontaneous seizures.

On the other hand a pathogenic role of immunity in epilepsies has long been suggested based on observations of the efficacy of immune-modulating treatments and, more recently, by the finding of inflammation markers including autoantibodies in individuals with a number of epileptic disorders. Clinical and experimental data suggest that both innate and adaptive immunity may be involved in epilepsy. Innate immunity represents an immediate, nonspecific host response against pathogens via activation of resident brain immune cells and inflammatory mediators. These are thought to contribute to seizures and epileptogenesis. Adaptive immunity employs activation of antigen specific B and T lymphocytes or antibodies in the context of viral infections and autoimmune disorders.

* Corresponding Author

This review focused first on the description of the interaction between the immune system and CNS peculiar aspects and relevance for the pathogenesis of immune–mediated diseases of the CNS, second, we offer an overview of the experimental evidence in experimental models of seizures to discuss how inflammation modulates epilepsy, and whether inflammation is always detrimental to cell survival. Such research has also sought to determine how inflammatory mechanisms might be harnessed to develop therapies for epilepsy and third we describe causal clinical evidences of various forms of human epilepsy in which CNS inflammation and markers of adaptive immunity have been described, also we describe some of the treatments used in pharmacoresistan epilepsy with probable autoimmune origin.

2. Overview of the immune system

The natural defences presented by an individual to any external agent are included in the immune system; this is generally divided into innate and adaptive immunity. Innate immunity is the first response presented against insult, that is triggered by physical, chemical or bacteriological damage, the latter is the most familiar and easier to reproduce by introducing systemic lipopolysaccharide or LPS, which is the substance that covers the outer membrane of Gram (-)bacteria (Condie, 1955; Rivest , 2000). For its study, innate immunity is divided into the afferent arm, which identifies or perceives to insult, and the efferent arm, which is how the infection is eradicated (Tracey, 2009). Several studies have shown that depending on the agent causing the damage, pathway, organ and even insult cells triggers a series of molecules for defence of the individual and the communication between immune system cells can lead to out both by direct contact between cells or by the involvement of soluble factors known as cytokines. This will differentiate the humoral components of the afferent arm (LBP, CD14, collectins, properdin, C3b, pentraxins) and efferent (cytokines, antimicrobial peptides, lysozyme, BPI, complement, lactoferrin, acute phase reactants) and cellular components of the afferent arm (TLRs, dectina-1, CD14, formyl peptide receptor or FMLP, NOD1, NOD2) and efferent (antimicrobial peptides, proteases, lipases, glycosidases, cell adhesion molecules, H_2O_2, hydroxyl radical, oxygen halides, nitric oxide, peroxynitrite, etc.) (Beutler, 2004; Vezzani, 2005).

Until recently, adaptive immunity was considered a type of immune response independent of the innate immune response; now it is known that both responses are intertwined, so the participation of dendritic cells, monocytes, macrophages, B lymphocytes and T, specialized molecules of immune histocompatibility, complex class I and II (MHC I and II) that are present during the innate response, are the beginning of the adaptive response (Iwasaki, 2010). In this type of response antigen recognition is carried by the specific antigen-presenting cells (APCs) and antigen receptors. In the adaptive immune response; it is identified two ways: the conventional adaptive immunity in jawed vertebrates and unconventional characteristic of jawless vertebrates.

The first is mediated by immunoglobulins (Ig) and T cell receptors (TCRs) (Fig 1). Low-affinity IgM antibodies circulate in the blood prior to encountering pathogens, however, high-affinity IgG and IgA antibodies are required to inactivate toxins, neutralize viruses, and promote the clearance of microorganisms (Li, 2004). Prior to antigen exposure, the initial generation of a diverse antibody repertoire is achieved early in B-lymphocyte development by the successful rearrangement of the V, D, and J gene. This recombination process depends on the recognition of recombination signal sequences (RSSs), which flank the segmental elements and create extensive variation in the receptor structure at junctional (joining) interfaces. V(D)J rearrangement form of somatic recombination occurs in the progenitors of B and T cells and is mediated by recombination-activating gene 1 (RAG1) and RAG2, which function in a lymphocyte- and site-specific recombinase complex and are supported by ubiquitous DNA repair factors (Fig 1A)(Gellert, 2002). The Immunoglobulins function first as membrane-bound receptors on B cells and their precursor cells, and they are selected for both antigen-binding specificity and affinity. A change in RNA splicing converts the membrane-bound receptor to a soluble product and is associated with the differentiation from receptor-expressing B cells to immunoglobulin-secreting plasma cells. A second wave of antibody diversification occurs through somatic hypermutation (SHM) (Fig. 1B) and/or gene conversion (GC) of the V region to generate high-affinity antigen binding sites (MacLennan, 1994). SHM is the predominant mechanism in mice and humans, whereas GC occurs in chickens and some other species (Weill and Reynaud 1996). In the same centroblast B cell, the heavy-chain V regions encoding the antigen binding sites are rearranged down the chromosome through class switch recombination (CSR) so that they can be expressed with one of the constant (C) region genes to carry out many different effector functions and be distributed throughout the body (Fig. 1C). Activation-induced cytidine deaminase (AID) mediates SHM, gene conversion and class-switch recombination (CSR).

The TCR is a clonotypic, membrane-bound receptor that binds peptide-MHC (pMHC). Similar to immunoglobulins, both classes of TCRs (αβ TCRs and γδ TCRs) are heterodimers in which a D segment is a rearranging component of one unit of the receptor heterodimer. The function of αβ TCRs relies on the polymorphic MHC class I and class II molecules expressed by antigen-presenting cells. By contrast, γδ TCRs function independently of MHC class I and class II molecules and it has been proposed that a forerunner of the rearranging antigen-binding receptors might have been a γδ TCR-like receptor (--12--). Genetically, TCRs are rearranged into α and β-chains from a selection of 176 variable (V), diversity (D), joining (J), and constant (C) genes on chromosomes 7 and 14. Random recombination of these genes generates only 5–10% of the potential diversity within the TCR repertoire; exonucleolytic activity, random N nucleotide additions at the V(D)J junctions (Cabaniols, 2001) and αβ chain pairing contribute the remainder (Fig 1). Theoretical TCR diversity in humans has been placed in the region of $10^{15} - 10^{20}$ unique structures (Davis, 1988; Lieber 1991; Shortman, 1990), with direct *in vivo* estimates greater than 2.5×10^7 unique structures (Arstila, 1999). Structurally, TCR α- and β-chains fold to expose six highly flexible complementary determining region (CDR) loops that can contact the pMHC binding face. The germline-encoded CDR1 and CDR2 loops, from the TRAV and TRBV genes, participate heavily in MHC contacts and occasionally peptide contacts. The variable CDR3 loops, which span the V(D)J joints, are key to TCR diversity and participate heavily in peptide contacts. TCRs dock with pMHC complexes in a roughly diagonal fashion, such that the CDR3α loops are placed over the peptide N-terminus and the CDR3β loops lie over the peptide C-terminus (Miles, 2010).

In unconventional adaptive immunity, the specific response to antigens of bacteria and blood cells is similar to cellular immunity and identified lymphocyte-like cells in organs and tissues (Alder, 2005). On the other hand humoral mediators are somatically derived variants of leucine-rich repeats or LRRs, termed variable lymphocyte receptors (VLRs), which are as efficient as V (D) J process. The mechanism of VLRs assembly seems to be driven by a copy choice mechanism of recombination that is based on sequence similarities of individual LRR segments rather than by specific recombination elements (Han, 2008; Nagawa, 2007).

Although immunoglobulins, TCRs, and VLRs are structurally unrelated and somatic variations generated through unrelated mechanisms, these molecules develop clonal specificity through somatic recombination, show evidence of specific cell lineage compartmentalization in receptor expression and can share common features in the recipient's immune regulation (Litman, 2010).

3. Immunology of the nervous system

The CNS has developed strategies to limit the entry of immune elements as well as to limit the emergence of immune activation with the tissue itself. Immune privilege in the CNS is partially dependent on the blood–brain barrier (BBB), which is designed to limit the entry of solutes and ions into the CNS(Carson et al.,2006). Exclusion from, and selective entry of compounds into the CNS takes place in the capillary venules. In contrast ,cell migration takes place at the post-capillary venules, where cell migration is controlled by adhesion molecules, cytokines and chemokines, and their receptors (Fig.2)(Owens et al., 2008). Not only the physical properties of the BBB, but also potentially damaging immune responses as such are regulated by the suppressive environment within the CNS. Both astrocytes and microglia play a major role in this regulation, while neurons are assumed to play a largely passive role being only the victims of immune responses. Microglia invade the brain early in development and take on a resting 'protective' role as sentinels, scattered uniformly throughout the CNS and forming a network of potential effectors cells. In contrast to peripheral macrophages that are highly effective at inciting pro-inflammatory responses, microglia take on an opposing role, limiting inflammation. This role is extended also to astrocytes, the first cells that CNS-infiltrating immune cells encounter. Astrocytes suppress T helper 1 (Th1) and T helper 2 (Th2) cell activation, the proliferation and effector functions of activated T cells, and possess a wide variety of molecular mechanisms to induce apoptosis in activated T cells. Contrary to the idea that neurons only play a passive role, many of their products (i.e. neuropeptides and transmitters), as well as the neuronal membrane proteins CD22, CD47, CD200, CX3CL1 (fractalkine), intercellular adhesion molecule (ICAM), neural cell adhesion molecule (NCAM), semaphorins and C-type lectins all regulate inflammation (Tian, 2009). In addition, neurons express low levels of major histocompatibility complex (MHC) molecules and actively promote T-cell apoptosis via the Fas–Fas ligand pathway (CD95-CD95L). Neuronal expression of the cannabinoid (CB1) receptor is also implicated in suppressing inflammation. CB1 knockout mice more readily develop experimental autoimmune encephalomyelitis (EAE), the autoimmune model of multiple sclerosis (MS). Neurons also favour the differentiation of T-regulatory cells, by providing a local microenvironment dominated by transforming growth factor-b1 (TGF-b1). Damaged neurons, however, are less able to maintain this protective shield, allowing further insults.

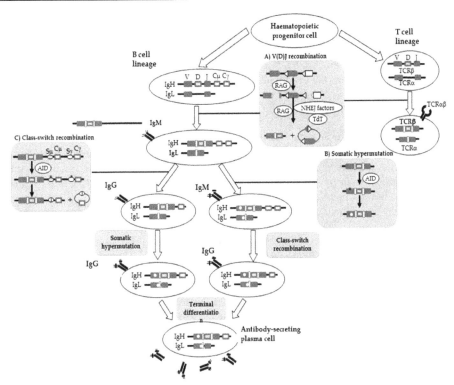

Fig 1. Conventional adaptative immune response in jawed vertebrates. A haematopoietic progenitor cell gives rise to distinct B and T cell lineages. During the development of Ig and TCR different recombination processes are involved. **A) V(D)J recombination.** In this process, RSSs (dark and white triangles) direct the RAG1–RAG2 recombinase complex to individual gene segments (dark and white boxes). The recombinase introduces two double-strand DNA breaks with blunt signal ends and hairpin-sealed coding ends. In the subsequent joining phase, TdT a template-independent DNA polymerase, adds random nucleotides to the junction of the gene elements, thereby increasing repertoire diversity dramatically; the RSSs are joined without further end processing and form excision circles. The key factors that facilitate each diversification step are NHEJ factors. Once functional DNA rearrangements occur, TCR sequences are unaltered. **B) Somatic hypermutation** is initiated by AID, which deaminates individual cytidines within the V(D)J exon of the immunoglobulin gene, leading to U:G mismatches (asterisk). Subsequent error-prone repair results in individual point mutations (white dot in the gene and white bar in the immunoglobulin molecules), and B cells with higher affinity for the original antigen are selected. **C) Class-switch recombination.** The AID creates U:G mismatches in the highly repetitive S regions (dark and white ovals) that are upstream of the exons encoding the constant regions of different isotypes. Error-prone repair leads to the generation of double-strand DNA breaks, excision of the intervening DNA (containing the Cμ exons) and joining of the remains of the S regions. The recombined, somatically mutated V(D)J region is then associated with Cγ, instead of Cμ. (Modified from Litman, 2010). **B and T cell lineages.** Immunoglobulin heavy and light chain: IgH and IgL; T cell receptor α and β chain: TCRα and TCRβ. **A) V(D)J recombination.** Variable, diversity,

joining genes: V(D)J; Recombination signal sequences: RSSs; Recombination activating gene 1 and 2: RAG1 and RAG2; Terminal deoxynucleotidyl transferase: TdT; Non-homologous end-joining: NHEJ. **B) Somatic hypermutation.** Activation-induced cytidine deaminase: AID. **C) Class-switch recombination.** Switch (S); Constant region for the Igμ isotype (Cμ) and a single representative downstream Cγ exon within the IgH locus.

4. Innate and adaptive responses in epilepsy

Despite the immune-privileged environment, it is clear that both innate and adaptive inflammatory responses do occur in the CNS. Activation of the innate immune system is a crucial first line of defense, to opsonize and clear apoptotic cells. Furthermore, innate immune responses recruit cells of the adaptive immune system by secreting various cytokines and chemokines that induce adhesion molecules on the BBB, and by inducing the expression of costimulatory molecules on microglia. Through conserved pattern-recognition receptors (PRRs), local CNS cells may be triggered to develop innate responses. Among these receptors are Toll-like receptors (TLRs), which bind highly conserved structural motifs either from pathogens (pathogen-associated molecular patterns, or PAMPs) or from damaged or stressed tissues (danger-associated molecular patterns, or DAMPs). Thus, not only invading micro-organisms, but also endogenous signals can switch on innate responses in the CNS. Some DAMPs, including heat shock proteins, uric acid, chromatin, adenosine and ATP, high mobility group box chromosomal protein 1 (HMGB-1), galectins and thioredoxin have adjuvant and pro-inflammatory activity. TLRs can be widely up-regulated during neurological disorders in varying patterns on microglia, astrocytes, oligodendrocytes and neurons (Bsibsi, 2002). When activated, TLRs are generally assumed to promote the production of pro-inflammatory cytokines, evoking a damaging environment that may contribute to neuronal damage. In vitro, Ab activates microglia through TLRs (Jackson et al., 2006, Okun et al., 2009;Letiembre et al.,2009). TLRs also aid the uptake of Ab and other aggregated proteins, thereby promoting their clearance from the CNS. Although in this manner, TLRs may seem to play a beneficial role in epilepsy it is currently unclear whether cellular activation by TLRs in another way may also contribute to epileptogenesis (Ravizza et al., 2011) . Therefore, rather than only playing a pathogenic role, several TLRs also play a role in repair during neurodegenerative disorders, under non-infectious conditions, suggesting that activation of at least some TLRs can also be used as a therapeutic strategy in CNS disorders(van Noort, 2007)

4.1 Experimental evidence

Due to advances in both structural and functional neuroimaging, as well as opportunities to perform invasive investigations of the human brain in an epilepsy surgery setting, an increasing amount of research on focal epilepsy is now utilizing patients and tissue obtained from patients. Nevertheless, parallel studies on patients and well validated equivalent animal models remain indispensable to circumvent difficulties in clinical research resulting from ethical limitations, cost, inadequate sampling, and absence of appropriate controls. The reliability of animal models in analysing epileptogenic mechanisms and testing the efficacy of antiepileptic drugs (AEDs) depends on how faithfully the epileptic phenomenology mimics ,both the clinical and EEG features of human seizures. Moreover, since human epilepsies are defined as pathological conditions characterized by the recurrence of epileptic

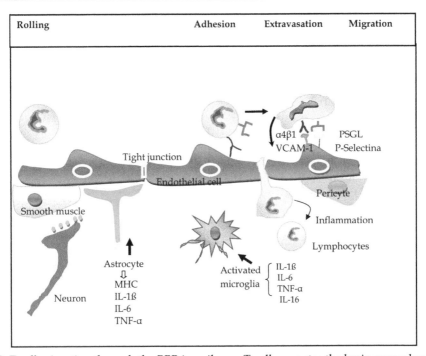

Fig. 2. T cell migration through the BBB in epilepsy. T-cell can enter the brain parenchyma by extravasation across the blood–brain barrier nonfenestrated endothelium and basal lamina. Antigen-presenting cells such as dendritic cells and macrophages are found in the subarachnoid space, in the perivascular space, and in the choroid plexus, whereas microglia are located in brain parenchyma; at these locations, these cells may encounter circulating CNS-borne antigens. The abnormal permeation across the barrier results in further, and perhaps distal, disruption of tight junctions, this time mediated by release of inflammatory mediators by both extravasated blood cells and activated microglia. Frank cellular immunoagression occurs if and when histocompatibility mechanisms are activated and antibody-mediated reactions occur. IL, interleukin; TNF, tumor necrosis factor; IFN, interferon; CSF, colony-stimulating factor; MHC, major histocompatibility complex, modify by Mix et al (2007) and Oby and Janigro (2006).

seizures only animals presenting with recurrent seizures can be defined as animal models of epilepsy. The acute experimental procedures designed to induce seizures, such as the injection of convulsant drugs, maximal electroshock etc., should therefore be referred to as animal models of seizures and not epilepsies unless they also induce a permanent epileptogenic. In this way the models have been described as **acute experimental seizure models**, in which seizures are induced by electrical stimulation, topical convulsants that block inhibition (e.g., penicillin, bicuculline, picrotoxina, pentylenetetrazol, strychnine), or topical convulsants that enhance excitation (e.g., carbachol, kainic acid). **Chronic models** of focal epilepsy can be induced with freeze lesions, partially isolated cortical slabs, metals (e.g., alumina, cobalt, tungstic acid, ferric chloride), kindling, tetanus toxin, anti-GM1 ganglioside antibodies, hippocampal sclerosis (kainic acid, pilocarpine, self-sustained status epilepticus), or focal dysplasia (neonatal freeze, prenatal radiation, MAM) (Engel, 2004).

Some of these epilepsy models in rodents trigger a prominent inflammatory response in brain regions recruited in the onset and propagation of epileptic activity; depending on the severity of the seizures, the inflammatory activity is affected in different ways (Minami, 1990;1991; Gahring, 1991;Jankowsky &Patterson, 2001; Kubera,2001; Oprica,2003; Turrin,2004). In models of temporal lobe epilepsy, the seizures produce changes in the function of the peripheral immune system. The thymus, for example, displays reduced weight, probably due to elevated corticosterone plasma levels during kainate-induced seizure; this steroid is induced during some kinds of stress or after a pathogenic infection. An increase in metabolic activity of splenocytes at the cellular level may be connected to enhanced phagocytic activity of macrophages (Kubera et al., 2001). The inflammatory response occurs during the 3 days following seizures. Although IL-1β, TNF-a, and IL-6 are expressed at very low levels in normal brain, their messenger RNA (mRNA) and protein levels are rapidly ($\leq$30 min) increased after the induction of seizures, declining to basal levels within 48–72 h from the onset of seizures. However, IL-1β is still up regulated in the brain 60 days after status epilepticus in rats with spontaneous seizures (Plata et al., 2000). The increase in interleukin (IL)-1β, IL-6 and TNF-α in microglia and astrocytes is followed by a cascade of downstream inflammatory events which may recruit cells of the adaptive immune system (Vezzani and Granata, 2005).

The kindled model exhibited a significant up-regulation of IL-1 β, IL-1RI, TNF-a and TGF-β1 mRNAs in several limbic brain regions. The overall profile of mRNA changes shows specificity of transcriptional modulation induced by amygdala kindling. The data support a role for cytokines and NPY in the adaptive mechanisms associated with generalized seizure activity (Gahring, 1997). Cytokine production is also induced in brain by audiogenic seizures(Lee, 2008). Production of proinflammatory molecules (a cytokine induced portfolio of genes that are established mediators of inflammation (Dinarello, 2000) is typically accompanied by the concomitant synthesis of anti-inflammatory mediators and binding proteins apt to modulate the inflammatory response, thus avoiding the occurrence of deleterious induction of genes that mediate inflammatory effects. In this respect, up regulation of IL-1–receptor antagonist (Ra), a naturally occurring antagonist of IL-1β, has been described after acute seizures, status epilepticus, and in kindling (Gasque ,1997; Gorter, 2006;Avignone ,2008). However, IL-1Ra and IL-1β are induced by seizures and IL-1Ra is produced with a delayed time course, differing from classic inflammatory reactions in which IL-1Ra is produced at 100- to 1,000-fold excess and concomitant with IL-1β production. Thus the brain is less effective than the periphery in inducing a crucial mechanism for rapidly terminating the actions of a sustained increase in endogenous IL-1β. Cytokine receptors in the CNS are expressed by neurons, microglia, and astrocytes. However, it is primarily microglia activation that has morphologic changes related to the seizures and inflammation; this is a complex process that includes changes in pharmacological and electrophysiological properties, migration, proliferation, and release of a variety of mediators. In the context of status epilepticus induced by kainate, microglia are activated within the same time course that is observed for neuronal degeneration (Hosokawa, 2003; Xiong,2003).

The immune response changes during all three phases of epileptogenesis. The genes related to immune response are induced during both acute and latent phases of epileptogenesis but also during the chronic phase (in CA3). Although the immune response was greater one week after status epilepticus, the levels of secreted phosphoprotein 1 (Spp1 or osteopontin), a glycoprotein that promotes macrophage migration, Hg2a (or CD74; H-2 class II histocompatibility antigen), proteasomes (Psmb9, macropain), toll-like receptor 4 (Tlr4), and tumor necrosis factor (Gorter,2006), also, the prostaglandin synthesis, illustrated by Cox-2 induction, was activated in the acute and chronic phases but not in the latent period, indicating that this process is related to the occurrence of seizure activity. Activation of prostaglandin receptors could increase intracellular calcium and subsequent glutamate release, which would increase excitability in the surrounding networks (Bezzi et al., 1998; Rozovsk et al.,1994)

An important component of the immune response is activation of the complement pathway. Although complement factors might invade the brain via a leaky BBB, part of the increased expression is likely to originate from activated glial cells (Ravizza et al., 2006;Vezzani, 2008). The complement system may be useful for eliminating aggregated and toxic proteins. However, overactivation of the complement system can also have damaging effects through the activation of microglia and proinflammatory cytokines. Interestingly, sequential infusion of individual proteins of the membrane attack pathway into the hippocampus of freely moving rats induces seizures as well as cytotoxicity (Ravizza et al., 2006).

The complement cascade is activated by three pathways: the classical, the alternative, and the lectin pathway; the lectin pathway leads to the formation of the C5b-C9 membrane attack protein complex (MAC). Complement activation in the CNS is increasingly recognized to be associated with exacerbation and progression of tissue injury in different degenerative and inflammatory diseases. Interestingly, sequential infusion of individual proteins of the membrane attack pathway (C5b6, C7, C8, and C9) into the hippocampus of awake, freely moving rats induces both behavioral and electrographic seizures as well as cytotoxicity, suggesting a role for the complement system in epileptogenesis. Rozowski and colleagues (1994) showed increased C1q and C4 mRNA in rat pyramidal neurons after systemic injection of convulsant doses of kainic acid in neuronal layers of limbic areas that are vulnerable to kainic acid-induced neurodegeneration (Vezzani, 2008); moreover, clusterin and C1q immunoreactivities were observed in both neurons and astrocytes, while increased immunoreactivities (as observed in vivo after seizures) were demonstrated following prolonged exposure of primary cultures of hippocampal neurons to glutamate. Additionally, with sequential infusion into the rat hippocampus the individual proteins of the MAC induced both behavioral and electrographic seizures as well as cytotoxicity (Ravizza et al, 2006).

In addition, there is prominent activation of the complement cascade during the epileptogenesis phase in the experimental model and in sclerotic hippocampi from a rat model of TLE and human TLE (Aronica et al., 2007). Interestingly, the expression of CD59, a complement inhibitor of the MAC, was increased in microglia, but only modestly in neurons, suggesting that in this cell population complement activation may be poorly controlled (Rozovsky et al., 1994). These findings are corroborated by clinical evidence showing that both IL-1β and IL-1 receptor type I (RI), NFkB and complex are overexpressed in lesional brain tissue of patients with diverse types of pharmacoresistant epilepsy (Sheng et al., 1994, Crespel et al., 2002)

4.2 Clinical evidence

From a clinical standpoint, a role of inflammation in the pathophysiology of human epilepsy is still hypothetical, although this possibility is supported by abundant evidence. The first insight into a role for inflammation in epilepsy originated from the demonstrated antiepileptic activity of select, powerful anti-inflammatory drugs, including steroids. Moreover, several reports showed increased markers of inflammation in serum, CSF, and brain resident cells in patients with epilepsy. For example, epileptic patients who have recently experienced tonic–clonic seizures display a proinflammatory profile of cytokines in plasma and CSF, consisting of higher IL-6 levels and a lower IL-1Ra–to–IL-1α ratio. Because the IL-6 concentration is much higher in CSF than in plasma (Pacifici et al., 1995; Peltola et al., ,1998) and the contribution of peripheral blood mononuclear cells (PBMCs) to increased plasma levels of cytokines is still unclear (Sheng et al., 1994), the most likely origin of CSF cytokines appears to be the brain. In the same way, Sinha et al. (2008) analyzed cytokine levels in patients with partial epilepsy, status epilepticus and some epilepsy syndromes. Compared to controls, the patient group showed detectable levels of the following cytokines in serum: IL-6, TNF-α, IL-2, IL-4, IFN-γ and IL-1β. Serial analysis during the seizure-free period revealed a decrease in cytokine levels: TNF-α (25% to 12.5%), IFN-γ (12.5%to 0%), IL-1 (25% to 0) and IL-2 (6.2% to 6.2%), IL-4 (18.8% to 0%) and IL-6 (18.8% to 6.2%). On the other hand, increased post-ictal serum cytokine levels were found in patients with several epilepsy syndromes. However, data collected using tissue of patients with TLE show that specific inflammatory pathways are chronically activated during epileptogenesis and that they persist in chronic epileptic tissue, suggesting that they may contribute to the etiopathogenesis of some types of epilepsy, such as TLE (Ravizza et al., 2008).

4.3 Temporal lobe epilepsy (TLE)

Temporal lobe epilepsy refers to both lesional and nonlesional epilepsies characterized by focal seizures arising from either the neocortex or the mesial temporal structures. One of these syndromes is TLE, associated with hippocampal sclerosis (HS), a histopathologic condition characterized by neuronal loss and gliosis, predominantly affecting the CA1 region and the dentate gyrus. Increased IL-1α expression in microglia-like cells (Aronica et al., 2007), TLE with hippocampal sclerosis, and astroglial, microglial, and neuronal (5/8 cases) expression of C1q, C3c, and C3d were observed, particularly within regions where neuronal cell loss occurs (Crespel et al., 2002). Bauer et al (2009) showed that patients with well-characterized TLE led to immediate and long lasting posictal increase in systemic IL-6 levels; however this rise of IL-6 was lacking in patients with hippocampal sclerosis. The authors in accord with Meador et al.,(2004) suggest the cerebral lateralization of immune functions. On the other hand, there was expression of proinflammatory molecules in neurons and glia in brain tissue obtained from patients surgically treated for drug-resistant epilepsies (Crespel et al., 2002; Maldonado et al., 2003). In particular, the genes involved in the biological process of immunity and host defense are highly overrepresented in HS TLE patients; the functional gene classes most affected are chemokines and neuropeptides (De Simoni et al.,2000; van Gassen et al., 2008). Evaluation of immunological parameters applied to different groups of epileptogenic focus localization has shown that the increase of CD8+ lymphocytes is limited to temporal and lateralized patients. Patients with extratemporal localization of focus, as well as psychogenic cases, show normal levels of immunological lymphocyte markers (Lorigados-Pedre., 2004). Thus, upregulation of these chemokines in the human TLE hippocampus may contribute not only to neuropathology, but also to epileptogenesis. Early up regulation of chemokines, for instance, after viral infection, may represent a common pathway linking the various predisposing factors in the etiology of TLE, such as trauma, febrile seizures, meningitis, encephalitis, and tumors.) These data show that specific inflammatory pathways are chronically activated during epileptogenesis and that they persist in chronic epileptic tissue, suggesting that they may contribute to the etiopathogenesis of TLE (van Gassen et al, 2008)

4.4 Rasmussen's encephalitis

Rasmussen's encephalitis serves as a prototype of inflammatory epilepsy. The autoimmune nature of this condition was suspected after the discovery of autoantibodies against the glutamate receptor GluR3, one of the AMPA (α-amino-3-hydroxy-5-methyl-4-isoxazolepropionic acid) subunits. Subsequently, anti-GluR3 antibodies were detected in other epilepsy syndromes, including early-onset noninflammatory focal epilepsy and catastrophic infantile epilepsy (Mantegazza et al., 2002). There is no effective medical treatment for Rasmussen's encephalitis, except perhaps steroids, which can be useful when given early in the course of the disease (Robitaille, 1991). Functional hemispherectomy has been the main procedure used to stop progression of the disease; in this way, the tissue could be examined and the progression of an inflammatory process confirmed. Pardo et al. (2004) describe the effect of disease duration on the burden of pathology. The greatest intensity of inflammation and microglial proliferation with nodule formation are generally seen in early states (Fig.3), followed by a decrease in the later stages. The intensity of inflammation, as represented by accumulation of T cells and microglial proliferation (Fig.3), has been reported to bear an inverse correlation with disease duration (Bauer et al., 2002; 2007). Different stages of inflammation may coexist in the same patient with a multifocal distribution, which is consistent with an ongoing and progressive immune-mediated process (Gahring et al., 2001;Neumann et al., 2002). CD8+ T cells are located in close opposition to degenerating neurons and may contribute to neuronal cell death via secretion of granzyme B, a strong activator of caspase-mediated apoptosis (He et al., 1998; Bien et al., 2002; 2005). Activated CD4+ T cells may also prime B cells to produce autoantibodies. The resulting autoantibodies may destroy neurons, either directly by excessive stimulation of receptor-mediated ion channels or indirectly by binding complement factors and leading to the formation of the MAC (Bien et al., 2002;2007) which can induce neuronal loss and seizures (Xiong et al., 2003). Epileptic activity may induce inflammatory mediators in microglia, astrocytes, neurons, and endothelial cells and may alter the properties and permeability of the BBB, thus facilitating the entry of components of the adaptive immune system and molecules usually excluded from the brain parenchyma. These phenomena may consolidate and perpetuate inflammatory reactions in the brain of an affected individual and exacerbate brain damage, thus contributing to brain atrophy. It is still unknown which mechanism ultimately leads to the autoimmune process: viral infection (Xiong et al., 2003), head trauma, or even seizures per se; knowledge of the factors that precipitate the disease can enable prevention of the future development of chronic epilepsy. These recent findings recall attention to the possibility that a viral antigen may act as the initiating event in the complex pathogenetic mechanism leading to brain damage in RE. A cytotoxic T-cell response is in fact compatible with a viral infection, and a viral infection could explain the peculiar hemispheric distribution with centrifugal expansion observed in RE. Previous studies failed to conclusively link a specific virus to RE, but this of course does not rule out the possible role of an unknown virus.

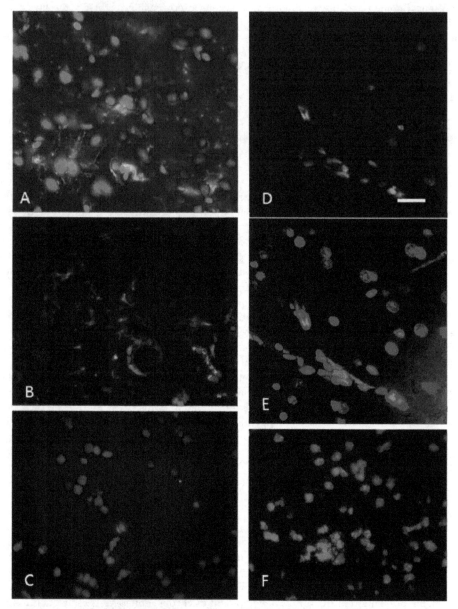

Fig. 3. Photomicrographs of activated microglia (HLA-Dr positive cells, green), A) nodules of microglia in Rasmussen syndrome, B) cortical dysplasia. Cytotoxic T lymphocytes (CD8 +, green) in dysplasia and TLE in (F). Coexpression in capillary of P-glycoprotein (green) and Cox-2 (red) in D and E in Rasmussen syndrome. (scale bar 20 μm D-F)

4.5 West syndrome (WS)

WS is an age-related epileptic encephalopathy with onset in the first year of life, featuring clustered spasms and hypsarrhythmia. It may occur in previously healthy children (cryptogenic WS) but more frequently is a symptom of different congenital or acquired diseases (symptomatic WS). Regardless of the etiology, WS patients benefit most from steroid treatment. Steroid efficacy, together with the possibility of spasm disappearance after viral infections (Hattori, 2001), has long been considered an index for an inflammatory or immune-mediated pathogenesis. A recent report (You et al., 2009). of increased serum levels of IL-2, TNF-*a*, and IFN-*a* in both cryptogenic and symptomatic WS reinforce this hypothesis. These cytokines are produced by monocytes and lymphocytes, and TNF-*a* is also produced by brain glial cells; all three have effects that may contribute to seizures and neuronal cell damage (Brunson et al., 1991). The presence of proinflammatory molecules in both cryptogenic and symptomatic WS patients suggests that cytokine changes are likely to be related to epilepsy rather than to the underlying etiology. However, symptomatic patients displayed a greater elevation of IL-2 levels, which varied depending on the underlying disorder (Prasad et al., 1996). If the extent of the inflammatory reaction depends also on the underlying disease, this could partly explain the different efficacies of steroid treatment in selected etiologic subgroups of symptomatic WS patients. For example, treatment with steroids and adrenocorticotropic hormone ACTH prevents patients with SW from developing Lenox-Gastau (Klein & Livingston, 1950). However, the mechanism underlying the anticonvulsant action of corticosteroids or ACTH remains elusive. Observations from animal models suggest that ACTH acts to repress infantile spasms by suppressing the level of endogenous corticotrophin releasing hormone (CRH) because stress receptors are located in areas of the brain known to be involved in seizure generation (Klein, 1950). It is postulated that the stimulation of synthesis of glucocorticoids that interact with CNS steroid receptors, which then influence voltage-dependent calcium channels, stimulates neurosteroid synthesis in glia and neurons that modulate GABAA receptors, down-regulating CRH, which has pro-convulsant activity in the immature brain, and immunomodulation (Joels, 1991)

4.6 Febrile seizures (FS)

FS are the most common cause of seizures in children, affecting 2 to 5% of children. The threshold to febrile seizures is dependent on body temperature, but the threshold varies with individuals and according to age and maturation (Millichap, 1959). A genetic susceptibility to inflammation may influence the threshold convulsive temperature. Seventeen to 30% of febrile seizure patients have a family history of febrile seizures (Millichap, 1959). A biallelic polymorphism in the promoter region of IL-1 at β the -511 position that can increase IL-1 β production occurs more frequently in patients with prolonged febrile convulsions (Virta et al., 2002; Kanemoto et al., 2003). In experimental animals, intraventricular injection of IL-1 β reduce the seizure threshold in 14-day old mice subjected to hyperthermia, while IL-1receptor knock-out mice have higher seizure thresholds, supporting the role of proinflammatory cytokines in triggering febrile seizures (Dubé et al., 2005)

Viruses are being increasingly implicated as causative agents of febrile seizures. Neurotropic viruses, such as the herpesviruses and influenza A, are commonly associated with febrile seizures in the United States and Asia (Hall et al., 1994; Chiu et al., 2001). Fever induced by viral infection is regulated by components of the immune response, particularly proinflammatory cytokines. Proinflammatory cytokines are higher in influenza-associated febrile seizures, further suggesting a causative role for cytokines in the pathogenesis of febrile seizures.

5. Anti-inflammatory treatments in epilepsy

Nearly 30% of epilepsy patients are refractory to conventional anti-epileptic drugs, and many alternative treatments have been tried to control epilepsy.(Prasad et al 1996). Immunotherapy, such as corticosteroids and ACTH, has been used to treat epilepsy since ACTH was first reported to have beneficial effects in the treatment of infantile spasms in 1950 (Klein, 1950 & Livingston,1950). For example there is no effective medical treatment for Rasmussen's encephalitis, except perhaps steroids,which can be useful when given early in the course of the disease(Bahi-Buisson et al., 2007), A long term follow-up of 11 Rasmussen's encephalitis patients who received steroids showed that 45% of patients had significant improvement of motor function and reduction of seizure frequency with disappearance of epilepsia partialis continua, while 55% patients had no benefit from steroid therapy and ultimately underwent hemispherotomy. Two initial responders to steroid treatment experienced progressive recurrence of seizures one to four years after the discontinuation of steroids and received a hemispherotomy. ACTH is a well-known effective treatment for infantile spasms that not only results in seizure control, but also improves both behavior and background EEG (Low, 1958). Meta-analysis reveals that ACTH is probably effective for short-term treatment of infantile spasms and leads to resolution of hypsarrhythmia (Mackay et al., 2004). Time to response is usually two weeks. Oral steroids can render 30 to 40% of patients seizure-free (Baram et al., 1996; Hrachovy et al., 1983). Further, early use of steroids is more effective; patients treated within one month of spasm onset had a better outcome than those treated after more than one month (Lombroso et al., 1983). The mechanism behind the anticonvulsant action of corticosteroids or ACTH remains elusive. Possibilities include (1) stimulation of glucocorticoid synthesis that interacts with CNS steroid receptors, which then influences voltage-dependent calcium channels; (2) stimulation of neurosteroid synthesis in glia and neurons that modulate GABAA receptors; (3) down-regulation of corticotrophin releasing hormone (CRH) that has proconvulsant activity in the immature brain; or (4) immunomodulation (Hrachovy et al.,1994; Baram et al., 1998; Reddy et al., 2000; Joëls, 2001).

On the other hand, various classes of specific anti-inflammatory drugs have been studied using models of status epilepticus or in kindling. The outcome measures were affected differently by inhibition of specific inflammatory pathways depending on the experimental model and the treatment schedule. For example non steroidal anti-inflammatory drugs (NSAIDs) NSAIDs act as inhibitors of constitutive COX-1 and inducible COX-2 enzymes. COX-2 selective inhibitors, such as celecoxib, parecoxib and SC58236, have been used to interfere with status epilepticus-induced epileptogenesis that was provoked either by electrical stimulation or systemic injection of pilocarpine in rats. These effects were observed under celecoxib treatment, thus a direct anticonvulsant action of this drug cannot be excluded.

Clinical phase	Drug/treatment	Animal models or Seizure type	Mechanism	References
Experimental (I)	Methanolic extract of *Asparagus pubescens*	PTZ-induced seizures	Inhibits inflammation and seizures	Nwafor et al., 2003
Experimental(I)	Aqueous and ethanolic extract of Solanum nigrum	Picrotoxin, pentylenetetrazole, and electroshocks induced seizures	Immunomodulatory activity	Jain et al, 2011., Ravi et al., 2009
Experimental(I)	Pralnacasan or VX-765	Kainic acid induced seizures	Interleukina converting enzyme/caspase 1 inhibitors and IL-1beta receptor antagonists	Vezzani et al., 2010
Experimental(I)	Naringin	kainic acid-induced status epilepticus in rats	Attenuated the TNF-α and malondialdehyde levels.	Golechha et al, 2011
Experimental(I)	Dexamethasone	Lithium and pilocarpine induced status epilepticus	IL-1 type 1 receptor antagonist and reduction in the number of circulating T-cells (CD3+)	Marchi et al, 2009
Experimental(I)	Naringin, a bioflavanoid	kainic acid (KA)-induced seizures	Antioxidant and anti-inflammatory activity.	Golechha et al., 2011
Experimental(I)	SC-58236, Celecoxib	electrically induced SE, Rat model of pharmacoresistant epilepsy	Selective inhibition of cyclooxygenase-2	Holtman et al., 2010, Schlichtiger et al, 2010
Experimental(I)	Minozac	Electroconvulsive shock	Suppression of proinflammatory cytokine	Somera-Molina et al., 2009; Chrzaszcz et al., 2010
Phase II/III	VX-765	Resistant partial epilepsy	ICE/caspase-1 blockade	Clinical trials gov.
In use	ACTH, prednisolone, and prednisone	Several epileptic syndromes	Antiinflammatory effects	Özkara Ç and Vigevano, 2011
In use	Dexamethasone, methylprednisolone and hydrocortisone	West, Landau-Kleffner or Lennox-Gastaut syndromes and Rasmussen encephalitis	Antiinflammatory effects and improvement of BBB integrity	Marchi et al., 2011
In use	Vigabatrin /and ACTH	Infantile spasms	Interfere with the cellular immune response	Ibrahim et al., 2010

Table 1. Immunotherapy treatments in epilepsy

Daily celecoxib treatment, starting 24 h post-status epilepticus for 42 days, resulted in reduction in the number and frequency of video-monitored spontaneous seizures (Jung, 2006). Other COX-2 inhibitors including nimesulide and rofecoxib, nonselective COX inhibitors such as paracetamol, naproxen, ibuprofen,mefenamic acid and indomethacin, and one selective COX-1 inhibitor SC560, have been tested in the kindling model of epileptogenesis, induced either by repetitive PTZ injections or by electrical stimulation. A significant delay in stage 5 seizure acquisition (i.e. delay in kindling development) was shown in NSAIDs-treated animals, with the exception of ibuprofen, which was found to be ineffective (Tanaka et al., 2009).

Three classical immunosuppressant agents have been used, namely cyclosporine A, FK-506 also known as Tacrolimus, and rapamycin. Their mechanisms of action include inhibition of T lymphocyte activation, although rapamycin alters multiple cellular functions by inhibiting mTOR kinase. Daily systemic injection of cyclosporine A or FK-506 during electrical amygdala kindling prevented the acquisition of stage 5 seizures in rats (Moia et al., 1994). Similar effects of FK-506 were shown in PTZ mkindling in mice(Singh, 2003). However, after drug withdrawal, stimulated animals showed stage 5 seizures, indicating that the treatments failed to inhibit epileptogenesis while providing anticonvulsant effects (Moia et al., 1994). Opposite effects were reported by Suzuki et al. (2001), showing acceleration of PTZ kindling in rats treated with FK-506. The pretreatment with VID-82925" kinase inhibitor molecule in 4-AP induced seizures model which revealed antiepileptogenic effect and it significantly suppressed the manifestation of epileptiform activity and was also effective against ictogenesis during the stable phase of focus (Gajda et al., 2011). Overall, these data indicate that the efficacy of immunosuppressant in kindling epileptogenesis is still controversial and requires further investigation, possibly using similar treatment protocols in the same kindling models. More consistent data are obtained in models of status epilepticus-induced epileptogenesis where T-cells do not appear to play a major role. Future studies are needed to target specific molecules involved in some of the pathways of the inflammatory process and to reduce adverse effects.

6. Concluding remarks

Accumulating evidence suggests that inflammatory and immune reactions may play an important role in promoting increased neuronal excitability, decreasing seizure threshold and is likely to be involved in the molecular, structural and synaptic changes characterizing epileptogenesis. Also, brain inflammation may contribute to the intractability of seizures and comorbidity in chronic epilepsy patients. Histologic analysis of the human brain from individuals with epilepsy of various etiologies strongly suggests the existence of a chronic inflammatory state in the brain almost invariably associated with neuronal loss, reactive gliosis, and activation of microglia. This observation, together with reports that anti-inflammatory drugs have anticonvulsant efficacy in some cases of drug-refractory epilepsies, suggests the possibility that chronic inflammation in the brain may be implicated in the etiopathogenesis of seizures and the associated long-term events. This hypothesis is supported by functional studies in experimental models of seizures, showing that some proinflammatory molecules exacerbate seizures, decrease the threshold for inducing convulsions, or cause seizures, per se.

Anti-inflammatory therapy may be particularly helpful when given during the latency period shortly after the initial neurologic insult, but prior to the onset of epilepsy, before permanent changes can occur in the neuronal aggregates that promote hyperexcitability and seizure spread. It is necessary to confirm with laboratory tests in serum and blood–cerebrospinal fluid to know the immune response of the epilepsy patient to give pharmacological therapy when the immune response is exacerbated. The causative role of inflammation in the pathogenesis of chronic intractable epilepsy needs to be established and requires further investigation from both the clinical and basic sciences. Pharmacological experiments in animal models suggest that antiepileptogenic effects might be achieved by interfering with specific pro-inflammatory pathways post-injury, although further studies are required to characterize the best targets and protocols for successful pharmacological intervention with limited side-effects.

7. Acknowledgment

This work was supported by National Council for Sciences and Technology grants (-52955-M and 98386) and Science and Technology Institute PIFUT -08/027

8. References

Alder MN, Rogozin IB, Iyer LM, Glazko GV, Cooper MD. & Pancer Z. (2005). Diversity and function of adaptive immune receptors in a jawless vertebrate. *Science*, 310,(5756), 1970-3. ISSN 0036-8075.

Aronica E, Boer K, van Vliet EA, Redeker S, Baayen JC, Spliet WG, van Rijen PC, Troost D, da Silva FH, Wadman WJ. & Gorter JA. (2007). Complement activation in experimental and human temporal lobe epilepsy. *Neurobiol Dis*, 26(3),497-511. ISSN 0969-9961.

Avignone E, Ulmann L, Levavasseur F, Rassendren F. & Audinat E. (2008). Status epilepticus induces a particular microglial activation state characterized by enhanced purinergic signaling. *J Neurosci*, 28(37), 9133–44. ISSN 0270-6474.

Bahi-Buisson N, Villanueva V, Bulteau C, Delalande O, Dulac O, Chiron C. & Nabbout R .(2007). Long term response to steroid therapy in Rasmussen encephalitis. *Seizure*, 1, 485-92. ISSN:1059-1311

Baram TZ, Mitchell WG, Tournay A, Snead OC, Hanson RA. & Horton EJ. (1996). High-dose corticotropin (ACTH) versus prednisone for infantile spasms a prospective, randomized, blinded study. *Pediatrics*, 97,375-9. ISSN 0031-4005.

Baram TZ. & Hatalski CG. (1998). Neuropeptide-mediated excitability: a key triggering mechanism for seizure generation in the developing brain. *Trends Neurosci*, 21, 471-6. ISSN 0166-2236.

Bauer J, Bien CG. & Lassmann H. (2002). Rasmussen's encephalitis a role for autoimmune cytotoxic T lymphocytes. *Curr Opin Neurol*, 15(2), 197–200. ISSN, 1350-7540.

Bauer J, Elger CE, Hans VH, Schramm J, Urbach H, Lassmann H. & Bien CG. (2007). Astrocytes are a specific immunological target in Rasmussen's encephalitis. *Ann Neurol*, 62,67–80. ISSN 0364-5134.

Bauer S, Cepok S, Todorova-Rudolph A, Nowak M, Koller M, Lorenz R, Oertel WH, Rosenow F, Hemmer B.& Hamer HM.(2009). Etiology and site of temporal lobe epilepsy influence postictal cytokine release. *Epilepsy Res*, 86, 82-88. ISSN 0920-1211

Beutler B. (2004). Innate immunity: an overview. *Mol Immunol,* 40(12), 845-59. ISSN 0161-5890.

Bezzi P, Carmignoto G, Pasti L, Vesce S, Rossi D, Rizzini BL, Pozzan T. &. Volterra A. (1998). Prostaglandins stimulate calcium-dependent glutamate release in astrocytes. *Nature,* 391,281–285. ISSN 0028-0836.

Bien CG, Bauer J, Deckwerth TL, Wiendl H., Wiestler OD, Schramm J, Elger CE. & Lassmann H. (2002). Destruction of neurons by cytotoxic T cells: a new pathogenic mechanism in Rasmussen's encephalitis. *Ann Neurol,* 51(3), 311–18. ISSN 0364-5134.

Bien CG, Granata T, Antozzi C, Cross JH, Dulac O, Kurthen M, Lassmann H, Mantegazza R. Villemure JG, Spreafico R. & Elger CE. (2005). Pathogenesis, diagnosis and treatment of Rasmussen encephalitis: a European consensus statement. *Brain,* 128(Pt 3), 454–471. ISSN 0006-8950

Bien CG, Urbach H, Schramm J, Soeder BM, Becker AJ, Voltz R, Vincent A. & Elger CE. (2007). Limbic encephalitis as a precipitating even in adult-onset temporal lobe epilepsy. *Neurology,* 69(12), 1236–44. ISSN 0028-3878.

Brunson KL, Khan N, Eghbal-Ahmadi M. & Baram TZ. (2001). Corticotropin (ACTH) acts directly on amygdala neurons to down regulate corticotropin-releasing hormone gene expression. *Ann Neurol,* 49(3), 304–12. ISSN 0364-5134.

Bsibsi M, Ravid R, Gveric D. & van Noort JM. (2002). Broad expression of Toll-like receptors in the human central nervous system. *J Neuropathol Exp Neurol,* 61(11), 1013–21. ISSN 0022-3069.

Cabaniols JP, Fazilleau N, Casrouge A, Kourilsky P, Kanellopoulos JM. (2001). Most alpha/beta T cell receptor diversity is due to terminal deoxynucleotidyl transferase. *J Exp Med,* 194(9), 1385–1390. ISSN 0022-1007

Carson MJ, Doose JM, Melchior B, Schmid CD. & Ploix CC. (2006). CNS immune privilege: hiding in plain sight. *Immunol Rev,* 213, 48–65. ISSN 0105-2896.

Chiu SS, Tse CY, Lau YL. & Peiris M. (2001). Influenza A infection is an important cause of febrile seizures. *Pediatrics,* 108(4), E63. ISSN 0031-4005.

Chrzaszcz M, Venkatesan C, Dragisic T, Watterson DM, & Wainwright MS. (2010).Minozac treatment prevents increased seizure susceptibility in a mouse "two-hit" model of closed skull traumatic brain injury and electroconvulsive shock-induced seizures. *J Neurotrauma,* 27(7), 1283-95.ISSN 0897-7151.

ClinicalTrials.gov. (2010). Study of VX-765 in subjects with treatmentresistant partial epilepsy. Available at http://clinicaltrials.gov/ct2/ show/NCT01048255.

Condie RM, Zak SJ. & Good RA. (1995). Effect of meningococcal endotoxin on the immune response. *Proc Soc Exp Biol Med,* 90(2), 355-60. ISSN 0037-9727.

Crespel A,Coubes P,Rousset MC, Brana C, Rougier A,Rondouin G,Bockaert J,Baldy-Moulinier M. & Lerner-Natoli M. (2002). Inflammatory reactions in human medial temporal lobe epilepsy with hippocampal sclerosis. *Brain Res,* 952(2), 159–69. ISSN 0006-8993.

Davis MM, Bjorkman PJ. (1988). T-cell antigen receptor genes and T-cell recognition. *Nature,* 334(6181), 395–402.ISSN 0028-0836

De Simoni MG, Perego C, Ravizza T, Moneta D, Conti M, Marchesi F, De Luigi A, Garattini S &Vezzani A. (2000). Inflammatory cytokines and related genes are induced in the rat hippocampus by limbic status epilepticus. *Eur J Neurosci,* 12(7), 2623-33. ISNN 0953-816X.

Dinarello CA. (2000). Proinflammatory cytokines. *Chest,* 118(2), 503–8. ISSN 0012-3692.

Dubé C, Vezzani A, Behrens M, Bartfai T. & Baram TZ. (2005). Interleukin-1beta contributes to the generation of experimental febrile seizures. *Ann Neurol,* 57(1), 152-5. ISSN 0364-5134.

Engel J Jr. (2004). Models of focal epilepsy. *Suppl Clin Neurophysiol,* 57, 392-9. ISSN 1567-424X.

Gahring LC, White HS, Skradski SL, Carlson NG. & Rogers SW. (1997). Interleukin-1alpha in the brain is induced by audiogenic seizure. *Neurobiol Dis,* 3(4), 263–9. ISSN 0969-9961.

Gahring L, Carlson NG, Meyer EL. & Rogers SW. (2001). Granzyme B proteolysis of a neuronal glutamate receptor generates an autoantigen and is modulated by glycosylation. *J Immunol,* 166(3), 1433–8. ISSN 0022-1767.

Gajda Z, Török R, Horváth Z, Szántai-Kis C, Orfi L, Kéri G, & Szente M.(2011). Protein kinase inhibitor as a potential candidate for epilepsy treatment. *Epilepsia,* 52(3), 579-588. ISSN0013-9580

Gasque P, Singhrao SK, Neal JW, Götze O. & Morgan BP. (1997). Expression of the receptor for complement C5a (CD88) is up-regulated on reactive astrocytes, microglia, and endothelial cells in the inflamed human central nervous system. *Am J Pathol,* 150(1), 31–41. ISSN 0002-9440.

Gellert, M. (2002). V(D)J recombination: RAG proteins, repair factors, and regulation. *Annu. Rev. Biochem,* 71, 101–132. ISSN 0066-4154.

Golechha M, Chaudhry U, Bhatia J, Saluja D, Arya DS. (2011).Naringin protects against kainic acid-induced status epilepticus in rats: evidence for an antioxidant, anti-inflammatory and neuroprotective intervention. *Biol Pharm Bull,* 34(3), 360-5. ISSN 0918-6158

Gorter JA, van Vliet EA, Aronica E, Breit T, Rauwerda H, Lopes da Silva FH. & Wadman WJ. (2006). Potential New Antiepileptogenic Targets Indicated by Microarray Analysis in a Rat Model for Temporal Lobe Epilepsy. *J Neurosci,* 26(43), 11083–110. ISSN 0270-6474.

Hall CB, Long CE, Schnabel KC, Caserta MT, McIntyre KM, Costanzo MA, Knott A, Dewhurst S, Insel RA. & Epstein LG. (1994). Human herpesvirus-6 infection in children. A prospective study of complications and reactivation. *N Engl J Med,* 331(7), 432-8. ISSN 0028-4793.

Han BW, Herrin BR, Cooper MD. & Wilson IA. (2008). Antigen recognition by variable lymphocyte receptors. *Science,* 321(5897), 1834-7. ISSN 0036-8075.

Hattori H. (2001). Spontaneous remission of spasms in West syndrome--implications of viral infection. *Brain Dev,* 23(7), 705–7. ISSN 0387-7604.

He XP, Patel M, Whitney KD, Janumpalli S, Tenner A. & McNamara JO. (1998). Glutamate receptor GluR3 antibodies and death of cortical cells. *Neuron,* 20(1), 153–63. ISSN 0896-6273.

Holtman L, van Vliet EA, Edelbroek PM, Aronica E, & Gorter JA. (2010).Cox-2 inhibition can lead to adverse effects in a rat model for temporal lobe epilepsy. *Epilepsy Res,* 2010; 91(1), 49-56. ISSN0920-1211

Hosokawa M, Klegeris A, Maguire J. & McGeer PL. (2003). Expression of complement messenger RNAs and proteins by human oligodendroglial cells. *Glia,* 42(4), 417–23. ISSN 089-1491.

Hrachovy RA, Frost JD Jr. & Glaze DG. (1994). High-dose, long-duration versus low-dose, short-duration corticotrophin therapy for infantile spasms. *J Pediatr*, 124(5 Pt 1),803-6. ISSN 0022-3476.

Hrachovy RA, Frost JD Jr., Kellaway P. & Zion TE. (1983). Double-blind study of ACTH vs prednisone therapy in infantile spasms. *J Pediatr*, 103(4), 641-5. ISSN 0022-3476.

Ibrahim S, Gulab S, Ishaque S, & Saleem T.(2010). Clinical profile and treatment of infantile spasms using vigabatrin and ACTH—a developing country perspective. *BMC Pediatr,*.10, 1,5-40.ISSN1471-2431-

Iwasaki A. & Medzhitov R. (2010). Regulation of adaptive immunity by the innate immune system. *Science*, 327(5963), 291-5. ISSN 0036-8075.

Jackson AC, Rossiter JP. & Lafon M. (2006). Expression of Toll-like receptor 3 in the human cerebellar cortex in rabies, herpes simplex encephalitis, and other neurological diseases. *J Neurovirol*, 12(3),229-34. ISSN, 1355-0284.

Jain R, Sharma A, Gupta S, Sarethy IP, & Gabrani R. (2011).Solanum nigrum: current perspectives on therapeutic properties. *Altern Med Rev*, 16(1),78-85. ISSN 10895159

Jankowsky JL. & Patterson PH. (2001). The role of cytokines and growth factors in seizures and their sequelae. *Prog Neurobiol*, 63(2), 125–49. ISSN 0301-0082.

Joëls M. (2001). Corticosteroid actions in the hippocampus. *J Neuroendocrinol*. 13(8),657-69. ISSN 0953-8194.

Jung H, K. Chu, S.T. Lee, J. Kim, D.I. Sinn, J.M. Kim, D.K. Park, J.J. Lee, S.U. Kim, M. Kim, S.K. Lee &. Roh J.(2006), Cyclooxygenase-2 inhibitor, celecoxib, inhibits the altered hippocampal neurogenesis with attenuation of spontaneous recurrent seizures following pilocarpine-induced status epilepticus. *Neurobiol Dis*, 23 237–246. ISSN0969-9961

Kanemoto K, Kawasaki J, Yuasa S, Kumaki T, Tomohiro O. & Kaji R. (2003). Increased frequency of interleukin-1beta-511T allele in patients with temporal lobe epilepsy, hippocampal sclerosis, and prolonged febrile convulsion. *Epilepsia*, 44, 796-9. ISSN0013-9580

Klein R. & Livingston S. (1950).The effect of adrenocorticotropic hormone in epilepsy. *J Pediatr*, 37, 733-42. ISSN0022-3476

Kubera M, Budziszewska B, Basta-Kaiml A, Zajicova A, Holan V. &Lasoń W.(2001).Immunoreactivity in kainate model of epilepsy. *Pol J Pharmacol*. 53(5), 541-5.

Letiembre M, Liu Y, Walter S, Hao W, Pfander T, Wrede A, Schulz-Schaeffer W. & Fassbender K. (2009).Screening of innate immune receptors in neurodegenerative diseases: a similar pattern. *Neurobiol Aging*, 30, 759–68. ISSN. 0197-4580

Lee CH, Hwang IK, Lee IS, Lee IS, Yoo KY, Choi JH, Lee BH. & Won MH. (2008).Differential immunoreactivity of microglial and astrocytic marker protein in the hippocampus of the seizure resistant and sensitive gerbils. *J Vet Med Sci*, 70(12), 1405–11 ISSN0916-7250

Li Z, Woo CJ, Iglesias-Ussel MD, Ronai D,&Scharff MD. (2004). The generation of antibody diversity through somatic hypermutation and class switch recombination. *Genes Dev*. 18(1),1-11. ISSN 0890-9369

Lieber MR. (1991). Site-specific recombination in the immune system. *FASEB J*, 5(14), 2934–2944.ISSN 0892-6638

Litman GW, Rast JP.& Fugmann SD. (2010).The origins of vertebrate adaptive immunity. *Nat Rev Immunol.*, 10(8), 543-53. ISSN 1474-1733

Lombroso CT. (1983). A prospective study of infantile spasms: clinical and therapeutic correlations. *Epilepsia*, 24, 135-58. ISSN0013-9580

Lorigados-Pedre L., Morales-Chacón L, Pavón-Fuentes N. Serrano-Sánchez T, Robinson-Agramonte MA, García-Navarro ME, & Bender-del Busto JE. (2004).Alteraciones inmunológicas en pacientes epilépticos asociadas a la localización del foco epileptogénico. *Rev neurol*, 39(2), 101-4. ISSN0210-0010 .

Low NL.(1958). Infantile spasms with mental retardation. II. Treatment with cortisone and adrenocorticotropin. *Pediatrics*, 22, 1165-9. ISSN0031-4005

Mackay MT, Weiss SK, Adams-Webber T, Ashwal S,Stephens D, Ballaban-Gill K, Baram TZ, Duchowny M, Hirtz D, Pellock JM, Shields WD, Shinnar S. & Wyllie E. (2004). Practice parameter: medical treatment of infantile spasms: report of theAmerican Academy of Neurology and the Child Neurology Society. *Neurology*, 62, 1668-81. ISSN0028-3878

MacLennan IC. (1994). Germinal centers. Ann Rev Immunol, 12, 117–139.ISSN 0732-0582

Maldonado M, BaybisM, NewmanD, Kolson DL, Chen W, McKhann G 2nd, Gutmann DH. & Crino PB.(2003). Expression of ICAM-1 TNF-alpha, NF kappa B, and MAP kinase in tubers of the tuberous sclerosis complex. *Neurobiol Dis*, 14(2), 279–90. ISSN0969-9961.

Marchi N, Granata T, Freri E, Ciusani E, Ragona F, Puvenna V, Teng Q, Alexopolous A, & Janigro D. (2011).Efficacy of anti-inflammatory therapy in a model of acute seizures and in a population of pediatric drug resistant epileptics. PLoS One, 6(3), 18200. ISSN-1932-6203

Mantegazza R, Bernasconi P, Baggi F, Spreafico R, Ragona F, Antozzi C, Bernardi G & Granata T (2002).Antibodies against GluR3 peptides are not specific for Rasmussen's encephalitis but are also present in epilepsy patients with severe, early onset disease and intractable seizures. J *Neuroimmunol*, 131(1-2), 179-85. ISSN 0165-5728.

Meador KJ,Loring DW, Ray PG, Helman SW, Vazquez BR. & Neveu PJ.(2004). Role of cerebral lateralization in control of immune processes in humans. *Ann Neurol*, 55, 840-844.ISSN 0364-5134

Miles JJ, Bulek AM, Cole DK, Gostick E, Schauenburg AJ, Dolton G, Venturi V, Davenport MP, Tan MP, Burrows SR, Wooldridge L, Price DA, Rizkallah P &, Sewell.(2010). Genetic and structural basis for selection of a ubiquitous T cell receptor deployed in Epstein-Barr virus infection. *PLoS Pathog*, 6(11), e1001198. ISSN 1553-7366

Millichap JG. (1959).Studies in febrile seizures. I. Height of body temperature as a measure of the febrile-seizure threshold. *Pediatrics*, 23 (1 Pt 1), 76-85. ISSN0031-4005.

Minami M, Kuraishi Y, Yamaguchi T, Nakai S, Hirai Y. & Satoh M. (1990). Convulsants induce interleukin-1 beta messenger RNA in rat brain. *Biochem Biophys Res Commun*, 171(2), 832–7. ISSN0006-291X

Minami M, Kuraishi Y, Satoh M. (1991). Effects of kainic acid on messenger RNA levels of IL-1 beta, IL-6, TNF alpha and LIF in the rat brain. *Biochem Biophys Res Commun*,. 176(2), 593–8. ISSN0006-291X

Mix E, Goertsches U, Zettl K. (2007). Immunology and neurology. *J Neurol*, 254, (Suppl 2). II/2–7. ISSN0340-5354

Moia, L.J. Matsui, Hde Barros, G.A. Tomizawa, K. Miyamoto K., Kuwata, Y. Tokuda, M.. Itano, T & Hatase O.(1994). Immunosuppressants and calcineurin inhibitors, cyclosporin A and FK506, reversibly inhibit epileptogenesis in amygdaloid kindled rat. *Brain Res*, 648, 337–341. ISSN 0006-8993

Nagawa F, Kishishita N, Shimizu K, Hirose S, Miyoshi M, Nezu J, Nishimura T, Nishizumi H, Takahashi Y, Hashimoto S, Takeuchi M, Miyajima A, Takemori T, Otsuka AJ. & Sakano H. (2007).Antigen-receptor genes of the agnathan lamprey are assembled by a process involving copy choice. *Nat Immunol*, 8(2), 206-13. ISSN 1529-2908

Neumann H, Medana IM, Bauer J. & Lassmann H. (2002).Cytotoxic T lymphocytes in autoimmune and degenerative CNS diseases. *Trends Neurosci*, 25(6), 313–9. ISSN 0166-2236

Nwafor PA, & Okwuasaba FK. (2003).Anti-nociceptive and anti-inflammatory effects of methanolic extract of Asparagus pubescens root in rodents. *J Ethnopharmacol*, 84(2-3),125-9. ISSN 0378-8741

Oby E. & Janigro D. (2006). The Blood–Brain Barrier and Epilepsy. *Epilepsia*, 47(11), 1761–74. ISSN 0013-9580

Okun E, Griffioen KJ, Lathia JD, Tang SC, Mattson MP. & Arumugam TV. (2009). Toll-like receptors in neurodegeneration. *Brain Res Rev*, 59, 278–92. ISSN 0165-0173

Oprica M, Eriksson C. & Schultzberg M. (2003).Inflammatory mechanisms associated with brain damage induced by kainic acid with special reference to the interleukin-1 system. *J Cell Mol Med*, 7(2), 127–40. ISSN 1582-1838.

Özkara Ç, & Vigevano F. (2011).Immuno- and antiinflammatory therapies in epileptic disorders. *Epilepsia*, 2011, 52 Suppl 3, 45-51. ISSN 0013-9580

Owens T, Bechmann I, Engelhardt B. (2008).Perivascular spaces and the two steps to neuroinflammation. *J Neuropathol Exp Neurol*, 67,1113–21. ISSN 0022-3069

Pacifici R, Paris L, Di Carlo S, Bacosi A, Pichini S. & Zuccaro P. (1995). Cytokine production in blood mononuclear cells from epileptic patients. *Epilepsia*, 36(4), 384–7. ISSN 0013-9580

Pardo CA, Vining EP, Guo L, Skolasky RL, Carson BS. & Freeman JM. (2004). The pathology of Rasmussen syndrome stages of cortical involvement and neuropathological studies in 45 hemispherectomies. *Epilepsia*, 45(5), 516–26. ISSN 0013-9580

Peltola J, Hurme M, Miettinen A. & Keränen T. (1998).Elevated levels of interleukin-6 may occur in cerebrospinal fluid from patients with recent epileptic seizures. *Epilepsy Res*, 31(2), 129–33. ISSN 0920-1211

Plata-Salamán CR, Ilyin SE, Turrin NP, Gayle D, Flynn MC, Romanovitch AE, Kelly ME, Bureau Y, Anisman H. & McIntyre DC. (2000). Kindling modulates the IL-1beta system, TNF-alpha, TGF-beta1, and neuropeptide mRNAs in specific brain regions. *Brain Res Mol Brain Res*, 75(2), 248–58. ISSN 0169-328X

Prasad AN, Stafstrom CF. & Holmes GL. (1996).Alternative epilepsy therapies : the ketogenic diet, immunoglobulins,and steroids. *Epilepsia*,37, Suppl 1, S81-95. ISSN 0013-9580

Rast JP, Anderson MK, Strong SJ, Luer C, Litman RT. & Litman GW.(1997).α, β, γ, and δ T cell antigen receptor genes arose early in vertebrate phylogeny. *Immunity*, 6 (1), 1-11. ISSN1074-7613

Ravi V, Saleem TSM, & Patel SS. (2009). Anti-inflammatory effect of methanolic extract of Solanum nigrum Linn berries. *Int J Appl Res Nat Prod*, 2,33-36. ISSN 1940-6223

Ravizza T, Boer K, Redeker S, Spliet WG, van Rijen PC, Troost D, Vezzani A. & Aronica E. (2006).The IL-1β system in epilepsy associated malformations of cortical development. *Neurobiol Dis*, 24, 128–43. ISSN 0969-9961

Ravizza T, Gagliardi B, Noé F, Boer K, Aronica E. & Vezzani A. (2008). Innate and adaptive immunity during epileptogenesis and spontaneous seizures: evidence from experimental models and human temporal lobe epilepsy. *Neurobiol Dis*, 29(1), 142-60. ISSN 0969-9961

Ravizza T, Balosso S. & Vezzani AM. (2011).Inflammation and prevention of epileptogenesis. *Neurosci lett*, 2011, 497, 223–230. ISSN 0304-3940

Reddy DS. & Rogawski MA. (2000).Enhanced anticonvulsant activity of ganaxolone after neurosteroid withdrawal in a rat model of catamenial epilepsy. *J Pharmacol Exp Ther*, 294, 909-15. ISSN 0022-3565

Rivest S, Lacroix S, Vallières L, Nadeau S, Zhang J. & Laflamme N. (2000).How the blood talks to the brain parenchyma and the paraventricular nucleus of the hypothalamus during systemic inflammatory and infectious stimuli. *Proc Soc Exp Biol Med*, 223(1), 22–38. ISSN 0037-9727

Robitaille Y. (1991).Neuropathologic aspects of chronic encephalitis. In: Andermann F Ed., Chronic encephalitis and epilepsy: Rasmussen`s syndrome. ISBN2-7420-0569-2, Boston:, Butterworth-Heinermann. Pp. 79-110.

Schlichtiger J, Pekcec A, Bartmann H, Winter P, Fuest C, Soerensen J, & Potschka H. (2010).Celecoxib treatment restores pharmacosensitivity in a rat model of pharmacoresistant epilepsy. *Br J Pharmacol*, 160(5), 1062-71. ISSN 0007-1188

Sheng JG, Boop FA, Mrak RE. & Griffin WS. (1994). Increased neuronal beta amyloid precursor protein expression in human temporal lobe epilepsy: association with interleukin-1 alpha immunoreactivity. *J Neurochem*, 63(5), 1872–9. ISSN 0022-3042.

Singh A., Kumar G., Naidu P.S. & Kulkarni S.K. (2003) Protective effect of FK506 (tacrolimus) in pentylenetetrazol-induced kindling in mice. *Pharmacol Biochem. Behav*, 75, 853–860. ISSN 0091-3057.

Sinhaa,S, ,Patil S, Jayalekshmyb V. & Satishchandraa P. (2008). Do cytokines have any role in epilepsy?. *Epilepsy Research*, 82, 171 − 176. ISSN 0920-1211.

Somera-Molina KC, Nair S, Van Eldik LJ, Watterson DM, & Wainwright MS.(2009). Enhanced microglial activation and proinflammatory cytokine upregulation are linked to increased susceptibility to seizures and neurologic injury in a 'two-hit' seizure model. *Brain Res*, 1282162-72. ISSN 0006-8993

Shortman K, Egerton M, Spangrude GJ, Scollay R. (1990). The generation and fate of thymocytes. *Semin Immunol*, 2(1),3–12. ISSN 1044-5323

Rozovsky I, Margan TE, Willoughby DA, Dugich-Djordjevich MM, Pasinetti GM, Johnson SA. & Finch CE.(1994). Selective expression of clusterin (SGP-2) and complement C1qB and C4 during responses to neurotoxins in vivo and in vitro. *Neuroscience*, 62(3), 741–58. ISSN 0306-4522

Stephens D, Ballaban-Gill K, et al.(2004). Practice parameter medical treatment of infantile spasms: report of theAmerican Academy of Neurology and the Child Neurology Society. *Neurology*, 62, 1668-81. ISSN 0028-3878

Suzuki K, Omura S., Ohashi Y., Kawai M., Iwata Y., Tani K., Sekine Y. Takei N. & Mori N (2001).FK506 facilitates chemical kindling induced by pentylenetetrazole in rats. *Epilepsy Res*, 46, 279–282. ISSN 0920-1211

Tanaka S, Nakamura, K. Sumitani F. Takahashi, R. Konishi, Itano T.& Miyamoto O. (2009). Stage and region-specific cyclooxygenase expression and effects of a selective COX-1 inhibitor in the mouse amygdala kindling model, *Neurosci Res*, 65, 79–87. ISSN 0077-7846

Tian L, Rauvala H.& Gahmberg CG. (2009). Neuronal regulation of immune responses in the central nervous system. *Trends Immunol*, 2009, 30, 91–9. ISSN 1471-4906

Tonegawa S. (1983).Somatic generation of antibody diversity. *Nature*, 302(5909), 575–81. ISSN 0028-0836

Tracey KJ.(2009). Reflex control of immunity. *Nat Rev Immunol*, 2009, 9(6), 418-28. ISSN 1474-1733

Turrin NP, Rivest S. Innate immune reaction in response to seizures: implications for the neuropathology associated with epilepsy. *Neurobiol Dis*, 2004, 16(2), 321–34. ISSN 0969-9961

Vezzani A. & Granata T. (2005).Brain inflammation in epilepsy: experimental and clinical evidence. *Epilepsia*, 46(11), 1724-43. ISSN 0013-9580

van Gassen KL, de Wit M, Koerkamp MJ, Rensen MG, van Rijen PC, Holstege FC, Lindhout D &de Graan PN (2008).Possible role of the innate immunity in temporal lobe epilepsy. *Epilepsia*, 49(6), 1055-65. ISSN 0013-9580

van Noort JM. (2007). Toll-like receptors as targets for inflammation,development and repair in the central nervous system. *Curr Opin Investig Drugs*, 8, 60–5. ISSN1472-4472

Vezzani A.(2008). Innate immunity and inflammation in temporal lobe epilepsy:new emphasis on the role of complement activation. *Epilepsy Currents*, 8(3), 75–7. ISSN 1535-7597

Vezzani A, Balosso S, Maroso M, Zardoni D, Noé F,& Ravizza T.(2010).ICE/caspase 1 inhibitors and IL-1beta receptor antagonists as potential therapeutics in epilepsy. *Curr Opin Investig Drugs*, 11(1),43-50. ISSN 1472-4472.

Visser L, Melief MJ, van Riel D, van Meurs M, Sick EA, Inamura S, Bajramovic JJ, Amor S, Hintzen RQ, Boven LA, 't Hart BA, & Laman JD. (2006).Phagocytes containing a disease-promoting Toll-like receptor/Nod ligand are present inthe brain during demyelinating disease in primates. *Am J Pathol*, 169, 1671–85. ISSN 0002-9440

Virta M, Hurme M. & Helminen M. (2002).Increased frequency of interleukin-1beta (-511) allele 2 in febrile seizures. *Pediatr Neurol*,26,192-5. ISSN 0887-8994

Weichhart,T. & Saemann M.D. (2009). The multiple facets of mTOR in immunity. *Trends Immunol*, 30, 218–226. ISSN 1471-4906

Weill JC, Reynaud CA. (1996). Rearrangement/hypermutation/gene conversion: When, where and why. *Immunol Today*, 17(2), 92–97. ISSN 0167-5699.

Xiong ZQ, Qian W, Suzuki K. & McNamara JO. (2003).Formation of complement membrane attack complex in mammalian cerebral cortex evokes seizures and neurodegeneration. *J Neurosci.* 23(9), 955–60 ISSN 0270-6474.

Yin L, Huseby E, Scott-Browne J, Rubtsova K, Pinilla C, Crawford F, Marrack P, Dai S. & Kappler JW. (2011).A single T cell receptor bound to major histocompatibility complex class I and class II glycoproteins reveals switchable TCR conformers. *Immunity*, 35(1), 23-33. ISSN 1074-7613.

You SJ, Kim HD. & Kang HC. (2009).Factors influencing the evolution of West syndrome to Lennox-Gastaut syndrome. *Pediatr Neurol*, 41(2), 111-3. ISSN 0887-8994

7

Plasma Exchange in Severe Attacks Associated with Neuromyelitis Optica Spectrum Disorder

Bonnan Mickael and Cabre Philippe

Service de Neurologie, Centre Hospitalier Universitaire Zobda Quitman, Fort-de-France,
French West Indies

1. Introduction

Neuromyelitis optica (NMO) is an inflammatory disorder restricted to the spinal cord and optic nerves. Contrary to multiple sclerosis (MS), relapses of NMO are often strikingly severe and most NMO patients present stepwise neurological impairments. NMO treatments are aimed to prevent the relapses with the administration of various promising immunosuppressive drugs. However, relapse treatment is still a tricky problem. Since the largely used steroid treatment usually fails to control severe attacks, specific add-on treatments have to be considered in order to limit the stepwise increase of residual impairment. Given that a strong humoral response characterizes NMO physiology, one might assume plasma exchange (PLEX) to be particularly well adapted in severe NMO relapses.

This chapter will analyze the relevant data of PLEX in the setting of NMO spectrum disorder. We will first outline the physiological grounds leading to the rationale of the PLEX treatment and the technical aspects of the procedure. Then we will assess the clinical results obtained in each type of attacks. Finally we will try to build an original concept linking the clinical results and the timing of PLEX onset with the dynamic of the inflammation inside the lesions.

2. Physiopathology of NMO

The physiopathology of demyelinating disorders is complex and may grossly be divided in two distinct parts: a cellular response implying lymphocytes, macrophages and granulocytes in NMO; and a humoral response involving many circulating components including antibodies, complement and cytokines which will be extravasated into the inflammatory sites where they will participate to the inflammatory cascade of events leading to the local lesion. We will briefly review the main physiopathological aspects of NMO and focus on the humoral response, which is especially suitable to be eliminated by PLEX upstream to the lesion.

2.1 Physiopathology of NMO lesions

2.1.1 Pathology

A characteristic pathological pattern has been described in NMO (Lucchinetti et al., 2002). Lesions are infiltrated by neutrophils and eosinophils and wall capillaries are hyalinized. A vasculocentric pattern of activated complement and immunoglobulin of IgG and IgM types is observed that mirrors the normal expression of AQP4. AQP4 expression is definitely reduced in normal appearing white matter and lost throughout the lesions. These modifications are the hallmark of NMO and could occur alone or associated with a wide range of lesions from mild demyelination to large necrosis. This pattern of lesion was classified in the pattern II of the Lassmann's classification of the inflammatory lesions (Lucchinetti et al., 2000, 2002).

Contrary to MS, T cells are rare in NMO lesions and probably had no major effect on the formation of the lesions (Saadoun et al., 2011). However T cells are probably involved upstream in physiopathological cascade in the earlier phases of the disease where a complex interplay leads to antigen sensitization and possibly in the initial opening of the blood-brain barrier (BBB) (Pohl et al., 2011).

2.1.2 Specific antibodies and their epitopes

The NMO-IgG antibody is an IgG1 directed against a surface epitope of the protein aquaporin-4 (AQP4) (Lennon et al., 2005). This antibody is detected with tissue-based immunofluorescence assays with a sensitivity and specificity for clinically defined NMO of more than respectively 60% and 90%. NMO-IgM theoretically coexits with NMO-IgG in about 10% of cases but significance is poorly known (Jarius et al., 2010a). Clinically diagnosed NMO patients share common clinical and evolutional characteristics according to the NMO-IgG status. Beyond the surrogate marker value of NMO-IgG, this marker is now used as a major diagnostic criterion (Wingerchuk et al., 2006) and delineates the *NMO spectrum disorders* that gather in a same entity both typical NMO and unusual or truncated clinical forms (Wingerchuk et al., 2007).

Astrocytes closely interact with endothelial cells to maintain the CNS BBB. These cells express AQP4 in the apical domain of the membrane feet expansions situated close to the surrounded blood vessels. They are generally found as single tetramers, closely arranged in orthogonal arrays. This transmembrane protein is critically involved in the homeostasis of the water in the brain and interfaces with blood vessels, especially in the clearance of free water. Loss of perivascular AQP4 in the basal state results in cellular swelling, ostensibly due to a failure to eliminate water generated from cellular metabolism (Amiry-Moghaddam et al., 2003). Thus in NMO, since the interaction of NMO-IgG and AQP4 leads to a functional knock-out phenotype of AQP4, edema develops as a result of functional impairment of AQP4 although BBB is expected to be still intact, which may explain the paradoxical lack of gadolinium enhancement in most NMO lesions. Apart from water homeostasis, the removal of AQP4 from astrocytes membrane is associated with an impaired homeostasis of glutamate via the loss of function of EAAT2, a major glutamate transporter associated with AQP4 in a macromolecular complex (Hinson et al., 2008). The disruption of glutamate homeostasis initiates an excitotoxic mechanism damaging oligodendrocytes and ultimately leading to demyelination (Marignier et al., 2010).

Virtually all the CNS astrocytes express AQP4, however some regions are enriched in AQP4. Those regions are the spinal cord gray matter, the posterior optic nerve, the floor of the fourth ventricle and the circum ventricular organs especially the area postrema, explaining the restriction of the sites of lesion characterizing NMO (Pittock et al., 2006a). Interestingly circumventricular organs are also the only sites of the CNS expressing fenestrated capillaries favoring local passive diffusion of circulating antibodies.

2.1.3 NMO-IgG and complement as key factors

Clinical activity may correlate with the underlying NMO-IgG titres. NMO-IgG detection is a strong predictor of recurrence after an initial spinal or optic attack (Jarius et al., 2008, 2010b; Weinshenker, et al 2006). In few patients, NMO-IgG was high during flares and became negative during the stabilized disease following treatment, and in contrary, an initially seronegative patient became positive during a further attack (Weinstock-Guttman et al., 2008). In the seminal work of Takahashi et al. (2007), NMO-IgG levels were positively correlated with both clinical severity (i.e. blindness) and radiological severity. Moreover a strong positive correlation was obtained between the NMO-IgG titres at the nadir of exacerbations and the spinal cord lesion length on MRI (Takahashi et al., 2007). In contrast, low NMO-IgG titres were observed during remission induced by immunosuppressive maintenance therapy (Jarius et al., 2008).

In vitro, the binding of NMO-IgG to the extracellular domain of AQP4 reversibly down-regulates its plasma expression. In the presence of active complement, this binding leads to strong complement activation and rapid cell destruction. NMO serum IgM is not AQP4-specific and abundant IgM deposits in the NMO lesions may have passively diffused after the BBB disruption by the seminal focal complement activation initiated by NMO-IgG (Hinson et al., 2007).

In an animal model of EAE with passive transfer of NMO-IgG, the transfer exacerbated EAE signs and the typical pathological characteristics were reproduced in treated rats (Kinoshita et al., 2009; Bradl et al., 2009). Direct injection of NMO-IgG in rat brains could reproduce the pathology but only when complement is coinjected (Saadoun et al., 2010)

The NMO-IgG ability to lesion AQP4-transfected cells in the presence of complement was assessed with serum drawn from patients with mild and severe attacks. The percentage of cells lesioned by complement was strongly higher in presence of sera from patients with severe attacks, although lesion induced by sera from patients with mild attacks did not differ from negative controls or MS patients (Hinson et al., 2009). Thus the severity of the disease may be partly determined by intrinsic NMO-IgG characteristics to activate the complement.

2.2 Proof of concept of PLEX in NMO

As we already described, NMO lesions are associated with a strong IgG, IgM and complement deposition, typical of the pattern II in Lassmann's classification. The NMO-IgG is involved in a complement-dependant toxicity against the astrocytes. All of these components -IgG, IgM, and complement- are targeted by plasma exchanges. By means of 5 exchanges, all the exchanged molecules will drop to less than 20% of their initial level. By this way, antibodies and complement, which are the core of the pattern II lesions, are excluded from the circulating pool and cannot migrate anymore to the lesions.

Although PLEX has long been used in various demyelinating disorders (Keegan et al., 2002), there is some clue that the pattern is a key determinant of PLEX efficiency. In a retrospective study, Keegan et al. (2005) reported that all the patients suffering from demyelinating disorders and improved by PLEX had a biopsy proven pattern II lesion. None of the patients with any other kind of lesion improved. However all these patients were MS without NMO-IgG and none were NMO (Keegan et al., 2005; Kale et al., 2009).

All the aforementioned findings stress that circulating NMO-IgG and complements are the two main actors of the NMO pathogeny and why clearing them from blood with PLEX should be appropriate for special benefits.

3. Plasma exchange procédure

3.1 Principles and goals

Basically, the goal of PLEX (or plasmapheresis) is to remove a given volume of patient's plasma containing harmful targeted substances and to reinfuse an artificial plasma substitute in its place -*the plasma exchange* (Brecher, 2002).

3.2 Technique

PLEX are carried on in a nephrology or a resuscitation ward. Two high flow rate accesses are mandatory: an input line from patient to device ('artery') and a return line from device to patient ('vein'). In continuous filtration, two needles are placed in both arms or groins in order to drawn out the blood of the body through an extracorporeal line connected to one needle, then blood is processed and reinfused continuously through the other needle. In case of discontinuous filtration, the separation and remixing are done in small batches through a single venous access in the groin where in and out cycles may alternate. Anticoagulation (citrate or heparin) is added to the blood pre-plasma filter to prevent from clotting. The removed blood is processed (*apheresis procedure*) in a cell separator that continuously separates plasma from cellular components (consisting of red and white blood cells and platelets) either by a centrifugation ring with permanent in and out flow, or by filtration through a porous membrane. Small molecules like cytokines as well as large molecules, such as albumin and immunoglobulin, are easily extruded from the blood compartment with a reported sieving coefficient >0.95 at a blood flow rate of 100 mL/min. The cleared cellular components are then combined with the replacement fluid (donor plasma or artificial albumin mixed with a saline solution) and returned to the patient through the needle in the other arm. A PLEX session is usually performed in 2 to 6 hours, depending on patient's height, weight, viscosity of the blood and technical parameters.

3.3 Kinetics of the target exchanged components.

All the targeted components are distributed in the interstitium (extra-vascular compartment) by variable part. Large molecular weight compounds equilibrate slowly between the vascular space and the interstitium. Calculations of the rate of removal are simplified to first order kinetics. The relation curve of the achieved concentration of a plasma component [C] after a unique exchange of a given plasma volume V is an exponential inverse: $[C] = [C_0].e^{-Y}$. The whole plasma volume can be approximated in an adult with the following formula:

Estimated plasma volume (liters)= 0.07 x weight (kg) x (1-hematocrit).

The larger volume of plasma exchanged during each session clears a larger amount targeted circulating component. An exchange of one body plasma volume leads to the immediate clearance of 50% of the circulating component. A 1.3 body mass volume exchange that removes about 72% of C is generally agreed. Beyond, the volume to process increases massively for too little gain. However, according to the distribution of C in the interstitium, the achievement of the clearance of C will necessitate the use of multiple PLEX sessions separated by the time necessary for the equilibration of C concentration between interstitium and vascular spaces. The number and frequency of sessions should be evaluated according to the biological characteristics of the components to remove (synthesis level, vascular distribution, diffusion ability). An empirically driven number of 4 to 6 sessions is usually scheduled. The durability of the immunomodulatory effect after PLEX is difficult to assess and will depend on the turnover rate of the targeted humoral components. Concomitant intensive immunosuppressive therapy (i.e. steroids, mitoxantrone, mycophenolate mofetil, rituximab) will be required to sustain the obtained depletive effect.

3.4 Risks and side effects

PLEX are contraindicated in case of ongoing infectious disease, precarious hemodynamics and active hemorrhage (heparin). Immediate side effects are related to the extracorporeal line: hemodynamic instability, vaso-vagal syndrome, numbness or tingling, venous puncture hazards with excessive local bleeding, septicemia or allergy. Since blood coagulation factors are all depleted by PLEX, hemostasis is affected in variable ways: first, a hypocoagulation state is immediately achieved by the global depletion of all the coagulation factors for half a day; at day 2, short life pro-coagulant factors are regained but antithrombin-III synthesis is delayed leading to a hypercoagulable state until day 3. Preventive anticoagulation with heparin is always required since the high risk of thrombosis. Persistently low fibrinogen levels have been described with the concomitant use of high dosage steroid infusion. In summary PLEX are generally well tolerated and now commonly and safely used.

4. PLEX in severe attacks

Various regimens of high doses of intravenous methylprednisolone are used in first line of treatment ranging from 3 g infused in 3 days, to 10 g in 5 to 10 days, depending on authors. There is no evidence in favor of one regimen or another and efficacy assessment has never been addressed. Moreover, even if steroids reduce the inflammatory cellular response by triggering apoptosis of lymphocytes, they are clearly not sufficient because poor outcomes are still a common issue even when steroid treatment is given immediately after onset. We wish to develop here the evidence for the effectiveness of PLEX that we have been largely using as an add-on therapy for more than 10 years.

Of note, steroids were always used to treat relapse. When used the same day as PLEX procedure, steroids were infused at the end of each PLEX session. However methylprednisolone pharmacokinetics is characterized by a short half-life and PLEX demonstrated to have no effect on steroids biodisponibility (Assogba et al., 1988; Stigelman et al, 1984).

4.1 Spinal attacks

PLEX proved to be efficient in central demyelinating diseases in a randomized sham-controlled study (Weinshenker et al., 1999, 2001). Keegan et al. (2002) reviewed the clinical data from 59 patients who received PLEX for inflammatory demyelinating diseases, including 10 NMO and 6 acute transverse myelitis (ATM) cases. A moderate or marked improvement was obtained in half of NMO and ATM patient groups. The late final outcome at one year was more or less obtained during the first month after treatment in both groups, without regard to success or failure of treatment (Keegan et al., 2002; Brunot et al., 2011). A small number of case reports and few small studies were reported with variable issues. Judging improvement is even more complex due to the subjective classification of improvement in mild/moderate/marked instead of a quantified clinical exam (Brunot et al., 2011; Keegan et al., 2002; Munemoto et al., 2011; Llufriu et al., 2009). Moreover the natural history of single spinal relapse in NMO has never been addressed, so any improvement bias after PLEX is inappreciable in the absence of a control group. Finally, most authors used PLEX as a rescue treatment given late after the onset. For example PLEX was delayed from onset by a mean of 33±30 days in Brunot et al. (2011) and a median of 30 days [6 to 90 days] in Llufiru et al. (2009).

Although a synergistic effect of steroids and PLEX was long expected due to their complementary action, none of these studies compared PLEX-treated attacks with conventional steroid treatment given alone with add-on PLEX-treated attacks.

We previously refined these results in a study of outcome after severe spinal attacks associated with NMO spectrum disorders (Bonnan et al., 2009a). We included 96 spinal attacks from 43 patients, divided in two groups: 1) a steroid-only group designed from historical patients treated with steroids alone; 2) an active group treated both with PLEX and steroids. Steroid infusion was started immediately after patient admission. PLEX decision was raised at the same time and started as soon as possible during the two days later. As a major difference with other groups, PLEX was never initiated as a delayed rescue treatment after a standard steroid treatment failure. Since PLEX therapy is mainly expected to minimize residual impairment, we used the ΔEDSS (calculated as the difference between residual and basal EDSS) as the main outcome.

If we except 5 PLEX delayed due to difficult medevac reasons, PLEX were initiated by a mean of 5.4 ± 3.1 days after attack onset with a median of 4 sessions.

There was no significant difference between the PLEX-treated and steroid-only groups for basal and acute EDSS (3.9 ± 2.9 vs 4.2 ± 2.9, and 7.9 ± 1.0 vs 8.0 ± 1.4; p=NS), however residual EDSS (5.1 ± 2.4 vs 6.8 ± 1.9, p<0.01) and mean ΔEDSS (1.2 ± 1.6 vs 2.6 ± 2.4, p<0.01) were significantly lower in the PLEX-treated group than in the steroid-only group.

Basal EDSS dramatically influenced therapy outcome as shown in Table 1. During the first attack, although acute EDSS were similar in both groups (7.6 ± 1.2 vs 7.1 ± 1.5, p=NS), ΔEDSS and residual EDSS were dramatically reduced in the PLEX-treated group (2.1 ± 1.9 vs 5.8 ± 2.0, p<0.01) given that acute EDSS was similar in this sub-group. In the two other sub-groups of basal impairment (EDSS 1.0 to 5.5 and EDSS ≥6.0), residual EDSS and ΔEDSS tended to be lower in PLEX-treated attacks but no statistical signification could be obtained due to the small size of these groups.

EDSS	St (n=17)	Basal EDSS null St+PLEX (n=7)	p	St (n=26)	Basal EDSS 1.0 to 5.5 St+PLEX (n=13)	p	St (n=24)	Basal EDSS ≥ 6.0 St+PLEX (n=9)	p
Basal	0	0	0.99	3.9±0.8	3.9±1.6	0.59	7.4±1.0	7.1±0.8	0.52
Acute	7.1±1.5	7.6±1.2	0.52	7.6±1.3	7.6±1.1	0.67	8.9±0.9	8.6±0.6	0.24
Residual	5.9±1.9)	2.1±1.9	<.01	5.8±1.6	5.1±1.1	0.21	8.5±1.1	7.6±1.0	0.05
ΔEDSS	5.9±1.9	2.1±1.9	<.01	2.0±1.5	1.2±1.6	0.10	1.1±0.8	0.5±0.8	0.11

Table 1. Disability measured as EDSS during spinal attacks stratified with basal impairment. St: steroid-only treated group; St+PLEX: steroid and PLEX-treated group. Values are given as mean±SD (from Bonnan et al., 2009a).

The classical Lazarus effect, defined as a very short-term dramatic improvement (Weinshenker et al., 2000), was rather unusual in our group but our study was not designed to analyse short-term improvement. The patients who experienced this effect have all received a very early treatment (less than 2 days). In Magana et al. (2011), patients who exhibited functional improvement did so within a median of 4 days (third PLEX), although a minority (6%) exhibited a delayed response (more than 2 months).

Minor side effects occurred in 24% of PLEX treated attacks and resulted in PLEX interruption once (84-year-old patient with pulmonary embolism).

In summary, PLEX-treated patients achieved a significantly better outcome after a spinal attack, especially if PLEX was given during the first attack. The exact effect of PLEX in previously impaired patients should be validated in a larger multicentric cohort. As PLEX proved to be a promising treatment in spinal attacks, it would now be unethical to design a study with a sham-treated control group.

Predictors of good outcome were studied in a large group of PLEX including 26 NMO patients (Bonnan et al., 2009a). The only good outcome predictor was normal or brisk reflexes in acute phase (Magana et al., 2011). Surprisingly a short PLEX delay was associated with a good outcome in a first study (Keegan et al., 2002) but had no effect in a second study, although one should remind that median PLEX delay (23 days) was delayed in this later compared to our group. The same PLEX response rate was obtained irrespective of NMO-IgG serostatus in our cohort and in the Mayo Clinic cohort (Magana et al., 2011).

As a practical consequence, faced with a patient suffering from a severe relapse, the knowledge of NMO-IgG status should not be required to start PLEX as soon as possible, since PLEX was found efficient in NMO-IgG negative patients.

4.2 Optic attacks

Visual impairment in NMO is very severe. We previously showed that an immediate unilateral blindness occurred in a third of patients after the first optic neuritis (ON), and generally two attacks are sufficient to cause a definitive loss of vision (Merle et al., 2007). Few PLEX were undertaken after ON and a quick dramatic recovery is usual as we also observed (Bonnan et al., 2009b; unpublished results). Depending authors, PLEX were used immediately (Bonnan et al., 2009b) or as a delayed add-on therapy (Schilling et al., 2006;

Watanabe et al., 2007a; Trebst et al., 2009; Yoshida et al., 2010). After pooling severe ON patients (acute visual acuity<1/10°) from available studies (Schilling et al., 2006; Ruprecht et al., 2004; Trebst et al., 2009) with ours (Bonnan et al., 2009b and unpublished results), data were gathered for 39 eyes. PLEX were given in median of 19 days in patients who recovered a visual acuity more than 1/10° (considered here as a treatment success) but 41 days in treatment failure. A clear effect of PLEX delay was observed since success rate was 8/8 (100%) during the first 11 days, than 4/7 (57%) from days 12 to 22, and 7/13 (53%) from days 23 to 73. Moreover, even when patients recovered, averaged residual VA tended to be lower in delayed PLEX patients (Figure 1).

Interestingly, the spontaneous recovery (>1/10°) after severe ON treated by steroids alone was about 40% in our cohort (from Merle et al., 2007), which is very close to the recovery obtained in the two last groups of late PLEX. In conclusion, strong clues support that PLEX change the outcome of severe ON only when they are given early, however broader studies are still lacking to confirm this hypothesis.

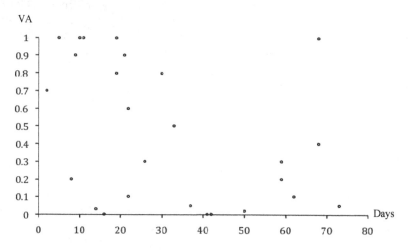

Fig. 1. Metanalysis of residual Visual Acuity as a function of PLEX delay (days) in severe ON attacks (acute VA<1/10°). See text.

4.3 Brain attacks

Apart from optico-spinal attacks, severe brain attacks are described in NMO, especially involving hypothalamus and medulla. Those lesions are usually severe and associated with blindness, central endocrine disorders or quadriplegia with respiratory failure. Brain lesions are common but are mostly asymptomatic (Pittock et al., 2006b). However symptomatic lesions involving supratentorial white matter are exceptional and extensive (Pittock et al., 2006b). Even if a favourable outcome after PLEX has been reported in a few severe cases (Viegas et al., 2009; Watanabe et al., 2009ab), comparative data are still lacking.

Posterior reversible encephalopathy syndrome (PRES) is an encephalopathy with consciousness and visual disturbances with rapidly reversible changes on MRI consistent with vasogenic edema. PRES are triggered by blood pressure instability or fluid stresses due to various causes. It seems to occur more often than coincidental in NMO patients: 5 out of 70 consecutive NMO-IgG patients evaluated at Mayo Clinic (Magana et al., 2009); 2 out of 5 in Hadassah Medical School, Israel (Eichel et al., 2008). Authors proposed that the auto-immune mediated disruption of the AQP4 water channel function may predisposes to PRES at comparable levels of acute illness (Magana et al., 2009). PLEX was involved as a trigger in one case with a good final outcome. In few cases, PLEX were implemented as curative treatment with an overall good outcome (Eichel et al., 2008; Magana et al., 2009).

5. Timing of PLEX: evolving to a key concept

Besides knowing PLEX are effective and safe, the central question remains: is PLEX necessary as-soon-as and as-often-as possible? Prospective, randomised, multi-centre clinical trials would be required to definitively answer the question. For most authors, to date PLEX are considered as an add-on rescue treatment after steroid failure. The European recommendation from EFNS is to start with an early steroid course no matter the severity (Sellner et al., 2010). Early escalation with PLEX is only recommended after a failure of a second course of steroids, that is to say that PLEX initiation may be postponed for more than a week. As we demonstrated before, PLEX efficiency is depends on the timing of initiation, ranging from immediate dramatic improvement (the *Lazarus effect*) to no effect according to whether they are given early or very late. We propose to regress to the dynamic of the inflammatory NMO lesions to explain why PLEX efficiency is strongly dependant of the timing of their onset.

5.1 Evidence for reversible dysfunction preceding irreversible tissue loss.

As we described above, the lesion is the consequence of a cascade of reversible events, susceptible to an external action. One could abruptly divide this cascade in two main points: a direct toxic action upon astrocytes and a bystander effect on oligodendrocytes and axons. Astrocyte dysfunction is initiated by the binding of NMO-IgG to the extracellular domain of AQP4 on the foot of the astrocyte membrane. In vitro, this binding reversibly down-regulates AQP4 plasma expression. The presence of fresh complement leads to a strong complement activation and a rapid cell destruction. IgG titres strongly correlates with the cytotoxic effect (Kalluri et al., 2010). By the other way, the removal of AQP4 from astrocytes membrane, due to internalization or cell death, impairs the clearance of free glutamate due to the dysfunction of the transporter EAAT2. The glutamate progressively accumulates and initiates an excito-toxic mechanism upon oligodendrocytes, ultimately leading to demyelination (Marignier et al., 2010).

The time sequence of these events was studied in lesions induced by direct mouse brain injection with NMO-IgG and complement (Saadoun et al., 2010). Loss of AQP4 and GFAP, and myelin breakdown were evident 7h following the injection. The inflammatory cells infiltration became evident later. Within 12h, axonal injury became prominent. By day 7, axonal loss and dying neurons were evident. Finally, one could suppose that a very early intervention targeting astrocytes dysfunction may prevent the progression to the bystander effect.

5.2 Evidence supporting an early treatment

The influence of treatment delay upon outcome has been addressed in a single study of first ON receiving steroid treatments (Nakamura et al., 2010). The outcomes were both visual acuity and the width of the retinal fibers layer evaluated with optic tomography (OCT). Patients were divided into two groups: one group with a good visual outcome, including a high residual visual acuity and high RFL; and a second group with a poor visual outcome in terms of low acuity and low RFL. Very interestingly, the two groups were similar in all the parameters except one: patients with a good outcome received steroids with a lower mean delay after ON onset, by a mean of 1.8±1.1 days compared to 7.8±3.8 in patients with a poor outcome. This study is the first proof that a delayed infusion of steroids is associated with a poorer outcome. A similar effect of treatment delay, although unknown, should be expected in spinal attacks. Even if no proof is yet available after a PLEX treatment, these clues could be gathered that early PLEX would improve the prognosis (see above).

In spinal attacks treated with PLEX, early initiation of treatment was one out of the predictors of good outcome (Keegan et al., 2002). In a larger study encompassing attacks from various demyelinating disorders, success rates were stratified by delay: improvement occurred in 83% when given before day 15, but fell to 43 after 2 months (Llufriu et al., 2009). Moreover the dramatically very short-term improvement, called Lazarus effect (Weinshenker et al., 2000), is sometimes observed after severe attacks receiving a very early treatment with PLEX and steroids. However, this earliness responsibility on the Lazarus effect remains elusive since no study is available on this rather unusual effect.

5.3 Lesion stages and PLEX action: 'time is cord and eyes'

In the light of the available data, we postulate a link between the staging of NMO lesion and the PLEX effect upon clinical and radiological outcome (Figure 2).

Stage 1 (first hours): acute attack provokes for hours an astrocyte dysfunction (by NMO-IgG binding on AQP4 leading to internalization) mainly expressed by an edema. This purely edematous lesion could be immediately reversible by the clearance of NMO-IgG preventing the loss of astrocytes and the excitotoxic cascade. Clinical and radiological recovery after PLEX is dramatic and explains the Lazarus effect. **Stage 2 (days):** the loss of EAAT2 induces an excitotoxic effect of glutamate on oligodendrocytes leading progressively to demyelination and axonal loss. Astrocytes loss initiates a self-sustained excitotoxic process henceforth independent from NMO-IgG persistence. Even if the extraction of NMO-IgG and complement by PLEX ends the astrocytes aggression. A variable amount of them has been already lost and excitotoxic effects upon oligodendrocytes are evident. Variable amount of tissue is lost as visible on MRI and recovery is incomplete. **Stage 3 (weeks):** atrocytes, oligodendrocytes and axonal loss is prominent, engulfed in large areas of necrosis. PLEX is almost useless. Neural tissue remains cavitated or atrophic on MRI and no recovery will be expected.

We propose to reconsider PLEX as a major part of the treatment of severe NMO attacks and suggest that PLEX could be given systematically in severe relapses of NMO, extended transverse myelitis or bilateral severe ON resistant to steroids. Moreover, when given they should be started as soon as possible with steroids.

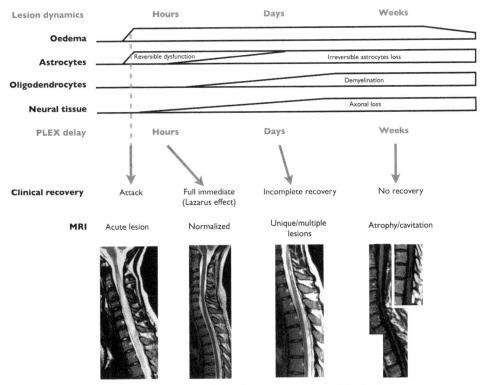

Fig. 2. Putative PLEX effect depending of the three main stages of the lesion.

6. PLEX as preventive treatment

Since NMO-IgG positivity is both predictive of attacks and severity, achieving a low concentration of plasmatic antibodies remains a goal to achieve. Besides immunosuppressive drugs, PLEX have been used to achieve a sustained depletion of NMO-IgG and complement. Favourable cases have been reported but studies are lacking (Miyamoto et al., 2009). Miyamoto et al. (2009) proposed to use PLEX as preventive treatment as an add-on therapy after immunosuppressive drugs failure.

7. Preventive treatments and future avenues

The natural history of NMO leads all the patients to a deep impairment in a stepwise fashion without progressive phase. In our study, 5 years after the onset, 70% of patients suffered from a unilateral loss of vision and almost half of them from a bilateral loss of vision (Merle et al., 2007). After 8 years, half of the patients had suffered from a severe myelitis and become chair-bound (Cabrera-Gomez et al., 2009). The mortality rate was very high before immunosuppressive drugs but dropped since they are largely used (Cabre et al., 2009). The exact role of recurring PLEX along the remaining attacks to tune the outcome to a low impairment has not yet been addressed but remains most probable considering this striking epidemiological change of mortality in French West Indies.

7.1 Immunosuppressive maintenance

Contrary to MS, cumulative evidence accumulates that interferon beta had no effect on activity rate and worsens some patients, especially in lupus-associated NMO (Uzawa et al., 2010). When IFN is compared to immunosuppressive drugs, a dramatic reduction of annualized relapse rate (ARR) is obtained (Papeix et al., 2007). Rituximab and mycophenolate mofetil were well tolerated and dramatically reduced ARR (Jacob et al., 2008; Jacob et al., 2009). A favorable action of mitoxantrone was reported in few cases (Weinstock-Guttman et al., 2006). In a group of 32 patients treated with mitoxantrone in our centre, a dramatic drop in ARR was obtained from a mean rate of 1.8 to 0.3 and sustained over 5 years (Cabre, personal communication). The choice in one these three drugs should mostly be driven by safety concerns since no comparative study or recommendation is readily available. Low dose steroids were reported to be effective in a few patients, however these data needs further studies with more patients. Various others treatments (cyclophosphamide, azathioprine, venous immuno-globulins) have been used in isolated cases where no general conclusion could be drawn upon ARR action. However cyclophosphamide is commonly used to treat lupus in overlapping cases of NMO (Polgar et al., 2011).

7.2 New strategies for the future

Since the lesion severity mostly depends on the initial and definitive depth of the loss of AQP4 and astrocytes, future treatments strategies may be directed upon AQP4 preservation. Small molecules or monoclonal antibodies could be used to prevent NMO-IgG binding to AQP4 and to block the physiopathological cascade upstream (Verkman et al., 2011; Yu et al., 2011). Another strategy may deplete pathogenic antibodies by apheresis using dedicated immunoadsorption systems as previously described in myasthenia gravis (Zisimopoulou et al., 2008) and in various extra neurological disorders. However the value of this technique is less clear in disorders like MS (De Andres et al., 2000; Moldenhauer et al., 2005) where pathology is broader than a specific antibody. No experience is yet available in the NMO setting. Lymphocytapheresis was successfully described in isolated cases of resistant attacks (Aguilera et al., 1984, Nozaki et al., 2006). A complementary approach may target the complement system with newly developed anti-complement recombinant antibodies at various levels, with preliminary promising results (Saadoun et al., 2010). Such future treatments may be aimed at preventing or curing the attacks. During attacks, neuroprotective treatments could be used to prevent the oligodendrocytes loss induced by the excitotoxic action of glutamate.

Animal models gave clues to dynamic mechanisms evolving over time and appear suitable to address the effect of those various early therapeutic interventions directed to halt or prevent ongoing lesions (Saadoun et al., 2010).

8. Conclusion

PLEX, in synergy with steroids, could be a major treatment of relapses, aimed at preventing cumulative disability. PLEX is a safe and efficient add-on therapy in NMO. Since PLEX proved to be effective regardless of NMO-IgG status, NMO-IgG status should not be required to initiate PLEX. These preliminary results suggest that PLEX may modify the short prognostic of NMO relapses. Immunosuppressive drugs are necessary to prevent further relapses but no recommendation is yet available.

Animal models have confirmed that mechanisms leading to lesion evolve over hours and days. Those models should be able to confirm that early therapeutic intervention directed to halt the ongoing lesions should be even more dramatic in an early narrow therapeutic window.

The next steps should be to concentrate upon large multicentric therapeutic trials in order to validate the therapeutic procedure. However we are aware that good trials against placebo could be difficult to accept since this is an extremely devastating disease. The take-away messages are: undertaking PLEX in severe relapses and the importance of starting treatment as soon as possible.

9. References

Aguilera AJ, Carlow TJ, Smith KJ & Simon TL. (1985). Lympho-cytaplasmapheresis in Devic's syndrome. *Transfusion*, Vol. 25, No. 1, pp. 54-6.

Amiry-Moghaddam M, Otsuka T, Hurn PD, Traystman RJ, Haug FM, Froehner SC, & al. (2003). An alpha-syntrophin-dependent pool of AQP4 in astroglial end-feet confers bidirectional water flow between blood and brain. *Proc Natl Acad Sci USA*, Vol.100, pp. 2106-11.

Assogba U, Baumelou A, Pecquinot MA, Raymond F, Durande JP, Lenoir G et al. (1988) Removal of prednisone and prednisolone during plasma exchange. *Ann Med Interne*, Vol. 139, pp. 38-9.

Bonnan M, Valentino R, Olindo S, Mehdaoui H, Smadja D & Cabre P. (2009). Plasma exchange in severe spinal attacks associated with neuromyelitis optica Spectrum disorder. *Mult Scler*, Vol.15, No. 4, pp. 487-92.

Bonnan M, Brasme H, Diaby MM, Vlaicu M, Le Guern V & Zuber M. (2009). Severe bouts of neuromyelitis optica: dramatic improvement after plasma exchanges. *Rev Neurol*, Vol.165, No. 5, pp. 479-81.

Bradl M, Misu T, Takahashi T, Watanabe M, Mader S, Reindl M, & al. (2009). Neuromyelitis optica: pathogenicity of patient immunoglobulin in vivo. *Ann Neurol*, Vol.66, No.5, pp. 630-43.

Brecher ME. Plasma exchange: why we do what we do. (2002). *J Clin Apher*, Vol.17, No.4, pp. 207-11.

Brunot S, Vukusic S, Fromont A, Couvreur G, Mousson C, Giroud M, Confavreux C & Moreau T. (2011). Plasma exchanges in severe and acute inflammatory demyelinating attacks of the central nervous system. *Presse Med*, Vol.40, No.5, pp. e271-8.

Cabre P, Gonzalez-Quevedo A, Lannuzel A, Bonnan M, Merle H, Olindo S, & al. (2009). Descriptive epidemiology of neuromyelitis optica in the Caribbean basin. *Rev Neurol*, Vol.165, pp. 676-83.

Cabrera-Gomez JA, Bonnan M, Gonzalez-Quevedo A, Saiz Hinajeros A, Marignier R, Graus F, & al. (2009). Neuromyelitis optica positive antibodies confer a worse course in relapsing-neuromyelitis optica in Cuba and French West Indies. *Mult Scler*, Vol.15, pp. 828-33.

de Andrès C, Anaya F & Gimenez-Rolden S. (2000). Plasma immunoadsorption treatment of malignant multiple sclerosis with severe and prolonged relapses. *Rev Neurol*. 2000, Vol.30, No.7, pp. 601-5.

Eichel R, Meiner Z, Abramsky O & Gotkine M. (2008). Acute disseminating encephalomyelitis in neuromyelitis optica: closing the floodgates. *Arch Neurol*, Vol.65, No.2, pp. 267-71.

Hinson SR, Pittock SJ, Lucchinetti CF, Roemer SF, Fryer JP, Kryzer TJ & Lennon VA. (2007). Pathogenic potential of IgG binding to water channel extracellular domain in neuromyelitis optica. *Neurology*, Vol.69, No.24, pp. 2221-31.

Hinson SR, Roemer SF, Lucchinetti CF, Fryer JP, Kryzer TJ, Chamberlain JL, Howe CL, Pittock SJ & Lennon VA. (2008). Aquaporin-4-binding autoantibodies in patients with neuromyelitis optica impair glutamate transport by down-regulating EAAT2. *J Exp Med*, Vol.205, No.11, pp. 2473-81.

Hinson SR, McKeon A, Fryer JP, Apiwattanakul M, Lennon VA & Pittock SJ. (2009). Prediction of neuromyelitis optica attack severity by quantitation of complement-mediated injury to aquaporin-4-expressing cells. *Arch Neurol*, Vol.66, pp. 1164-7.

Jacob A, Matiello M, Weinshenker BG, Wingerchuk DM, Lucchinetti C, Shuster E, Carter J, Keegan BM, Kantarci OH & Pittock SJ. (2009). Treatment of neuromyelitis optica with mycophenolate mofetil: retrospective analysis of 24 patients. *Arch Neurol*, Vol.66, No.9, pp. 1128-33.

Jacob A, Weinshenker BG, Violich I, McLinskey N, Krupp L, Fox RJ, Wingerchuk DM, Boggild M, Constantinescu CS, Miller A, De Angelis T, Matiello M & Cree BA. (2008). Treatment of neuromyelitis optica with rituximab: retrospective analysis of 25 patients. *Arch Neurol*, Vol.65, No.11, pp. 1443-8.

Jarius S, Aboul-Enein F, Waters P, Kuenz B, Hauser A, Berger T, Lang W, Reindl M, Vincent A & Kristoferitsch W. (2008). Antibody to aquaporin-4 in the long-term course of neuromyelitis optica. *Brain*, Vol.131, No.11, pp. 3072-80.

Jarius S, Franciotta D, Bergamaschi R, Wildemann B & Wandinger KP. (2010). Immunoglobulin M antibodies to aquaporin-4 in neuromyelitis optica and related disorders. *Clin Chem Lab Med*, Vol.48, No.5, pp. 659-63.

Jarius S, Frederikson J, Waters P, Paul F, Akman-Demir G, Marignier R, Franciotta D, Ruprecht K, Kuenz B, Rommer P, Kristoferitsch W, Wildemann B & Vincent A. (2010). Frequency and prognostic impact of antibodies to aquaporin-4 in patients with optic neuritis. *J Neurol Sci*, Vol.298, No. 1-2, pp. 158-62.

Kale N, Pittock SJ, Lennon VA, Thomsen K, Roemer S, McKeon A & Lucchinetti CF. (2009). Humoral pattern II multiple sclerosis pathology not associated with neuromyelitis Optica IgG. *Arch Neurol*, Vol.66, No.10, pp. 1298-9.

Kalluri SR, Illes Z, Srivastava R, Cree B, Menge T, Bennett JL, Berthele & Hemmer B. (2010). Quantification and functional characterization of antibodies to native aquaporin 4 in neuromyelitis optica. *Arch Neurol*, Vol.67, No.10, pp. 1201-8.

Keegan M, Pineda AA, McClelland RL, Darby CH, Rodriguez M & Weinshenker BG. (2002). Plasma exchange for severe attacks of CNS demyelination: predictors of response. *Neurology*, Vol.58, No.1, pp. 143-6.

Keegan M, Konig F, McClelland R, Bruck W, Morales Y, Bitsch A, Panitch H, Lassmann H, Weinshenker B, Rodriguez M, Parisi J & Lucchinetti CF. (2005). Relation between humoral pathological changes in multiple sclerosis and response to therapeutic plasma exchange. *Lancet*, Vol.366, No.9485, pp. 579-82.

Kinoshita M, Nakatsuji Y, Kimura T, Moriya M, Takata K, Okuno T, Kumanogoh A, Kajiyama K, Yoshikawa H & Sakoda S. (2009). Neuromyelitis optica: Passive transfer to rats by human immunoglobulin. *Biochem Biophys Res Commun*, Vol.386, No.4, pp. 623-7.

Lennon VA, Kryzer TJ, Pittock SJ, Verkman AS & Hinson SR. (2005). IgG marker of optic-spinal multiple sclerosis binds to the aquaporin-4 water channel. *J Exp Med*, Vol.202, No.4, pp. 473-7.

Llufriu S, Castillo J, Blanco Y, Ramio-Torrenta L, Rio J, Valles M, Lozano M & al. (2009). Plasma exchange for acute attacks of CNS demyelination: Predictors of improvement at 6 months. *Neurology*, Vol.73, pp. 949-53.

Lucchinetti CF, Mandler RN, McGavern D, Bruck W, Gleich G, Ransohoff RM, Trebst C, Weinshenker B, Wingerchuk D, Parisi JE & Lassmann H. (2002). A role for humoral mechanisms in the pathogenesis of Devic's neuromyelitis optica. Brain, Vol.125, No.7, pp. 1450-61.

Lucchinetti C, Brück W, Parisi J, Scheithauer B, Rodriguez M & Lassmann H. (2000). Heterogeneity of multiple sclerosis lesions: implications for the pathogenesis of demyelination. *Ann Neurol*, Vol.47, No.6, pp. 707-17.

Magana SM, Matiello M, Pittock SJ, McKeon A, Lennon VA, Rabinstein AA, Shuster E, Kantarci OH, Lucchinetti CF & Weinshenker BG. (2009). Posterior reversible encephalopathy syndrome in neuromyelitis optica spectrum disorders. *Neurology*, Vol.72, No.8, pp. 712-7.

Magana SM, Keegan BM, Weinshenker BG, Erickson BJ, Pittock SJ, Lennon VA & al. (2011). Beneficial plasma exchange response in central nervous system inflammatory demyelination. *Arch Neurol*, Vol.68, pp. 870-8.

Marignier R, Nicolle A, Watrin C, Touret M, Cavagna S, Varrin-Doyer M, Cavillon G, Rogemond V, Confavreux C, Honnorat J & Giraudon P. (2010). Oligodendrocytes are damaged by neuromyelitis optica immunoglobulin G via astrocyte injury. *Brain*, Vol.133, No.9, pp. 2578-91.

Merle H, Olindo S, Bonnan M, Donnio A, Richer R, Smadja D & Cabre P. (2007). Natural history of the visual impairment of relapsing neuromyelitis optica. *Ophthalmology*, Vol.114, No.4, pp. 810-5.

Miyamoto, K. & Kusunoki, S. (2009). Intermittent plasmapheresis prevents recurrence in neuromyelitis optica. *Ther Apher Dial*, Vol.13, pp. 505-8.

Moldenhauer A, Haas J, Wascher C, Derfuss T, Hoffmann KT, Kiesewetter H & Salama A. (2005). Immunoadsorption patients with multiple sclerosis: an open-label pilot study. *Eur J Clin Invest*, Vol.35, No.8, pp. 523-30.

Munemoto M, Otaki Y, Kasama S, Nanami M, Tokuyama M, Yahiro M, Hasuike Y, Kuragano T, Yoshikawa H, Nonoguchi H & Nakanishi T. (2011). Therapeutic efficacy of double filtration plasmapheresis in patients with anti-aquaporin-4 antibody-positive multiple sclerosis. *J Clin Neurosci*, Vol.18, No.4, pp. 478-80.

Nakamura M, Nakazawa T, Doi H, Hariya T, Omodaka K, Misu T, Takahashi T, Fujihara K & Nishida K. (2010). Early high-dose intravenous methylprednisolone is effective in preserving rétinal nerve fiber layer thickness in patients with neuromyelitis optica. *Graefes Arch Clin Exp Ophthalmol*, Vol.248, No.12, pp. 1777-85.

Nozaki I, Hamaguchi T, Komai K & Yamada M. (2006). Fulminant Devic disease successfully treated by lymphocytapheresis. *J Neurol Neurosurg Psychiatry*, Vol.77, No.9, pp. 1094-5.

Papeix C, Vidal JS, de Seze J, Pierrot-Deseilligny C, Tourbah A, Stankoff B, Lebrun C, Moreau T, Vermersch P, Fontaine B, Lyon-Caen O & Gout O. (2007). Immunosuppressive therapy is more effective than interferon in neuromyelitis optica. *Mult Scler*, Vol.13, No.2, pp. 256-9.

Pittock SJ, Weinshenker BG, Lucchinetti CF, Wingerchuk DM, Corboy JR & Lennon VA. (2006). Neuromyelitis optica brain lesions localized at sites of high aquaporin 4 expression. *Arch Neurol*, Vol.63, No.7, pp. 964-8.

Pittock SJ, Lennon VA, Krecke K, Wingerchuk DM, Lucchinetti CF & Weinshenker BG. (2006). Brain abnormalities in neuromyelitis optica. *Arch Neurol*, Vol.63, No.3, pp. 390-6.

Pohl M, Fischer MT, Mader S, Schanda K, Kitic M, Sharma R, Wimmer I, Misu T, Fujihara K, Reindl M, Lassmann H & Bradl M. (2011). Pathogenic T cell responses against aquaporin 4. *Acta Neuropathol*, Vol.122, No.1, pp. 21-34.

Polgar A, Rosa C, Muller V, Matolcsi J, Poor G & Kiss EV. (2011). Devic's syndrome and SLE: challenges in diagnosis and therapeutic possibilities based on two overlapping cases. *Autoimmun Rev*, Vol.10, No.3, pp. 171-4.

Ruprecht K, Klinker E, Dintelmann T, Rieckmann P & Gold R. (2004). Plasma exchange for severe optic neuritis: treatment of 10 patients. *Neurology*, Vol.63, No.6, pp. 1081-3.

Saadoun S., Waters P., Bell BA., Vincent A., Verkman AS. & Papadopoulos MC. (2010). Intra-cerebral injection of neuromyelitis optica immunoglobulin G and human complement produces neuromyelitis optica lesions in mice. *Brain*, Vol.133, pp. 349–61.

Saadoun S, Waters P, Macdonald C, Bridges LR, Bell BA, Vincent A & al. (2011). T cell deficiency does not reduce lesions in mice produced by intracerebral injection of NMO-IgG and complement. *J Neuroimmunol*, Vol.235, pp. 27-32.

Schilling S, Linker RA, Konig FB, Koziolek M, Bahr M, Muller GA & al. (2006). Plasma exchange therapy for steroid-unresponsive multiple sclerosis relapses: clinical experience with 16 patients. *Nervenarzt*, Vol.77, pp. 430-8.

Sellner J, Boggild M, Clanet M, Hintzen RQ, Illes Z, Montalban X, Du Pasquier RA, Polman CH, Sorensen PS & Hemmer B. (2010). EFNS guidelines on diagnosis and management of neuromyelitis optica. *Eur J Neurol*, Vol.17, No.8, pp. 1019-32.

Stigelman WH Jr, Henry DH, Talbert RL, (1984) Townsend RJ. Removal of prednisone and prednisolone by plasma exchange. *Clin Pharm*, Vol.3, pp. 402-7.

Takahashi T, Fujihara K, Nakashima I, Misu T, Miyazawa I, Nakamura M, Watanabe S, Shiga Y, Kanaoka C, Fujimori J, Sato S & Itoyama Y. (2007). Anti-aquaporin-4 antibody is involved in the pathogenesis of NMO: a study on antibody titre. *Brain*, Vol.130, No.5, pp. 1235-43.

Trebst C, Reising A, Kielstein JT, Hafer C & Stangel M. (2009). Plasma exchange therapy in steroid-unresponsive relapses in patients with multiple sclerosis. *Blood Purif*, Vol.28, No.2, pp. 108-15.

Uzawa A, Mori M, Hayakawa S, Masuda S & Kuwabara S. (2010). Different responses to interferon beta-1b treatment in patients with neuromyelitis optica and multiple sclerosis. *Eur J Neurol*, Vol.17, No.5, pp. 672-6.

Verkman AS, Ratelade J, Rossi A, Zhang H & Tradtrantip L. (2011). Aquaporin-4: orthogonal array assembly, CNS functions, and role in neuromyelitis optica. *Acta Pharmacol Sin*, Vol.32, pp. 702-10.

Viegas S, Weir A, Esiri M, Kuker W, Waters P, Leite MI & al. (2009). Symptomatic, radiological and pathological involvement of the hypothalamus in neuromyelitis optica. *J Neurol Neurosurg Psychiatry*, Vol.80, pp. 679-82.

Watanabe S, Nakashima I, Miyazawa I, Misu T, Shiga Y, Nakagawa Y, Fujihara K & Itoyama Y. (2007). Successful treatment of a hypothalamic lesion in neuromyelitis optica by plasma exchange. *J Neurol*, Vol.254, No.5, pp. 670-1.

Watanabe S, Nakashima I, Misu T, Miyazawa I, Shiga Y, Fujihara K & Itoyama Y. (2007). Therapeutic efficacy of plasma exchange in NMO-IgG-positive patients with neuromyelitis optica. *Mult Scler*, Vol.13, No.1, pp. 128-32.

Weinshenker BG, O'Brien PC, Petterson TM, Noseworthy JH, Lucchinetti CF, Dodick DW, Pineda AA, Stevens LN & Rodriguez M. (1999). A randomized trial of plasma exchange in acute central nervous system inflammatory demyelinating disease. *Ann Neurol*, Vol.46, No.6, pp. 878-86.

Weinshenker BG. (2001). Plasma exchange for severe attacks of inflammatory demyelinating diseases of the central nervous system. *J Clin Apher*, Vol.16, No.1, pp. 39-42.

Weinshenker BG, Wingerchuk DM, Vukusic S, Linbo L, Pittock SJ, Lucchinetti CF & Lennon VA. (2006). Neuromyelitis optica IgG predicts relapse after longitudinally extensive transverse myelitis. *Ann Neurol*, Vol.59, No.3, pp. 566-9.

Weinshenker BG. (2000). Plasma exchange for acute attacks of demyelinating disease: detecting a Lazarus effect. *Ther Apher*, Vol.4, No.3, pp. 187-9.

Weinstock-Guttman B, Ramanathan M, Lincoff N, Napoli SQ, Sharma J, Feichter J & Bakshi R. (2006). Study of mitoxantrone for the treatment of recurrent neuromyelitis optica (Devic disease). *Arch Neurol*, Vol.63, No.7, pp. 957-63.

Weinstock-Guttman B, Miller C, Yeh E, Stosic M, Umhauer M, Batra N, Munschauer F, Zivadinov R & Ramanathan M. (2008). Neuromyelitis optica immunoglobulins as a marker of disease activity and response to therapy in patients with neuromyelitis optica. *Mult Scler*, Vol.14, No.8, pp. 1061-7.

Wingerchuk DM, Lennon VA, Lucchinetti CF, Pittock SJ & Weinshenker BG. (2007). The spectrum of neuromyelitis optica. *Lancet Neurol*, Vol.6, No.9, pp. 805-15.

Wingerchuk DM, Lennon VA, Pittock SJ, Lucchinetti CF & Weinshenker BG. (2006). Revised diagnostic criteria for neuromyelitis optica. *Neurology*, Vol;66, No.10, pp. 1485-9.

Yoshida H, Ando A, Sho K, Akioka M, Kawai E, Arai E, Nishimura T, Shinde A, Masaki H, Takahashi K, Takagi M & Tanaka K. (2010). Anti-aquaporin-4 antibody-positive optic neuritis treated with double-filtration plasmapheresis. *J Ocul Pharmacol Ther,* Vol.26, No.4, pp. 381-5.

Yu X, Green M, Gilden D, Lam C, Bautista K & Bennett JL. (2011). Identification of peptide targets in neuromyelitis optica. *J Neuroimmunol,* Vol.236, No.1-2, pp. 65-71.

Zisimopoulou P., Lagoumintzis G., Kostelidou K., Bitzopoulou K., Kordas G., Trakas N. & al. (2008) Towards antigen-specific apheresis of pathogenic autoantibodies as a further step in the treatment of myasthenia gravis by plasmapheresis. *J Neuroimmunol,* Vol. 201-2, pp. 95-103.

8

Glial and Axonal Pathology in Multiple Sclerosis

Maria de los Angeles Robinson-Agramonte[1], Alina González-Quevedo[2]
and Carlos Alberto Goncalves[3]
[1]International Center for Neurological Restoration,
[2]Institute of Neurology and Neurosurgery,
[3]Federal University of Rio Grande del Sur. Porto Alegre,
[1,2]Cuba
[3]Brazil

1. Introduction

The central nervous system (CNS) consists of a series of complex structures which comprise cellular elements with basic communication functions and elaboration of information as part of their role in the process of biological adaptation and maintenance of homeostasis [Hickey WF, 2001].

1.1 Mayor components of the CNS

The major components of the CNS; neurons and neurites, microglias, astrocytes, ependymal cells and oligodendrocytes, establish all an important interrelationship, vital to the brain maintenance homeostasis. Ependymal cells lay around layers of astrocytes, which in turn envelop neurons, neurites and vascular elements. In addition, the normal CNS parenchyma contains blood vessels and resident macrophages. Glial cells, as they possess no conventional synaptic contacts, differ from neurons mainly establishing a rich interrelationship with other CNS components. The neuroglia, brain interstitial element, is recognized as including three groups of glial cells: 1) macroglias, such as astrocytes and oligodendrocytes,2) microglia and 3) ependymal cells.

Regarding glial function, the astrocytes are involved in glutamate uptake, repair and transport, and are part of the blood brain barrier (BBB). Studies conducted by Reese and Karnowosky [1967] indicate that the astrocyte end-feet provide little resistance to molecule movement, and that the blockage of their passage into the brain occurs at the endothelial-cell-lining blood vessels. In this case, endothelial cells forming for brain vascular endothelium, play an important role in the communication between the CNS and the periphery, this latter understood as intravascular space.

Oligodendrocytes are the myelin producing cells within the CNS and are potentially highly vulnerable to immune mediated damage, since they share together with the myelin sheath many molecules with affinities to elicit specific T and B cell responses, which lead to their destruction. Oligodendrocytes do not express class I or II MHC molecules, but a wide profile of cytokine receptors, both pro-inflammatory and regulatory which have been found on this cell-type, suggesting their innate and adaptive ability to participate in immune response.

Microglial cells, the most interesting and enigmatic CNS type cells, play a role in phagocytosis and inflammatory response in the CNS. Under normal conditions these cells seem to be in a resting state, becoming a very active macrophage during the disease, and constituting the major effector cell in immune-mediated damage in the CNS. An explosive activity in the field of microglia cell-research conducted in the past 15 to 20 years has led to the identification of microglia as a highly efficient accessory and effector cell of the immune system. Microglia expresses class II MHC antigen upon activation [Perry & Gordon, 1997] in the absence of a T cell response, which suggests that major histocompatibility complex (MHC) antigen expression may represent a marker of activation and/or a state of immunological competence. Microglia are also major producers of a large number of proinflammatory cytokines with well-known effects on T cells [Perry & Gordon, 1997]. All the previous information supports a wide glial involvement in brain internal homeostasis maintenance that plays a major role in the regulatory function of barrier systems.

1.2 Brain neurovascular unit

The blood-brain barrier (BBB) system, located between the intravascular space and the brain tissue, constitutes a phenomenon of selective permeability and reduced exchange of products between the blood and the nervous system. It is a characteristic of brain capillaries and is regulated by the cells that form the neurovascular unit (NVU) [Becher et al, 2006; Nathanson & Chun, 1990; Seyfert & Faultish, 2003] and the dynamics of cerebrospinal fluid (CSF) flow [Becher et al, 2006; Seyfert & Faultish, 2003]. NVU refers to the dynamic exchange among the cellular elements forming these barriers in the brain; there is a regional specialized interface between the neural tissue and the blood [Neutwelt et al, 2008].

The NVU is formed by: 1) The CSF-blood barrier, site of immunological communication between the CSF and intravascular space, which favours antigenic recognition and lymphocyte activation at this level [Bigio, 1995; Nathanson & Chun, 1990a; Redzic et al, 2005]; 2) The meningeal barrier, that is, the aracnoid membrane, bordering the duramater, where the CSF drains to the dural venous sinuses, the olfactory nerve and the carotid sheaths[Nag S. 2003]; 3) the BBB, constituted by the brain vascular endothelium, regulates the entrance of molecules and supply of nutrients to the brain, as well as preserving the ionic homeostasis in the brain environment [Petty & Lo, 2002]; 4) the blood-nerve barrier, which surrounds the axon tangles and includes the endothelial membrane of the endoneural capillary and the perinerium [Hemmer, 2004]; 5) the blood–retinal barrier, formed by the retinal endothelial capillary and the retinal tissue, like BBB; 6) the blood-labyrinth barrier, which has as anatomical reference the endolymph-blood and endolymph-perilymph barriers.These capillaries are lined with endothelial cells that are joined by tight junctions and physiologically form the blood–labyrinth barrier that is essential for sensitive auditory function; and 7) the blood-spinal cord barrier - with a greater permeability than the BBB - which communicates with the periphery through the nerve roots plexus [Haukins & Davis , 2005].

For centuries, the BBB, the lack of conventional lymphatic drainage and low response to aloantigens inoculated in the CNS, were arguments to consider this compartment as a privileged site. Nevertheless, today it is well known, that there is no such privilege, but rather the main differences of the immune response in the brain, regarding the periphery, are in the kinetics and the degree of regulation of the different stages of the immune response at this level, which will take place under the functional control of the immune response and influence of cellular mediators acting in a regulated quantitative and temporally balanced sequence[Fisher & Gage, 1993].

In normal conditions, neurons are unable to interact with T-cells, via MHC expression antigens, however, neurons possess unique antigenic proteins, which are normally sequestered by the BBB from the circulating immune system, making the CNS vulnerable to immune-mediated damage. On the other hand, there is increasing evidence on the ability of astrocytes to act as accessory cells of the immune system, as a facultative phagocyte able to interact with lymphocytes, since astrocytes express class II MHC antigens, essential molecules for antigen presentation to T helper cells. Astrocytes are also able to synthesize cytokines like interleukin 1, interferon γ and tumor necrosis factor, among others. During inflammation, the mechanism of selective transport displayed by endothelial cells (EC) is disrupted and endothelial tight junctions display altered permeability with subsequent edema within and around neighboring astrocytes. Evidence of the immunological role of microglia in demyelinating diseases like Multiple Sclerosis, as well as evidences of their putative role as a major effector-cell of immune mediated cell damage at this level has been well established.

1.3 Astrocytes as dynamic regulators of neuronal functional activity

One of the main functions of astrocytes is the uptake of neurotransmitters released from nerve terminals. But astrocytes can also release neuroactive agents, including transmitters, eicosanoids, steroids, neuropeptides and growth factors [Anderson & Swanson, 2000]. The regulation and mechanism (or mechanisms) of astrocyte-mediated release of neuroactive compounds are for most agents poorly defined. Release of glutamate appears to be the primary mechanism by which astrocytes modulate synaptic transmission [Kang, 1998].

In addition, astrocytes might serve neurons not so much as servants but as parents – both literally, as a developmental source of new neurons, and figuratively, as the regulators and judges of neuronal behaviour and activities. Simply stated, astrocytes command neurons what to do, besides keeping their environment clean. Interactions among astrocytes, neurons and endothelial cells define the gliovascular unit.

BBB is a diffusion barrier that regulates the exchange of molecules between the two tissues. The primary seal of the blood–brain barrier is formed by endothelial tight junctions. Astrocytes enwrap the vasculature with a large number of endfeet covering the vessel wall, although their role in BBB is poorly defined, they do not have a barrier function in the mammalian brain [del Zoppo & Hallenbeck, 2000]. Several factors released by astrocytes might be important for the induction and maintenance of the blood–brain barrier, as manifested by the appearance of endothelial tight junctions in cells ensheathed by astrocytic endfeet. Several investigators have studied this issue and have identified agents released by astrocytes, including transforming growth factor-a (TGFa) and glial-derived neurotrophic factor (GDNF), that support the formation of tight junctions in cultured endothelial cells [Abbott, 2002].

In general, the interactions between the barriers conforming the neurovascular unit, constitute the base of pathological events involved in neurological diseases, with inflammatory, neurodegenerative or autoimmune components as in MS, neuromyelitis optica (NMO), posterior uveitis, CNS vasculitis, cerebral ischemia, Alzheimer´s disease, among others [Brown, 2001] and at the same time they derive from transduction signals, disruption and assembling of the BBB in pathological conditions [Friese & Fugger, 2005]. As an extension of surveys on neuroaxonal loss and inflammatory demyelination in MS, this chapter focuses on the involvement of immune factors in axonal and neuronal neurodegeneration and summarizes concepts on immune-mediated axoneuronal dysfunction and highlights the potential pathways amenable to therapeutic interventions.

This chapter will focus on the physiopathology of Multiple Sclerosis with special emphasis on glial pathology, information on viral diseases and their relationship in its physiopathology, as well as on current therapeutic aspects.

2. Multiple Sclerosis

2.1 Heterogeneity in Multiple Sclerosis

Multiple Sclerosis (MS) is a primary inflammatory demyelinating autoimmune disease affecting the CNS and the peripheral nervous system (PNS). Recent results suggest a degenerative and hemodynamic profile in this disease, which arises from the evidence of early axonal damage [Kira, 2007; Porras-Betancourt et al, 2007] and stenotic changes in the extracranial vessels that modify the NVU [Rose & Carlson, 2007].

MS is included among the 50 neurological autoimmune diseases that affect approximately 75 x10[6] persons in the world [Lucchinetti et al, 2000], it is more frequent in women between 20 and 40 years of age and it constitutes the major cause of neurological disability in young adults [Martinez et al, 2005; Martinez-Yélamo et al, 1998].

Neuropathology of MS shows periventricular vascular impairment and leukocyte infiltration directed toward the myelin sheath and axon [Babbe et al, 2000; Forman et al, 2006; Jiang & Chess, 2006; Komek, 2003; Neumann et al, 2002]. Inflammation leading to progressive focal tissue damage and early axonal damage in MS could explain the current paradox concerning the temporal sequence of events that mediate axoneuronal damage in this disease, as well as the influence of immunomodulating therapy on the rate of relapses [Coles et al, 2006; Pittock et al, 2004], the persistence of oligoclonal response in the CSF and response against neurofilament proteins observed previous to demyelination. These are features that support the primary degenerating character of the disease.

MS is a prototype of neurodegenerative disease affecting primarily the axons and myelin in the CNS and the PNS. In spite of the fact that it is a disease which was described more than a century ago, the mechanism triggering the immunological reaction against myelin antigens remains unknown. Loss of myelin is accompanied by an impairment of nerve conduction leading to varied symptoms observed in this disease, that follow the formation of demyelinating plaques present in different parts of the brain and spinal cord.

It has been suggested that MS occurs as a consequence of an inflammatory response induced by the interaction of immune, environmental and genetic factors, which lead to demyelination, oligodendrocyte death, gliosis, axonal damage and neurodegeneration. In this sense, three aspects are of interest in the neuropathological approach of the disease: heterogeneity, viral or immune-environmental hypothesis and the axoneuronal degeneration that occurs in early stages of the disease.

MS displays a great heterogeneity that manifests itself not only in the immunogenetic pattern and the clinical forms of presentation, but also in the neuropathology, diagnosis and therapeutic response. Different authors have referred to these aspects [Bielekova et al, 2005; Lim et al, 2005] that could be defined as a) clinical neuropathological heterogeneity and b) heterogeneity related to the interpretation of neurobiological findings with respect to the diagnosis and clinical course of the disease.

Heterogeneity due to the influence of genetic and immuno-environmental factors in MS

The influence of genetic and immune-environmental factors in MS ranges from the geographic north-south distribution gradient of the disease, with a higher prevalence in developed countries, to the hygienic hypothesis [Cabre et al, 2005].

From a genetical point of view, MS displays a dominant poligenic character, with an incidence 20 to 50 times higher in first-degree relatives as compared with the general population and more than 100 genes reported. [Mirsattari et al, 2001]. Nevertheless, the highest individual genetic susceptibility is linked to MHC genes, with a distinctiveness for HLA DR 15* aplotypes in those exhibiting a more benign course, and HLA DR4 for those with a progressive form of the disease. Also, studies in monozygotic twins show a concordance of 25% and for dizygotic twins of less than 5%[Hillert, 2006; Lisak, 2006; Wingerchuck & Kantarci, 2007].

Other genes reported in MS include transcription genes of MHC class II, complement system, cytokines such as IL 17 e IL 17R, IL 1R, TNFp75R, GFAP, TNFα, TNFβ, TNFαR, beta linfotoxin, adhesion molecules (CD11a, CD18, CD49, β7-Integrin, transcripts for T-cells (TCR α), NK cells, B cells and proteases involved in antigen processing [Camerona, 2009; Gandhi , 2008]. The other hypothesis has strong supporters, due to the autoimmune character of the disease and the inflammatory and excitotoxic axonal degenerative reaction underlying the demyelinating process.

Clinical heterogeneity and neuropathology in MS

Clinical heterogeneity of MS is a consequence of the brain and spinal cord regions where plaques are located and the relapse rate - the latter is a very important element in the progression of the disease. From a clinical point of view, MS displays 4 clinical forms of presentation:1) relapsing-remitting MS, characterized by episodic exacerbations (relapses)followed by partial or complete recovery in approximately one month, and periods of clinical stability (remission); 2) primary progressive MS that displays a chronic progressive course, with no relapses; 3) secondary progressive MS characterized by relapses that progress in time, with less exacerbations, more incomplete recovery and irreversible disability; and 4) benign MS, which does not display a secondary progressive phase, or does not accumulate a significant disability until several decades after the onset of the disease [Fox et al, 2006; Lee et al, 2007; McDonald et al, 2001].

In all cases, MS clinical forms overlap, along with the neuropathological patterns described for the disease [Luchinetti, 2007]. In RR-MS an inflammatory pattern prevails, while in the progressive form a degenerative pattern prevails.Changes in the disability scale also correspond to clinical findings and imaginological changes in MRI studies. Although other factors are involved in the heterogeneous and multiorgan character of MS, all converge with the clinical picture to characterize the disease´s behavior individually.

Clinical and diagnostic heterogeneity

This aspect refers to the heterogeneity the disease management introduces in the interpretation of neurobiological variables, that allow the establishment of criteria from a prognostic point of view of the clinical course of MS, specifically for the immunological evaluation of CSF and MRI studies [Chabas, 2010; Villar, 2005].

The persistence of an oligoclonal response in the CSF of MS patients indicates the presence of a chronic inflammatory process with confirmatory value in this disease. CSF oligoclonal banding is an immunological feature not only of MS, but also of other neuroinflammatory diseases, including neuromyelitis optica.

The oligoclonal pattern that prevails in the CSF of MS patients is the presence of oligoclonal bands in CSF, but not in serum [Andersson, 1994, Correales, 2004, Falip, 2001]. It is suspected that autoantibodies can exacerbate inflammation and neurodegeneration in patients with MS, but which antigens intrathecal oligoclonal IgG recognize and how the autoimmune response is induced are still unknown [Meinl, 2008].

Heterogeneity is also associated with specific oligoclonal patterns in specific clinical forms. Thus, in the majority of cases, with primary progressive MS, a pattern of CSF and serum oligoclonal bands with additional bands in CSF is also found. On the other hand, oligoclonal bands directed to myelin lipids have been detected in RR-MS, secondarily progressive MS, but not in primary progressive MS [Camerona, 2009, Villar, 2005].

The presence of oligoclonal bands in the CSF has been considered a prognostic tool for the clinical management of these patients. Heterogeneity has also been introduced in the concordance of CSF analysis and the results of the MRI studies. According to Barkhof's criteria, different lesión patterns have been reported in patients positive or negative for CSF oligoclonal bands [Sospedra, 2009]. A lower frequency of infratentorial lesions have been reported in the MRIs of MS patients who are negative for oligoclonal bands and a higher frequency of juxtacortical lesions in patients with CSF oligoclonal bands. These associations are important in order to acquire a better comprehension and management of these patients based on the topography of the MRI lesions and their relation with the immunological response in the CSF [Sospedra & Martin, 2009].

2.2 Multiple Sclerosis pathology

2.2.1 Pathogenic mechanisms inducing Multiple Sclerosis

The oligoclonality and specificity of autoreactive T-cells suggest that myelin protein peptides are the activating antigens predominating in MS, whose essential attributes allow them to bind the T-cell receptor related with the structure of the lateral chain of the variable region of MHC Ag. Actually, it has been stated that the degeneration of the T-cell receptor´s ligand specificity is a main mechanism through which infectious agents can cause MS [Lee et al, 2007; Levin et al, 2010].

Among the pathogenic viruses in humans, those which induce persistent infection are relevant in MS as the triggering element of the autoimmune process that damages myelin. Herpes virus is of particular interest due to its neurotrophism, ubiquitous nature and tendency to produce latent recurrent infection. In general, there are 3 mechanisms through which viral agents can induce MS: a) molecular mimicry, b) "bystander" activation, and c) recognition of cryptic antigens [Lu et al, 2011; Levin et al, 2010].

a. Molecular mimicry

Considering the viral agents involved in the pathogenesis of MS, 83% of the patients show high titers of IgG antibodies for Epstein Barr´s virus [Barnett, 2006; Wingerchuck, 2006]. The molecular mimicry hypothesis is based on the structural similarity between myelin basic protein (MBP) peptide and Epstein Barr virus peptide, followed by the activation of autoreactive T-cells for myelin and the subsequent loss of the axon´s myelin [Haahr & Hollsberg, 2006; Maghzi et al, 2010].

b. Bystander activation

Autoreactive T-cells are also activated by unspecific inflammatory events. These events can depend on the specific recognition of exposed self-antigens due to tissue damage induced by viruses, by the autoreactive immunocompetent cell´s receptor or by independent recognition of viral antigens via autoreactive T/B cell´s receptor. In this case, 3 mechanisms have been proposed: activation by superantigens, action of pro-inflammatory cytokines derived from viral persistence and activation by Toll- like receptors [Fujinami et al, 2006; McCoy et al, 2006].

Activation by superantigens

This mechanism involves the exposure to superantigens (superAgs), toxins derived from viral agent induced relapses. This was demonstrated in the EAE model by interaction with specific T-cell clones for MBP expressing the βV TCR chain [Torkildsen et al, 2006].

Superantigens, are active mitogens, mostly all small basic proteins (20-30 kD), that induce a response by binding to the MHC Ags´ lateral part, which is not the usual location. Binding does not take place through the polymorphic trimolecular complex or binding Ag site, but laterally, at a specific sequence coded by genes of the βV TCR chain. After MHC-II and TCR bind, aggregation of the receptor and cellular activation follows. Contrary to what conventionally occurs, superAgs are not processed by the antigen-presenting cells, nor are they presented in the restricted MHC self-antigens context [Fujinami et al, 2006; McCoy et al, 2006].

Viral persistence and activation mediated by inflammatory cytokines

As a consequence of persistent viral infection, virus infected antigen-presenting cells (APC), present viral peptides to T $CD4^+$ and $CD8^+$ cells together in the context of MHC class antigens. The activation of these cells induces the production of INFγ and the differentiation of T-cells via IL-12. T CD4 effector - cells secrete more INFγ and IL-12 that stimulates the T-cells differentiation to effectors, secreting more mediators like INFγ and TNFα. Activated macrophages also, secrete TNFα, nitric oxide and other reactive oxygen species that damage the infected cells and other bystander non-infected cells, to be phagocytized by macrophages and dendritic cells who process and present self-antigens to T CD4 and CD8 autoreactive cells, destroying the tissue´s infected self-cells via perforins, among other mechanisms [Lassmann, 2011]. The resulting cellular detritus are captured and processed by APC and presented to autoreactive CD8-T lymphocytes who display an autoimmune reaction. In this manner, the pro-inflammatory cytokines and chemokines secreted during the infection mediate the damage, becoming activators of the T CD8 cells specific for viral antigen and autoreactive inductors of the autoimmune process [Pender: 2011]. In this case the activation and differentiation of T CD8 cells occurs in an unspecific way [Becher et al , 2007; Haahr & Hollsberg, 2006].

On the other hand, the CNS antiviral polyspecific immune response in MS, has become a potential tool to evidence chronic autoimmune response in these patients [Cohrs, 2007]. This hypothesis has been supported by the reports showing that more than 80% of people with MS display humoral intrathecal response against neurotrophic viruses (herpes simplex, measles, rubella and varicela zoster, among others). The combined response against these neurotrophic viruses in the CNS of MS patients, was coined by Reiber et al as MRZ reaction, and many others groups have disagreed on the diagnostic value of this detection from CSF analysis in more than 90% of MS patients [Colleen et al, 2006; Correales, 2004; Jarius, 2008, Jarius et al, 2009; Luchinetti, 2007], since a similar frequency of this autoimmune chronic reaction was observed in other neurological diseases [Jarius, 2008; Jarius et al, 2009]. The MRZ reaction has also been reported in NMO patients, although in a lower frequency than in MS, and it has been useful to establish a differential diagnosis between both demyelinating diseases [Jarius, 2008]. Other MRZ reaction results were reported in tropical regions with variations regarding the previous reports [Robinson et al, 2001; Robinson et al, 2007]. In this case, a lower response to rubella virus was observed in the CNS in a smaller series of patients regarding varicela zoster and measles virus. The later showed a neurotrophic virus response similar to those reported by Reiber et al in German MS persons [Reiber et al, 1998].

We could think that a reliable interpretation of these last findings probably comes from different epidemiological factors in the two countries, or that a previous contact with this neurotrophic virus could be necessary for a detectable intrathecal polyspecific MRZ antibody response, either by immunization or native infection. In this case, as rubella is a mild disease, it may be under-reported, even in areas where reporting has been mandatory for years. As it has been previously stated [Cooper & Alford, 2001], antibodies to rubella in people under 35 years of age is as low as 30% in tropical countries like Trinidad or Panama, compared with more than 80% in Europe or the USA [Cooper & Alford, 2001]; thus, the results found in Cuban patients could be comparable for our region without the influence of any additional factor.

Activation by Toll- like receptors

Although the role of innate – immunity involves native protection and maintenance of homeostasis, in some circumstances, it could result in a destructive autoimmunity via toll – like receptor (TLR), or unspecific mechanisms due to the action of lysozime, lactoferrin, oxidative stress or the recognition of molecular structures expressed in non – infected cells with an inhibitory effect on the immune response (NK cells, complement proteins and family receptors of type C lectins, among others [Frischer; 2009]. The TLR is expressed in a wide range of immune and non-immune cells like microglias, oligodendrocytes and astrocytes, which act as centinels, a) by recognition of a conserved molecular pattern associated with pathogens or b) generating pro-inflammatory signals that influence the adaptive immune response [Chauhan & Marriott, 2007].

It is believed that this mechanism initiates the lesion, previously preceded by peripheral activation. The LPS binding TLR4 increase cytokine expression and oxygen reactive species inducing peripheral autoreactive T cell activation and where an inappropriate TLR signal can contribute to MS development [Kielian; 2005]. In this way, the increased expresion of TLR on dendritic cells inhibit the immunosupresor effect of regulatory T cells CD4+/CD25+ on autoreactive T cells vía IL 6, causing loss of peripheral tolerance. The increase of exacerbations around viral infections in MS supports this hypothesis.

Cryptic Antigens

Cryptic or sequestered antigens are exposed as a consequence of myelin loss, induce an antibody response against them, causing reactive changes within the neuron cellular body and axon, blocking the interaction of oligodendrocyte precursors with the axon and consequently promoting remyelination and axonal repair [Devries, 2006; Magliozzi et al, 2010].

2.2.2 Mechanism involving the axoneuronal degeneration in MS

The investigation of neurodegeneration in MS has received the highest priority in the last few years, establishing a multifactorial process involving myelin loss, immune-mediated histotoxicity, decreased trophic support, mitochondrial damage, metabolic-energetic changes, and altered signalling [Ghafourifar, 2008; Klawiter & Cross, 2007; Lindberg et al, 2008; Sobel, 1998].

It is commonly accepted that the initial activation of the T cell system takes place in the systemic immune compartment outside the CNS, where T lymphocytes encounter a specific autoantigen presented in the context of MHC class II molecules [Neumann et al, 2002] and the simultaneous delivery of additional co-stimulatory signals, such as B7-1 (CD80) and B7-2 (CD86), on the cell surface of antigen presenting cells. Such autoreactive T cells may reside quiescently at this level, until an external trigger - most likely a viral infection- renders these cells active to develop their auto aggressive potential.

The degree of neurological impairment seems to be determined by the extent of axonal loss, which is proposed to be the final step in the pathogenesis of the MS lesions. However, so far it remains unclear: (a) whether axonal injury is the result of an active destructive process targeting the axon; (b) if it occurs as a result of increased vulnerability of demyelinated axons or as part of a bystander effect; or (c) if axonal degeneration takes place as a physiological response to permanent demyelination inhibiting the extrinsic trophic signal to axons [Luchinetti. 2007].

Pathogenic events involved in axoneuronal degeneration

Two main pathogenic events must be considered as the cause of axoneuronal damage leading to irreversible discapacity in MS: a) damage of the myelin oligodendrocytic unit and b) the axoneuronal neurodegeneration process.

Damage of the myelin oligodendrocytic unit

Indirect effect of T cells can also mediate damage to the myelin-oligodendrocytic unit. Autoreactive T lymphocytes activated from the periphery get into the CNS by degradation of the brain vascular endothelial cells. Th1 lymphocytes expressing adhesion molecules such as VLA-4 y LFA-1, release cytokines and metalloproteinases MMP2/9 that acting at the BBB level, induce an increase of its permeability. The later, linked with a higher integrin expression (V-CAM /I-CAM) induced by INFγ and TNFα, facilitate the migration of activated T cells into the CNS. Once in the CNS, these activated T-cells release cytokines – such as INFγ- which induces activation and differentiation of others autoreactive T cells resting in the Tho state, to transform into effector cells, activating microglias, resident macrophages in the CNS and Tγδ cells, thus contributing to the damage. Recently it has also been postulated that T cell regulators can transform into Th-17 effector cells, contributing to a major lesional effect on the myelin-oligodendrocytic unit [Ishizu , 2010]. Figure 2 shows the mechanisms related with the indirect effect of T lymphocytes and microglia in the damage of the myelin-oligodendrocyte unit.

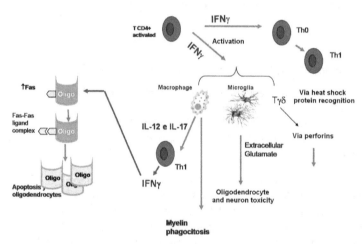

Fig. 1. Pathogenic mechanism, involving damage of the myelin oligodendrocytic unit. Microglia interfere the oligodendrocyte repopulation and mediate their toxicity and death with the main intervention of cytokine like IFNγ and TNFα.

Microglia also cause a toxic effect on oligodendrocytes and neurons via extracellular glutamate and nitric oxide secretion, while Tγδ cells induce direct oligodendrocyte damage, via perforine. INFγ- activated macrophages are also induced to secrete cytokines such as IL-12 and IL 17 that induce Th1 cells to secrete more INFγ. INFγ then induces the expression of Fas molecules on the oligodendrocyte surface promoting a Fas-Fas ligand interaction, followed by oligodendrocyte apoptotic death, Fig 1. Thus, the microglia, main mediator of glial –neuron interaction becomes a binding point between the innate and adaptative immune systems. In acute inflammation, microglia act as antigen presenting cells (APC), and contribute to antibody clearance and elimination of myelin detritus after clinical relapse. However, during the chronic phase of a pathological condition like MS, this cell type contributes to irreversible damage. Glial-derived INFγ, also interferes with the vitality, recruitment and function of OPC, interfering with complete remyelination at lesion sites.

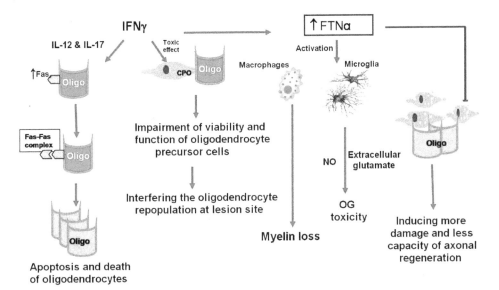

Fig. 2. Indirect T cell effect, on the myelin-oligodendrocytic unit in MS. Microglia also, causes a toxic effect on oligodendrocytes and neurons via extracellular glutamate and nitric oxide secretion. Th1: T-helper-1 cells.

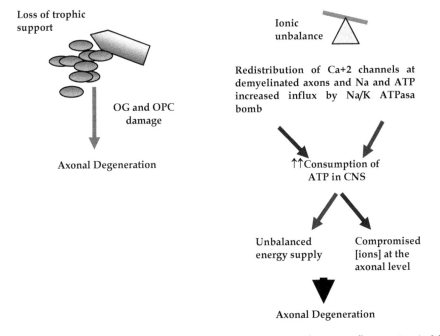

Fig. 3.Axonal damage mediated by mechanisms independent of active inflammation in MS. OG; oligodendrocyte, OPC: oligodendrocyte precursor cells.

On the other hand, damage to the myelin-oligodendrocytic unit occurs as a consecuence of an increased vulnerability of demyelinated axons to immune attack, a reduced trophic support, since myelination provides an extrinsic trophic signal to axons. Fig 3 shows the mechanisms leading to axonal damage independent from active inflammation: loss of trophic factors and ionic and energetic unbalance, Fig 3.

Neuronal damage in MS results from two insults: on one side mediated by microglia, via IL 1beta, TNFα, IL 6 and NO, all neurotoxic to neurons which are functionally compromised by hypoxic damage, and on the other side due to an excess of extracellular glutamate, oligodendrocyte toxicity, and axonal loss. Gene transcripts for TNF and IL 6 with an impact on the pathophysiology of MS have been identified in the margins and center of the active lesions, but not in the inactive lesions [Jack et al, 2007].

Axoneuronal degeneration in MS

Loss of trophic support in MS pathophysiology: Reduced inflammation occurring during the course of chronic demyelination suggests the existence of mechanisms not related to active inflammation as being responsible of continuous axonal loss and progressive and irreversible inability. It has been acknowledged that this is due to the loss of trophic support derived from oligodendrocyte damage, which is necessary for axonal survival independent from compact myelin (Fig 4).

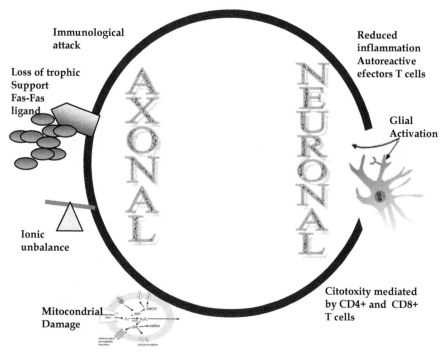

Fig. 4. Mechanism involved in the axoneuronal degeneration process. Neuroaxonal loss represents the major pathophysiological element correlating with clinical disability. The figure summarizes the mechanisms causing demyelination and axoneuronal degeneration in MS and their combined contribution to disease progression and irreversible inability.

Ionic unbalance in MS pathophysiology: Ionic unbalance –as a result of compensatory changes to restore nervous conduction following demyelination- can induce long term axonal degeneration. Therefore, the redistribution of Na channels on demyelinated axons restores the action potential, neuronal function and increases Na and ATP influx, via the Na/K ATPase pump to maintain the ionic gradient, which is necessary for neurotransmission. Both processes are highly energy consuming, leading to energetic unbalance, altered axonal ion concentrations and subsequent neurodegeneration (Fig4).

Antibodies to Cytoskeletal Proteins: Neurofilaments are a group of cytoskeletal proteins expressed in neuronal cells and axons. Neurodegenerative disorders like Alzheimer's disease and Parkinson's disease are characterized by accumulation of NF proteins leading to abnormalities in axonal transport and an impending neuronal loss [Amor et al, 2010; Arumugam et al, 2008]. Antibodies to axonal cytoskeletal proteins may be markers of axonal damage, as well as important contributors to neurodegeneration and clinical disability in MS. CSF levels of antibodies against the NFL correlate with disease duration, clinical disability, IgG index, and the degree of cerebral atrophy measured by MRI [Bartos et al, 2007; Eikelenbom, 2003]. Although elevated levels of NFL-specific antibodies are present in sera of patients with PP-MS, these antibodies are also increased in sera of patients with other neurological diseases [Bartos et al, 2007; Huizinga, 2008].

Although there is no confirmed evidence to establish that antineurofilament antibodies themselves contribute to mayor neuroaxonal damage, experimental models provide supportive evidence [Amor et al, 2010]. Immunization of mice with NFL triggers the development of a CNS disease characterized by axonal damage, paralysis, and spasticity [Huizinga et al, 2008]. Furthermore, microinjections of anti-kinesin or anti-dynein antibodies cause impairment of the anterograde and retrograde NF transport in cultured neurons [Theiss et al, 2005] and induce the formation of long and branched mitochondrial structures redistributed to the nuclear periphery. These intracellular changes are associated with altered calcium homeostasis, apoptosis, and neurodegeneration [Arumugam et al, 2009]. Antibodies to neurofilaments and possibly to other cytoskeletal proteins are produced during tissue damage in MS. Experimental data support that these antibodies may gain access to their intracellular target and cause changes in axonal transport, mitochondrial distribution and calcium homeostasis, and thus contribute to apoptosis and neurodegeneration [Vishkina & Kalman, 2008].

Criteria based on evidence regarding the role of Ab-mediated autoreactivity to neurofilament proteins in MS has been controversial [Silber et al, 2002; Bartos et al, 2007; Bartos el al, 2007a; Bejartmar & Trapp, 2003; Semra et al, 2002; Eikelenboom et al, 2003]. Bartos et al for example, detected increased intrathecal IgG and IgM antibodies against the medium subunit of neurofilaments (NFM) in patients with all subtypes of MS [Bartos et al, 2007; Bartos et al, 2007a] while Silber et al [2002] maintained the relevance of autoantibody to NFL in CSF as progression markers in MS. Unexpectedly, anti-NFM antibody levels appeared to be higher in the serum than in CSF, possibly related to NF antigen leakage from the CNS to the peripheral blood, or to the higher concentration of plasma cells in the blood. Alternatively, anti-NFM antibodies may be triggered by exogenous antigens and molecular mimicry in the peripheral blood [Bartos et al, 2007; Bartos et al, 2007a; Bejartmar et al, 2003; Eikelenboom et al, 2003; Semra et al, 2002; Silber et al, 2002].

Besides these considerations, the evaluation of axonal markers from CSF analysis, have shown different results; some experiences considering these biomarkers promissory for monitoring progression and/or relapsing rate in MS. So, a study in patients published by Eikelenboom et al, reported a significant correlation between intrathecal production of NFLP antibody in CSF and cortical atrophy and more recently a significant relationship between NFLP antibody index and relapsing rate was observed in patients bearing MS [Eikelenboom et al 2003; Robinson, 2010]. Fig 5 shows a study conducted in a group of 26 Cuban MS patients with different clinical forms of the disease. The evaluation of Ab reactivity to NFLP in CSF was significantly correlated with the relapsing rate, denoting an association between both clinical and biological parameters. These results are interesting since they show another aspect of the idiotipic response in MS, and its possible insertion not only from the view point of the pathogenic mechanism of the disease, but also as a useful clinical tool, at least to predict or monitor treatment response.

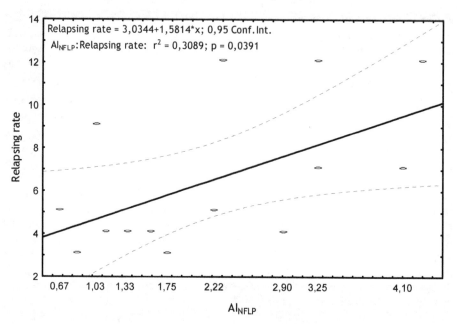

Fig. 5. Statistical analysis between AI_{NFLP} and relapsing rate in MS patients showed a significant correlationship between both parameters. * Spearman´s correlation test, p<0.05. AI_{NFLP}: Antibody index to neurofilament light protein. AI_{NFLP}: NFLP CSF/NFLP Serum / IgG CSF/IgG serum.

2.3 Autoimmunity contributing to glial pathology in MS

Neurodegeneration in MS occurs in response to a multifactorial process involving loss of myelin protection by immune-mediated histotoxicity, decreased trophic support, mitochondrial damage, metabolic changes and altered signaling [Ghafourifar et al, 2008; Lindberg et al, 2008]. Nevertheless, different neuronal targets have been identified as causing neuronal dysfunction, following a humoral immune mechanism in MS which can be classified as neuronal surface molecules, intracellular enzymes, signaling molecules and chaperones, nuclear antigens and cytoskeletal protein among others (Vyshkina & Kalman, 2008 |. On the other hand, it has been suggested that microglial responses are tailored in regional and insult-specific manners [Carson et al, 2007]. The most recognizable role of microglia in brain defense is as a scavenger of cellular debris by phagocytosis, as occurs in the event of infection, inflammation, trauma, ischemia, and neuronal death [Kraft & Harry, 2011]. However, it is well known that, not only do microglia dynamically survey the CNS to clear damaged cellular debris, but they are also capable of initiating a rapid and specific response to subtle changes in the microenvironment. Different types of neuronal pathology and other activating stimuli clearly elicit differing responses from brain-resident microglia [Colton & Wilcock, 2010; Rivest, 2009], evidencing the autoimmune process that leads to brain damage as occurs in MS.

B cells and autoimmunity in MS

B cells are involved in multiple immune pathways including the presentation of antigenic determinants and the expression of costimulatory signals for T lymphocytes, immunoglobulin production, secretion of cytokines, and recruitment of T cells into the CNS. The B-cell lineage is represented by B lymphocytes (CD19þ, CD138), plasma blasts (CD19þ, D138þ), and plasma cells (CD19_, CD138þ; all detectable in CNS and CSF. In MS most of these cells express memory phenotypes, CD27þ positive. A relevant contribution of humoral autoimmunity in myelin loss has been proposed in demyelinating diseases with a prominent intervention of complement molecules and Ab itself [Lucchinetti et al, 2000; Serafini et al, 2010]. Thus, immunological and molecular results have repeatedly been reported by differents groups in this field, all of them directed towards the characterization of the cellular arm of autoimmunity.

Mechanisms leading to autoimmune B-cell activation may be initiated by CD4 T helper type 2 (TH2) lymphocytes and their soluble inflammatory products (eg. interleukins 4, 5 and 13) followed by an antigen-specific expansion of clones either in the peripheral circulation or in the damaged CNS tissue, where intracellular proteins are released. As it was expressed earlier in this chapter, bystander activation describes a non-antigen-specific activation of T or B cells usually mediated by soluble inflammatory products of nearby immune cells, while the humoral immune system appears to be more successful in breaking anti-neuronal tolerance than the cellular system, and has greater pathogenic significance supporting the involvement of the humoral immune response in MS-related neurodegeneration [Huizinga et al, 2008].

From a molecular view point, data also support the involvement of B lymphocytes and their products in MS. Intrathecal production of immunoglobulins with an oligoclonal electrophoretic distribution pattern is a hallmark of the disease. Clonally expanded autoreactive B cells in the CSF and CNS have increased VH mutation rates concentrated in the complementarity determining regions. VH sequences expressed in plaques are absent in the peripheral blood [Owens et al, 2001]. B-cell heavy and light chain editing, a mechanism to prevent autoimmunity by the replacement of elements in rearranged immunoglobulin genes after the re-expression of recombination activating genes —RAG1/RAG2, is inefficient in MS, a fact which is suggested by the detection of autoreactive B cells with unsuccessfully edited receptors in the CSF [Lambracht-Washington et al, 2007; O'Connor et al, 2007] These observations suggest that CNS antigen-specific and clonally expanded B cells present in CNS and CSF of MS patients exhibit complex molecular characteristics and intraclonal diversity.

Neuroaxonal targets of humoral autoimmunity in MS and EAE have been identified in the CNS during the process of demyelination. Immunoglobulins produced by activated B cells in the CNS and CSF target numerous self-antigens including components of CNS myelin such as myelin basic protein, proteolipid protein, myelin-associated glycoprotein, and myelin oligodendrocyte glycoprotein [Dutta & Trapp, 2007]. A great number of papers discuss the involvement of myelin-specific antibodies in the development of demyelination and disease progression and although not uniformly, the use of some of these antibodies as biomarkers is accepted as a support to the diagnosis or to monitor disease activity and course [Amor et al, 2007; Lutterotti et al, 2007]

Anti-Neuronal Antibodies in MS

Antibodies to a variety of intracellular molecules including enzymes, signaling molecules, HSPs, and nuclear proteins are detected in MS and other inflammatory and neurological disorders. The production of these antibodies may be related to bystander immune activation and epitope spreading during tissue injury, as was referred before, although their pathogenic significance remains uncertain in some cases.

Antibodies Targeting Neuronal Cell-Surface Molecules: Neuronal cell-surface antigen molecules in the surface membrane of myelinated axons are normally hidden from the immune system, and only become exposed after demyelination becoming antigenic and inducing the production of neuron-specific antibodies. IgG and IgM antibodies binding to the surface of a neuronal cell line were found in 70% of sera from patients with secondary progressive (SP)-MS and in 25% of sera from patients with relapsing-remitting (RR)-MS [Kraft & Harry, 2011] . This finding may indicate the spreading of autoimmunity to neuronal antigens as a consequence of CNS expansion and tissue damage.

Axolemma-enriched fractions: Antibodies to axolemma-enriched fractions (AEF) of the CNS are also present in CSF and sera of MS patients, [Zaffaroni, 2003].From in vitro assays, there is evidences that these antibodies damage neurites and prevent neuronal outgrowth. The production of anti-axolemma and anti-myelin IgGs appears to be independent. Criteria to consider antiaxolemmal IgG antibodies as markers of axonal damage are based on these observations [Zaffaroni, 2003].

Neurofascin: One of the targets in antibody-mediated axonal injury is the cell-adhesion molecule neurofascin. The 186 kDa neuronspecific isoform of neurofascin (NF186) is involved in the clustering of voltage gated Na channels at Ranvier´s nodes, while the 155 kDa glial-specific isoform (NF155) is required for the proper assembly of paranodal junction, targeting the interaction sites between myelin and axon. Early in the disease course and preceding demyelination, changes in the distribution of NF155 have been observed in MS lesions [Vyshkina1 & Kalman, 2008]. Maier et al [2007] showed that the NF155-levels were reduced, suggesting that NF155 is subject to protein degradation in the lesions. On the other hand, studies in sera showed levels significantly higher in patients with chronic progressive forms of MS compared to other inflammatory neurological diseases. At the same time, studies in vitro showed that antibodies to neurofascin inhibit axonal conduction and that NF155-specific antibodies cross-react with NF186-transfected cells at the nodes of Ranvier possibly initiating axonal injury and accelerating disease progression [Mathey et al, 2007]. Neurofascin-specific antibodies can also inhibit remyelination by binding to NF155 expressed on the surface of oligodendrocytes. In vivo experiments revealed that antibodies to neurofascin and complement can selectively target nodes of Ranvier, cause axonal injury, and trigger disease exacerbation in EAE [Mathey et al, 2007].

Anti ganglioside antibodies: It is well known that gangliosides are glycolipids with sialic residues in the outer layer of cell membranes, particularly enriched in the membranes of neurons. Experimental data reveal that antiganglioside antibodies can disrupt the BBB, create neuromuscular block by binding to neuronal gangliosides at the neuromuscular junction and inhibit axonal regeneration after peripheral nerve injury in mice [Amor et al, 2010],. Increased levels of anti-GM3 (monosialoganglioside) antibodies can be found in sera of a great proportion of patients with progressive forms of MS (56.3%) in primary progressive (PP)-MS and in 42.9% of SP-MS vs 2.9% in RR-MS and 14.6% in OND. Anti-GD2 (disialo-ganglioside)-like IgM autoantibodies were detected in sera of 30% of MS patients, and a positive correlation of anti-GD2-like IgM reactivity with neurological disability was observed [*Kanda et al, 2000*]. The increased prevalence of GD2-specific IgM antibodies in SP-MS (47.8%) compared to RR-MS (24.2%) and PP-MS (26.7%), also suggests the involvement of these antibodies in inflammation-induced neurodegeneration [Marconi et al, 2006]. It should be emphasized; that it is not clear whether anti-ganglioside antibodies can cause or result from axonal damage, and whether they may definitely function as putative markers of neurodegeneration in MS.

In general, these data suggest that antibodies specific to neuronal cell-surface molecules are produced during demyelination, and that they may themselves contribute to glial pathology or axonal injury in MS. These antibodies can activate complement and exert cytotoxicity, provide binding sites for the Fc receptors on macrophages and microglial cells, interrupt axon–myelin interaction, inhibit axonal conduction and outgrowth, disrupt the BBB, and alter oligodendrocyte functioning. Correlation of the antibody titers with the severity of disability offers an opportunity of using these neuronal cell-surface antibodies as biomarkers.

Antibodies to Intracellular Molecules: Arrestins, glutamate decarboxylase and nuclear antigens

MS patients show a high prevalence of autoreactivity to intracellular antigens such as neuron-specific enolase (metabolic enzyme), b-arrestin and retinal arrestin among others. So, antibody reaction to arrestins, a family of multifunctional, intracellular proteins that regulate signal transduction and the activity of G-protein-coupled receptors, has been reported in MS; while b-arrestin-1 enhances the expression of antiapoptotic Bcl2 that may control the development of both MS and EAE. Anti-b-arrestin-specific antibodies and antibodies to retinal arrestin can be found in sera of patients with MS. [Gorczyca et al, 2004]. B-Arrestin-1-knockout mice are more resistant, and b-arrestin-1 transgenic mice are more susceptible to EAE [Frederick & Miller, 2007; Shi et al, 2007].

Immunity to glutamate decarboxylase (GAD), an enzyme that converts glutamate into the inhibitory neurotransmitter aminobutyric acid (GABA), can also be detected in MS. GAD is expressed in various cell types including neurons, and its activity is reduced in sera of MS patients. Serum anti- GAD65 antibodies are present in 10% of MS patients [Hermitte et al,

2000]. Anti-GAD antibodies have also been associated with systemic autoimmune disorders, such as type 1 diabetes, although without a clear understanding of the pathogenic significance [Taplin & Barker, 2008]. Elevated antinuclear antibodies (ANA) in sera of MS patients have been reported at varying frequencies (2.5–81%) depending on the methodological approaches [Ferreira et al, 2005; Roussel et al, 2000]. In contrast, the ANA titers are low (between 1:40 and 1:100) in sera of MS patients, who also often have low-affinity IgG antibodies to multiple other nuclear and cytoplasmic epitopes. [Ferreira et al, 2005; Roussel et al, 2000; Lu & Kalman, 1999]. These data suggest that detection of ANA and related antibodies in MS may result from a nonspecific immune activation.

Furthermore, these observations support that B cells may contribute directly or indirectly to MS development. Removal of immunoglobulins from the peripheral blood by plasmapheresis appears to be beneficial in the subgroup of patients with type II lesions [Keegan et al, 2005] and depletion of CD20 B cells by rituximab results in a significant reduction in the number of enhancing MRI lesions. The latter intervention, however,does not exert its beneficial effects by directly affecting the immunoglobulin pool, but by depleting memory B cells and altering antigen presentation, T-cell activation, or T-cell recruitment into the CNS [Hauser et al, 2008].

Autoimmunity and Glutamate-Mediated Neurotoxicity

Glutamate is a neurotransmitter released by neurons into the synaptic space where it binds to its postsynaptic receptors. Elevated levels of extracellular glutamate can lead to the death of neurons, astrocytes and oligodendrocytes [Matute et al, 2006]. Excitotoxic tissue damage mediated by glutamate has been described in a number of neurologic diseases (eg stroke, traumatic injury, neurodegeneration) including MS [Vercellino et al, 2007].

Glial cells and neurons express various types of glutamate excitatory amino-acid transporters (EAAT1–EAAT5). The reuptake of glutamate appears to be impaired in MS due to the downregulation of EAAT1 and EAAT2 molecules in white matter and cortical lesions[Vercellino et al, 2007]. Glutamate levels in the CSF are higher during relapses than remissions, and correlate with disease severity [Sarchielli et al, 2003.) These observations suggest that inflammation upsets the balance of glutamate release and re-uptake, and the excessive glutamate may escalate tissue injury in MS.

Glutamate toxicity may be further enhanced by altered receptor expression and signaling.Two main subtypes of glutamate receptors have been identified: ionotropic, coupled directly to membrane ion channels; and metabotropic, coupled to G proteins. The ionotropic receptors are divided into three subtypes based on their selective agonists: N-methyl-D-aspartate (NMDA), a-amino-3-hydroxy-5-methyl-4-isoxazolepropionate (AMPA), and kainate [Lipton & Rosenberg, 1994]. An elevated expression of subunit 1 of AMPA receptor (GluR1) on oligodendrocytes at the borders of active plaques, and subunit 3 of AMPA receptor (GluR3) and metabotropic glutamate receptors (mGluR) on reactive astrocytes in MS lesions have also been reported. Activated microglia and macrophages are immunopositive for NMDA receptor subunit 1 (NR1) in plaques and may also play a role in Ca-dependent injury of oligodendrocytes and neurons. NMDA receptor antagonists, memantine, amantadine, and MK-801 reduce neurological deficits in EAE, and the blockade of AMPA receptors by antagonists, also ameliorate clinical signs of EAE. [Bolton & Paul, 1997; Smith et al, 2000; Stys & Lipton, 2007; Wallstrom 1996].

Antibodies targeting glutamate receptors may have agonist or antagonist effects. Agonists usually cause excitotoxicity and complement-mediated cell death [Groom et al, 2003]. Anti-GluR3 antibodies are implicated in epilepsy syndromes but not in MS. In summary, these observations suggest that glutamate homeostasis is being upset in inflammatory lesions of MS, where the concentration of glutamate is increased, at least in part, due to a decreased re-uptake. In addition, anti-glutamate receptor antibodies are associated with inflammatory and neurodegenerative disorders, like MS, often correlating with clinical improvement.

Induction of Central Nervous System Autoimmunity by Th17 lymphocyte in MS

T-helper cells classically divide into two functional subsets including: Th1 and T-helper-2 (Th2); each one with a distinct activity of transcription factor and pattern of cytokine-secretion phenotype [Mosmann et al, 1986.]. Th1 cells produce IFN-γ, TNF-β and interleukin-10 (IL-10), and mediate cellular immune responses against tumor cells, intracellular viruses and bacteria via macrophages and cytotoxic T-cell activation. In addition, Th1 cells drive cell-mediated response leading to tissue damage and drive humoral immune responses to Ig2a subclasses. Innate immune cells, through STAT6 signals, secrete IL-4 that induces the transformation of naïve CD4+ T cells into Th2 cells, leading to the expression of transcription factor GATA3. This cascade of events in turn results in the production of IL-4, IL-5, IL-13, IL-21 and IL-31, important for host defense against helminths and contribute to the pathogenesis of asthma and allergy [Monteleone et al, 2008; Steinman, 2007; Wilson et al, 2009]. Other T-cell subsets that co-express CD4 and CD25 are Th3 cells, or regulatory T (TREG) cells, which regulate both Th1 and Th2 cell function, and maintain homeostasis of the immune system [Vojdani & Lambert, 2011]. TREG cells can develop from thymic CD4+ T-cell precursors in the presence of IL-2 and TGF-β, which are termed natural TREG cells. TREG cells produce low levels of IL-2 and IFN-γ, but produce high levels of IL-10, IL-35 and TGF-β, suppressing immune responses to self-antigens and preventing autoimmune disease by two different immunoregulatory immunosuppressive or antiinflammatory cytokines, IL-10 and TGF-β, Fig 6.

More recently, a specific T-cell subset, termed Th17 cell, that secretes a cytokine called IL-17, has been identified. This cell develops from naïve CD4+ T cells in response to IL-6, IL-23, TGF-β and IL-1β. IL-6 and IL-23 activate STAT3, which increases the expression of RORγt and RORγ transcription factors, promoting the expression of IL-17A, IL-17F, IL-21 and IL-22. These cells, important for host defense against extracellular bacteria, are also involved in mediating autoimmune diseases [Chung & Dong, 2009; Stockinger & Veldhoen, 2007]. The immunopathogenic activities of Th17 cell in inflammation and autoimmunity has been linked to a growing list of cancers, autoimmune and inflammatory diseases such as rheumatoid arthritis, systemic lupus erythematosus, multiple sclerosis, asthma, psoriasis, systemic sclerosis, chronic inflammatory bowel disease and allograft rejection [Chung & Dong, 2009; McGeachy et al, 2009; Steinman, 2007].

Th1 and Th2 effector molecules antagonize the development of Th17 cells, which are responsible for destructive tissue pathology in autoimmune diseases including neuroinflammation; whereas, naïve CD4 cells in the presence of IL-12 and transcription factors, such as T-bet and STAT4, become Th1 cells, which express IL-12R and produce IFN-γ. Naïve CD4 cells in the presence of IL-4, GATA-3 and STAT6 become Th2 cells, which produce IL-4. Finally, naïve CD4 cells in the presence of TGF-β, IL-23 and transcription factor RORγt become IL-17-producing Th17 cells [Batten et al, 2006; Cheung et al, 2008].

As it was previously mentioned, the pathogenic contribution of Th1, Th2 and Th17 lymphocytes to autoimmune disorders has been reported both in systemic and in neurological diseases [Zheng et al; 2007]. IL-17-producing T-helper cells play an important role in the induction of neuroimmune diseases, like MS and its animal model called experimental autoimmune encephalomyelitis (EAE) [Iwakura & Ishigame, 2006.]. This observation is based on the detection of IL-17 levels in both the plaques and cerebrospinal fluid of MS patients [Ishizu et al, 2005].

It has been established that IL-17 is a proinflammatory cytokine that stimulates epithelial, fibroblast and endothelial cells to a produce other inflammatory chemokines and cytokines, including macrophage inflammatory protein (MIP)-2, monocyte chemoattractant protein (MCP-1), granulocyte-colony stimulating factor (G-CSF) and IL-6 and synergizes with IL-1β and TNF-a, to induce more chemokine expression [Vojdani & Lambert, 2011].

Also, microglia is known either as antigen presenting cells and effector cells and is involved in inflammatory demyelination of the CNS. It was shown that treatment of microglia with IL-17 upregulated microglia production of IL-6, MIP-2, nitric oxide, neurotrophic factors and adhesion molecules. In a similar way IL-1β and IL-23 may induce microglial IL-17 production, contributing to neuroimmune pathology in MS [Kawanokuchi et al, 2008]. An additional support to this hypothesis came from the experience in mice injected with specific antibodies against IL-17, which resulted in inhibition of chemokine expression, whereas overexpression of IL-17 in lung epithelia resulted in chemokine production and leukocyte infiltration [Vojdani & Lambert, 2011].

In MS, the location and distribution of CNS lesions under the influence of genetic susceptibility is determinant for clinical outcome and disease course and suggests that T-cell immune response specificity influences the sites of inflammation. A recent study published by Stromnes et al in 2008, demonstrated that T-cells specific to MBP epitopes generate two different populations of helper cells, Th17 and Th1 [Stromnes et al, 2008]. Notably, the Th17 to Th1 ratio of infiltrating T-cells determines that inflammation in the brain parenchyma occurs when the ratio of Th17 to Th1 cells is much greater than one, triggering a disproportionate increase of IL-17 in the brain that results in inflammation, Fig.6. At the same time, these results indicate that Th17, Th1 and their ratio, are main mechanisms regulating cell infiltration into the brain parenchyma.

Stromnes´ group also considered that a differential regulation of inflammation in the brain with a Th17:Th1 ratio >1, and in the spinal cord with a Th17: Th1 ratio <1, indicates that Th1 cells play a significant pathologic role in spinal cord autoimmunity [Stromnes et al, 2008]. It was concluded that IL-17 produced by Th17 cells is the major regulator of CNS autoimmunity. So, IL-17, deemed as the most pathogenic cytokine in inflammatory neuroimmune and autoimmune disorders, induces the activation of matrix metalloproteinase-3 (MMP-3) and recruits neutrophils to the site of inflammation, which also activates MMPs, proteases and gelatinases, contributing to BBB breakdown and a further enhancement of neutrophil recruitment. This increase in protease activity, which attracts a significant number of monocytes and macrophages to the inflammatory sites, with a subsequent citokine secretion and glial activation, reinforces the eventual myelin and axonal damage [Tester et al, 2007]. Thus, it is possible to consider that under CNS inflammatory conditions, microglia, which act as antigen presenting cells, produce IL-1β

and IL-23 and act in an autocrine manner, via IL-17 expression in microglia and IL-17-induced activation of MMP-3, contributing to neuroimmune pathology in MS.

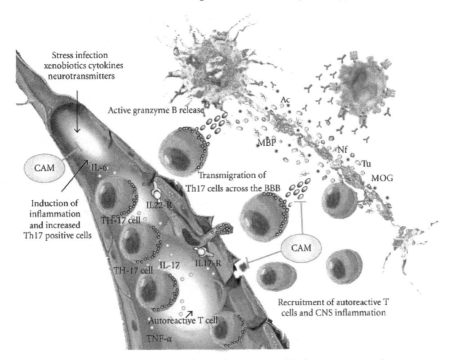

Fig. 6. The role of Th17 lymphocytes in the pathogenesis of inflammatory and neuroimmunological disorders. Environmental factors' induction of inflammatory response, production of cytokines and increase in the number of Th17 positive cells in circulation. Expression of IL-17 and IL-22 receptors on blood-brain barrier endothelial cells result in the binding of Th17 cells to BBB tight junctions. This disrupts the tight junctions, and the Th17 cells then transmigrate across the BBB, setting the stage for the killing of neurons by the release of granzyme B. CAM protocols may be used to block the inflammatory cascade induced by infection. CAM: Complementary alternative medicine, BBB; blood brain barrier. Taken from: The Role of Th17 in Neuroimmune Disorders: Target for CAM Therapy. Part II. In Hindawi Publishing Corporation Evidence-Based Complementary and Alternative Medicine, Volume 1-7, 2011.

Induction of BBB Disruption and Neuroinflammation mediated by IL 17 in MS

The BBB is composed of two layers: the microvascular endothelial cells and the glia limitans formed by glial foot processes [Maes et al 2007]. The perivascular space between the endothelial cells and astrocytes is populated by macrophages, which behave like immature dendritic cells [Vojdani & Lambert, 2011]; thus factors able to open the epithelial barrier will destroy both the BBB and neural tissue [Maes et al 2007; Maes et al, 2008].

Since microglia play a significant role in MS, to further strengthen the role of IL-17 in CNS inflammation, microglia were treated with IL-17. Treatment with IL-17 upregulated the microglial production of IL-6, MIP-2, nitric oxide, adhesion molecules and neurotrophic factors [Kawanokuchi et al, 2008]. Since it is known that IL-17 can be secreted by microglia in response to IL-1β or IL-23, these results strongly suggest that the cells co-expressing IL-17, IL-22 and granzyme B through the action of IL-17 and IL-22, play a significant role in the induction and breach in the BBB and its permeabilization to circulating CD4+ lymphocytes and soluble molecules resulting in CNS inflammation [Vojdani & Lambert, 2011]. The role of Th17 lymphocytes in the pathogenesis of inflammatory and neuroimmunological disorders is shown in Figure 6. This role of Th17 cells and the IL-17 produced by them in neuroinflammation could make these novel CD4 cells a suitable target for treatment in demyelinating diseases like MS.

Therapies towards BBB repair and the inhibition of lymphocyte transmigration can reduce neuro-inflammation, and at the same time, could be relevant since resident microglia and astrocytes, play an important role in the initiation and progression of immune responses induced by pathogen invasion or their antigens [Chauhan and Marriott ; 2007]. So, infections associated with high levels of inflammatory cytokines including IL-1β, IL-6, TNF-a and IL-17 in the CNS may result in neurological dysfunction. In this case, microglia and astrocytes via TLR and nucleotide-binding domain promote the recruitment and antigen-specific activation of infiltrating leukocytes [Rock et al.; 2004; Kielian; 2005].

Accumulated evidence has shown that substance P (SP), the most abundant tachykinin in the brain, also plays an important role in the inflammatory immune responses at peripheral sites [Vojdani & Lambert, 2011]. Neuropeptide SP, with its high affinity receptor NK-1R is expressed on microglia and can also modulate the function of myeloid cells, such as dendritic cells and macrophages via a high affinity receptor called neurokinin-1 (NK-1). SP with NK- 1R activate the transcription factor NF-κB, which facilitates the production of key proinflammatory cytokines such as TNF-a, IL-6 and IL-17, and also reduce the production of immunoregulatory cytokines (TGF-β, IL-10) by macrophages; thereby further exacerbating inflammation [Vojdani & Lambert, 2011]. The mechanism of bacterial antigens inducing the neuronal SP production and it's binding to SP receptors, result in cytokine production and brain inflammation. Furthermore, products, such as SP receptor antagonists for the inhibition of NF-κB, or minocycline, a-Lipoic acid, resveratrol [Aebischer & Kato; 2007; Lampl et al, 2007] or quercetin [Sternberg et al, 2008], which are known to be effective in the repair of BBB damaged by infections, may represent important new therapeutic strategies to combat potentially disabling consequences of inflammation within the brain.

2.4 Current perspective on treatment in MS

Further evidence to support the importance of neurodegeneration in MS is obtained from clinical data showing only a partial success of the available disease-modifying drugs (interferons, Glatiramer Acetate, monoclonal antibodies to antigenic determinants expressed on T lymphocytes, among others), which impede activation and migration of inflammatory cells via the BBB, but have no direct effect on the degenerative processes in the CNS. [Antel & Miron, 2008; Bergamaschi et al, 2006; De Jager , 2007; Miron et al, 2008; Weinstock-Guttman, 2006].

The research community has clarified the underlying biology of MS and shown great promises for developing an improved therapy. Areas of research that hold promise in the near future include: 1) the development of drugs that block the movement of myelin-attacking T cells from the bloodstream into the brain, 2) engineering drugs that specifically inhibit the damaging T cells or antibodies, 3) finding approaches that promote remyelination (myelin ro treatment in MS repair), which may allow individuals to regain function and 4) studies of MRI, immune, and genetic variables that improve our ability to predict the disease course, and tailor or engineer therapy to individuals with MS.

Trials of stem cell transplantation, with the goal of repopulating oligodendrocytes, are underway in people with MS. Remyelination may also be promoted by blocking leucine rich repeat and Ig domain-containing, Nogo Receptor-interacting protein 1 (LINGO-1), a protein on the surface of neurons that inhibits differentiation of precursor oligodendrocytes into mature cells. Antibody blockade of LINGO-1 has shown promise in an animal model of MS [Loeb, 2007]. Neurotrophins are protein factors produced by CNS cells that support neuronal growth, survival and differentiation [Azoulayet al, 2008]. In MS, secretion of the neurotrophin brain-derived neurotrophic factor is low and dysregulated [Mi et al, 2009] and BDNF is therefore also being considered as a therapeutic target. Current MS therapeutics are moderately effective for modifying disease during its relapsing-remitting phase. There are a number of oral and parenteral agents that target developing inflammation, and several are likely to be approved for treatment of RRMS within the next few years. These therapies will likely more effectively control RRMS but will also carry greater known and, as yet, unknown safety risks. These risks and benefits will have to be weighed carefully against the efficacy and proven safety of the IFNs and Glatiramer acetate. Furthermore, none of the anti-inflammatory therapies currently in late stage of development are likely to benefit patients with SPMS and PPMS. Development of effective neuroprotective and neurorestorative therapies are needed in order to benefit patients with progressive MS.

3. Conclusion

Since MS shows a great heterogeneity, the influence of multiple etiopathogenic factors could be considered as the main cause of this behavioral pattern. Nevertheless the well established hypothesis on the aetiology and pathogenic mechanisms described for this disease are not enough, at least to explain the wide clinical variations in response to treatment. From this view point, it is true that serious contributions have been achieved, but more protocols must be conducted for a major understanding of MS pathology, as well as for a more effective response to treatment.

4. References

Abbott NJ 2002 .Astrocyte–endothelial interactions and blood–brain barrier permeability. J. Anat. 2009, 629–638.

Aebischer P and. Kato A C. 2007. Playing defense against Lou Gehrig's disease. *Scientific American*, 297: 86– 93.

Amor S, Giovannoni G. 2007 Antibodies to myelin oligodendrocyte glycoprotein as a biomarker in multiple sclerosis—are we there yet? Mult Scler, 13:1083–1085.

Amor S, Puentes F, Baker D & van der Valk P. 2010. Inflammation in neurodegenerative diseases. Immunology, 129: 154–169.

Anderson, C.M. and Swanson, R.A. 2000 Astrocyte glutamate transport: review of properties, regulation, and physiological functions. Glia 32: 1–14.

Anderson, M, Alvarez-Cermeño, J, Bernardi, G & Cogato, I. 1994. Cerebro Spinal fluid in the diagnosis of multiple sclerosis: a consensus report. J Neurol Neurosurg Psych, 57: 897-902.

Antel JP & Miron VE. 2008. Central nervous system effects of current and emerging multiple sclerosis-directed immuno-therapies. Clinical Neurology and Neurosurgery 110: 951-957 .

Arumugam TV, Woodruff TM, Lathia JD, Selvaraj PK, Mattson MP, Taylor SM. 2009 Neuroprotection in stroke by complement inhibition and immunoglobulin therapy. Neuroscience.

Azoulay D, Urshansky N, Karni A. 2008Low and dysregulated BDNF secretion from immune cells of MS patients is related to reduced neuroprotection. *J Neuroimmunol,* 195:186-193.

Babbe, H, Roers, A & Waisman, A. 2000. Clonal expansion CD8+ T cells dominate the T cell infiltrate in active multiple sclerosis lesions as shown by micromanipulation and single cell polymerasa chain reaction. J Exp Med, 192: 393-404.

Barnett M.H. &, Sutton I. 2006. The pathology of multiple sclerosis: a paradigm shift. Curr Opin Neurol , 19: 242-47.

Bartos A, Fialova L, Soukupova J, Kukal J, Malbohan I & Pitha J. 2007 Antibodies against light neurofilaments in multiple sclerosis patients. Acta Neurol Scand,116: 100-7.

Bartos A, Fialova L, SoukupovÃ¡ J, Kukal J, Malbohan I & Pitha J. 2007a. Elevated intrathecal antibodies against the medium neurofilament subunit in multiple sclerosis. J Neurol, 254: 20-25.

Batten M., Li J., Yi S et al. 2006. Interleukin 27 limits autoimmune encephalomyelitis by suppressing the development of interleukin 17-producing T cells. Nature Immunology, 7: 929-936.

Becher B, Bechmann, I & Greter, M. 2006. Antigen presentation in autoimmunity and CNS inflammation: how T lymphocytes recognize the brain. J Mol Med; 84: 532-43.

Bejartmar C, Trapp B.D. 2003. Axonal degeneration and progressive neurologic disability in multiple sclerosis. Neurotox Res , 5: 157-64.

Bergamaschi R, Kappos L, Antel J, Comi G, Montalban X, O'Connor P, et al. 2006. Oral Fingolimod (FTY720) for Relapsing Multiple Sclerosis. N Engl J Med; 355: 1124-40.

Bielekova, B, Kadom, M & Fisher, E. 2005 MRI as a marker for disease heterogeneity in Multiple sclerosis. Neurology, 65: 1071-76.

Bigio, MR. 1995. The ependyma. A protective barrier between brain and cerebrospinal fluid. Glia; 14:1-13.

Bolton C, Paul C. MK-801 limits neurovascular dysfunction during experimental allergic encephalomyelitis. J Pharmacol Exp Ther 1997; 282: 397-402.

Brown K.A. 2001. Factors modifying the migration of lymphocytes across the blood-brain barrier. Int Immunopharmacol, 1: 2043-62.

Cabre P, Signate,A, Olindo, S; Merle,H ; Caparros-Lefebvre, D, et al. 2005. Role of return migration in the emergence of multiple sclerosis in the French West Indies. Brain, 128: 2899-2910.

Camerona EM; Spencera S; Lazarinia, J; Harpa, CT; Wardb,ES; et al.2009. Potential of a unique antibody gene signature to predict conversion to clinically definite Multiple Sclerosis. J Neuroimmunol, 213: 123-130.

Carson, M.J.; Bilousova, T.V.; Puntambekar, S.S.; Melchior, B.; Doose, J.M.; Ethell, I.M. 2007. A rose by any othername? The potential consequences of microglial heterogeneity during CNS health and disease. Neurotherapeutics, 4: 571-579

Chabas, D; Ness, J; Belman, A; Yeh, EA; Kuntz, N; Gorman, MP; et al. 2010. Younger children with MS have a distinct CSF inflammatory profile at disease onset. Neurology, 74: 399-405.

Chauhan V S & Marriott I. 2007. Bacterial infections of the central nervous system: a critical role for resident glial cells in the initiation and progression of inflammation. Curr Immunol Rev, 3: 133-143.

Cheung P.F.Y., Wong C.K., and Lam C.W.K. 2008. Molecular mechanisms of cytokine and chemokine release from eosinophils activated by IL-17a, IL-17f and IL-23: implication for Th17 lymphocyte-mediated allergic inflammation. J Immunol 180: 5625-35.

Chung Y. & Dong C. 2009. Don't leave home without it: the IL- 23 visa to TH-17 cells. Nat Immunol, 10: 236-38.

Cohrs RJ, Gilden DH. 2005. Prevalence and abundance of latently transcribed varicella-zoster virus genes 17. Nature Immunol 6: 1133-41.

Coles AJ, Cox, A, Le Page, E. 2006. The window of therapeutic opportunity in multiple sclerosis: Evidence for monoclonal antibody therapy. J Neurol, 253: 98-108.

Colleen MK, Burns BA, and KevinAA. 2006. Does rubella immunity predict méasles immunity? A serosurvey of pregnant women.Infectious Disease Obstetrics and Gynecology. Clinical Study. Hindawi Publishing Corporation. pp. 23.

Colton C.A.; Wilcock, D.M. 2010. Assessing activation states in microglia. CNS Neurol. Disord. Drug Targets, 9: 174-191.

Cooper LZ, Alford CA. 2001. Rubella. In: Remington JS, Klein, JO, eds. Infectious diseases of the fetus and newborninfant. London: W.B. Saunders; 347–87.

Correales J. 2004. Oligoclonal bands and antibody response in multiple sclerosis.In: Focus on Multiple sclerosis Research. Frank Columbus (ed): pp. 37-65.

De Jager, PL & Hafler, DA. 2007. New therapeutic approaches for multiple sclerosis. Annu Rev Med, 58:417-432.

Del Zoppo, GJ & Hallenbeck, JM 2000. Advances in the vascularpathophysiology of ischemic stroke. Thromb. Res. 98: 73–81.

Departamento de análisis de datos. 2004. Dirección nacional de estadística y registros médicos. Ministerio de Salud Pública de Cuba, Havana City, Cuba.

Devries HG 2006. Cryptic axonal antigens and axonal loss in multiple sclerosis. Neuroch Res, 29:1999- 2004.

Dutta R, Trapp BD. Pathogenesis of axonal and neuronal damage in multiple sclerosis. Neurology 2007. 68(Suppl 3): S22–S31.

Eikelenboom MJ, Petzold A, Lazeron RHC, Silber E, Sharief M, Thompson EJ; et al. 2003 Neurofilament light chain antibodies are correlated to cerebral atrophy. Neurology, 60: 219-23.

Falip M; Tintore, M; Jardi, R; Duran, I; Link; H & Montalban, X. 2001.Utilidad clínica de las bandas oligoclonales. Rev Neurol, 32: 1120-24.

Ferreira S, D'Cruz DP, Hughes GRV. 2005. Multiple sclerosis, neuropsychiatric lupus and antiphospholipid syndrome: where do we stand? Rheumatology (Oxford); 44: 434–442.

Fisher LJ & Gage, F.H. 1993. Grafting in the mammalian central nervous system. Physiol Rev, 73: 583-16.

Forman, ME; Racke, KM & Raine, SC. 2006. Multiple Sclerosis- the plaque and its pathogenesis. N Eng J Med, 354: 942-55.

Fox RJ, Bethoux F, Goldman MD, Cohen JA. 2006. Multiple sclerosis: advances in understanding, diagnosing, and treating the underlying disease. Cleve Clin J Med, 73: 91-102.

Frederick TJ, Miller SD. 2007. Arresting autoimmunity by blocking beta-arrestin-1. Nat Immunol; 8: 791–792.

Friese, MA & Fugger, L. 2005. Autoreactive CD8+ T cells in multiple sclerosis: a new target for therapy? Brain, 128: 1747–63.

Frischer J M, Bramow S, Dal-Bianco A, Lucchinetti CF,Rauschka H, Schmidbauer M, Laureen H, Sorensen PS & Lassmann H. 2009. The relation between inflammation and neurodegeneration in multiple sclerosis brains. Brain, 132; 1175–1189.

Fujinami RS, von Herrath MG, Christen U, Whitton JL. 2006. Molecular mimicry, bystander activation, or viral persistence: infections and autoimmune disease. Clin Microbiol Rev, 19: 80–94.

Gandhi, KS, McKay FC, Schibeci SD, Arthur JW, Heard RN, StewartGJ & Booth DR. 2008. BAFF is a Biological Response Marker to IFN-β Treatment in Multiple Sclerosis. J Inter & Cytok Res 28: 529–540.

Ghafourifar P, Mousavizadeh K, Parihar MS, et al. Mitochondria in multiple sclerosis. 2008. Front Biosci 13: 3116–3126.

Gorczyca WA, Ejma M, Witkowska D, et al. 2004. Retinal antigens are recognized by antibodies present in sera of patients with multiple sclerosis. Ophthalmic Res; 36: 120-123.

Groom AJ, Smith T, Turski L Xiong ZQ, Qian W, Suzuki K, et al. 2003. Formation of complement membrane attack complex in mammalian cerebral cortex evokes seizures and neurodegeneration. J Neurosci; 23: 955-960.

Haahr S, Hollsberg P. 2006. Multiple sclerosis is linked to Epstein-Barr virus infection. Rev Med Virol, 16: 297-10.

Haukins, BT & Davis, TP. 2005. The blood-brain barrier/neurovascular unit in health and disease. Pharmacol Rev, 57: 173-85.

Hauser SL, Waubant E, Arnold DL, , et al. 2008. Hermes Trial Group. B-cell depletion with rituximab in relapsing-remitting multiple sclerosis. N Engl J Med; 358: 676–688.

Hemmer, B, Cepok, S, Zhou, D & Sommer, N. 2004. Multiple sclerosis – a coordinated immune attack across the blood brain barrier. Current Neurovasc Res; 1: 141-50.

Hermitte L, Martin-Moutot N, Boucraut J, et al. 2000. Humoral immunity against glutamic acid decarboxylase and tyrosine phosphatase IA-2. J Clin Immunol; 20: 287-293.

Hickey, WF. 2001. Basic principles of immunological surveillance of the normal central nervous system. Glia, 36: 118–24.

Hillert J. 2006. Multiple sclerosis: postlinkage genetics. Clin Neurol Neurosurg , 108:220-2.

Huizinga R, Linington C, Amor S. 2008. Resistance is futile: antineuronal autoimmunity in multiple sclerosis. Trends Immunol ; 29: 54–60.

Ishizu T, Osoegawa M., Mei F.-J. et al, 2005. Intrathecal activation of the IL-17/IL-8 axis in opticospinal multiple sclerosis. Brain, 128: 988–1002.

Ishizu, KJ. 2009. Intrathecal activation of the IL-17-IL-8 axis in opticospinal multiple sclerosis. Pharmacol Res, 128: 207-09.

Iwakura Y. & Ishigame. 2006. The IL-23/IL-17 axis in inflammation. J Clin Invest, 116: 1218-22.

Jack, C; Jack, A, Wolfgang B & Tanja K. 2007. Contrasting Potential of Nitric Oxide and Peroxynitrite to Mediate Oligodendrocyte Injury in Multiple Sclerosis. GLIA 55: 926-934.

Jarius S, Eichhorn P, Jacobi C, Wildemann B, Wick M, Voltz R. 2009. The intrathecal, polyspecific antiviral immune response: Specific for MS or a general marker of CNS autoimmunity? J Neurol Sci, 280: 98-100.

Jarius S. 2008. Polyspecific, antiviral immune response distinguishes multiple sclerosis and neuromyelitis optica. Nature Clin Pract Neurol; 4: 524.

Jiang, H & Chess, L. 2006. Regulation of immune response by T cell. New Engl J Med 354: 1166-76.

Kanda T, Iwasaki T, Yamawaki M, et al. 2000. Anti-GM1 antibody facilitates leakage in an in vitro blood-nerve barrier model. Neurology; 55: 585-87.

Kawanokuchi J, Shimizu K., Nitta A. et al. 2008. Production and functions of IL-17 in microglia. J Neuroimmunol, 194: 54-61.

Kang, J. 1998 Astrocyte-mediated potentiation of inhibitory synaptic transmission. Nat. Neurosci, 1: 683-92.

Keegan M, Kónig F, McClelland R, et al. 2005. Relation between humoral pathological changes in multiple sclerosis and response to therapeutic plasma exchange. Lancet; 366: 579-82.

Kielian T, Esen N and Bearden E. D. 2005. Toll-like receptor 2 (TLR2) is pivotal for recognition of S. aureus peptidoglycan but not intact bacteria by microglia. GLIA, 49: 567-76.

Kira J. 2007. Etiology of multiple sclerosis. In: Multiple Sclerosis for the Practicing Neurologist. Theodore (ed). pp. 1-6, Demos Medical Publishing LLC, Vol 5, New York.

Klawiter, EC & Cross, AH. 2007. B cells: no longer the nondominant arm of multiple sclerosis. Curr Neurol Neurosci Rep; 7: 231-238.

Komek, BL. 2003. Neuropathology of multiple sclerosis-new concepts. Brain Res Bull, 61: 321-26.

Kraft AD & Harry GJ. 2011. Features of Microglia and Neuroinflammation Relevant to Environmental Exposure and Neurotoxicity Int. J. Environ. Res. Public Health, 8: 2980-3018

Lambracht-Washington D, O'Connor KC, Cameron EM, et al. 2007. Antigen specificity of clonally expanded and receptor edited cerebrospinal fluid B cells from patients with relapsing remitting MS. J Neuroimmunol; 186: 164-76.

Lampl Y, Boaz M, Gilad R, et al. 2007. Minocycline treatment in acute stroke: an open-label, evaluator-blinded study. Neurology, 69: 1404-10.

Lassmann H, Niedobitek G,Aloisi F, & Middeldorp JM. 2011. Epstein–Barr virus in the multiple sclerosis brain: a controversial issue — report on a focused workshop held in the Centre for Brain Research of the Medical University of Vienna, Austria. Brain: 134: 2772-86.

Lee, MA, Palace D, Palace J. 2007. The diagnostic and differential diagnostic in multiple sclerosis.In: Multiple Sclerosis for the Practicing Neurologist Theodore E (ed). New York: Demos Medical Publishing, LLC, Vol 5, p. 33-50.

Levin LI, Munger KL, O'Reilly EJ, Falk KI, Ascherio A. 2010, Primary infection with Epstein-Barr virus and risk of multiple sclerosis. Ann Neurol; 67: 824-30.

Lim, ET, Sellebjerg, F, Jensen, CV, Altmann, DR, Grant, D & Keir, G. 2005 .Acute axonal damage predicts clinical outcome in patients with multiple sclerosis. Mult Scler ,11: 532-6.

Lindberg RL, Achtnichts L, Hoffmann F, et al. 2008. Natalizumab alters transcriptional expression profiles of blood cell subpopulations of multiple sclerosis patients. J Neuroimmunol; 194: 153-64.

Lipton SA, Rosenberg PA. 1994. Excitatory amino acids as a final common pathway for neurologic disorders. N Engl J Med; 330: 613-22.

Lisak, PR. 2007.Neurodegeneration in multiple sclerosis.Defining the problem. Neurology 2007; 68: S5-S12.

Loeb JA. 2007. Neuroprotection and repair by neurotrophic and gliotrophic factors in multiple sclerosis. Neurology; 68(Suppl 3): 38-54.

Lovato L, Willis SN, Rodig SJ, Caron T, Almendinger SE, Howell OW, et al. 2011. Related B cell clones populate the meninges and parenchyma of patients with multiple sclerosis. Brain; 134: 534-41.

Lu F, Kalman B. 1999. Autoreactive IgG to intracellular proteins in sera of MS patients. J Neuroimmunol; 99:72-81.

Lu J, Murakami M, Verma SC, Cai Q, Haldar S, Kaul R, et al. 2011. Epstein-Barr virus nuclear antigen 1 (EBNA1) confers resistance to apoptosis in EBV-positive B-lymphoma cells through upregulation of survivin. Virology; 410: 64-75.

Lucchinetti, C, Brück W, Scheithauer B, Rodriguez M Lassman H. 2000, Heterogeneity of multiple sclerosis lesions: implications for the pathogenesis of demyelination. Ann Neurol, 47: 707-17.

Luchinetti CF. 2007. Advances in the neuropathology of multiple sclerosis: evolving pathogenesis insight. Continuum Lifelong Learning. Neurology 13: 86-116.

Lutterotti A, Berger T, Reindl M. 2007. Biological markers for multiple sclerosis. Curr Med Chem; 14:1956-65.

Maes M, Kubera M., and Leunis JC. 2008. The gut-brain barrier in major depression: intestinal mucosal dysfunction with an increased translocation of LPS from gram negative enterobacteria (leaky gut) plays a role in the inflammatory pathophysiology of depression. Neuroendocrinol Letters, 29: 117-24.

Maes M, Coucke F, and Leunis JC. 2007. Normalization of the increased translocation of endotoxin from gram negative enterobacteria (leaky gut) is accompanied by a remission of chronic fatigue syndrome. Neuroendocrinol Letters, 28: 739-44.

Maghzi AH, Marta M, Bosca I, Etemadifar M, Dobson R, Maggiore C, et al. 2010. Viral pathophysiology of multiple sclerosis: a role for Epstein-Barr virus infection? Pathophysiology; 18: 13-20.

Magliozzi R, Howell OW, Reeves C, Roncaroli F, Nicholas R, Serafini B, et al. 2010. A gradient of neuronal loss and meningeal inflammation in multiple sclerosis. Ann Neurol; 68: 477-93.

Maier O, Baron W, Hoekstra D. 2007. Reduced raft-association of NF155 in active MS-lesions is accompanied by the disruption of the paranodal junction. Glia; 55: 885–95.

Marconi S, Acler M, Lovato L, et al. 2006. Anti-GD2-like IgM autoreactivity in multiple sclerosis patients. Mult Scler; 12: 302–08.

Martinez, A; Mas, A; de las Heras, V; Arroyo, R; Fernandez-Arquero, M; de la Concha, EG et al. 2005. Early B-cell Factor gene association with multiple sclerosis in the Spanish population. BMC Neurol, 5: 19-22.

Martinez-Yélamos, S, Ballabriga, J, Martinez-Yélamos, A, Hernandez, JJ & Arbizu, T. 1998. Evolución y pronóstico de la esclerosis múltiple. Medicine; 7: 4333-37.

Mathey EK, Derfuss T, Storch MK, et al. 2007. Neurofascin as a novel target for autoantibody-mediated axonal injury. J Exp Med; 204: 2363–72.

Matute C, Domercq M, Sanchez-Gomez MV. 2006. Glutamate-mediated glial injury: mechanisms and clinical importance. Glia; 53: 212–24.

McCoy, L; Tsunoda, I & Fuginami, RS. 2006. Multiple sclerosis and virus induced immune responses: autoimmunity can be primed by molecular mimicry and augmented by bystander activation. Autoimmunity, 39: 9-19.

McDonald, W, Compston, A, Edan, G, Hangtung, H, Lublin, F, McFarland H et al. 2001. Recommended diagnostic criteria for multiple sclerosis. Ann Neurol , 50: 121-27.

McGeachy M. J., Chen Y, Tato C.M et al. 2009. The interleukin 23 receptor is essential for the terminal differentiation of interleukin 17-producing effector T helper cells in vivo. Nat Immunol, 10: 314–24.

Meinl E, Krumbholz M, Derfuss T, Junker A,Hohlfeld R. 2008. Comparmentalization of inflammaion in the CNS:A major mechanism driving progressive multiple sclerosis. J Neurol Sci; 274: 42-44.

Mi S, Miller RH, Tang W, Lee X, Hu B, Wu W, Zhang Y, Shields CB, Zhang Y, Miklasz S, Shea D, Mason J, Franklin RJ, Ji B, Shao Z, Chédotal A, Bernard F, Roulois A, Xu J, Jung V, Pepinsky B. *2009*. Promotion of central nervous system remyelination by induced differentiation of oligodendrocyte precursor cells. *Ann Neurol*; 65: 304–15.

Miron VE, Jung CG, Kim HJ, Kennedy TE, Soliven B &. Antel JP. 2008. FTY720 Modulates Human. Oligodendrocyte Progenitor Process Extension and Survival Ann Neurol; 63: 61–71.

Mirsattari, SM, Johnston, J, McKenna R, et al. 2001. Aborigenals with multiple sclerosis HLA types and proedominance of neuromyelitis óptica. Neurology, 56: 317-23.

Monteleone G., Pallone F, & MacDonald T.T. 2008. Interleukin- 21: a critical regulator of the balance between effector and regulatory T-cell responses. Trends Immunol, 29: 290–94.

Mosmann T. R.; H. Cherwinski, M.W.; Bond, M.A.; Giedlin, & Coffman R.L. 1986. Two types of murine helper T cell clone. I. Definition according to profiles of lymphokine activities and secreted proteins. J Immunol, 136: 2348–57.

Nag, S. 2003. Pathophysiology of blood brain barrier breakdown. Methods Mol Med, 89: 97-111.

Nathanson, JA & Chun, LYL. 1990. Possible role of the choroid plexus in immunological communication between the brain and periphery. BB Johansson, Ch Owman, H Widner (Eds). In. Pathophysiology of the blood brain barrier, Elsevier Science Publisher, pp. 501 505.New York.

Nathanson, JA, Chun, LYL. 1990a. Immunological function of the blood- cerebrospinal fluid barrier. Proc Natl Acad Sci. USA, 86: 1684-88.

Ness, JM; Chabas, D; Sadovnick, AD; Pohl, D; Banwell, B & Weinstock-Guttman, B. 2007. Clinical features of children and adolescents with multiple sclerosis. Neurology, 68; 37-45.

Neumann, H, Medana, IM, Bawer, J & Lassmann, H. 2002. Cytotoxic T lymphocyte in autoimmune and degenerative CNS diseases. Trends Neurosci, 25: 313-19.

Neutwelt, E, Abbott, NJ , Abrey, L, Banks, W A, Blakley, B, Davis, T, et al. 2008. Strategies to advance translational research into brain barriers. Lancet Neurol; 7: 84-96.

O'Connor KC, Cameron EM, et al. 2007. Antigen specificity of clonally expanded and receptor edited cerebrospinal fluid B cells from patients with relapsing remitting MS. J Neuroimmunol; 186: 164–76.

Owens GP, Burgoon MP, Anthony J, et al. 2001. The immunoglobulin G heavy chain repertoire in multiple sclerosis plaques is distinct from the heavy chain repertoire in peripheral blood lymphocytes. Clin Immunol; 98: 258–263.

Pender MP. 2011. The essential role of Epstein-Barr Virus in the pathogenesisof multiple sclerosis. Neuroscientist, 17: 351–67.

Perry, V H & Gordon, S. 1997. Microglias and macrophages. In: Immunology of the nervous system, R W Keane and WE Hickey (eds), pp (155-172) Oxford University Press,New York.

Petty, MA & Lo, HE. 2002. Junctional complexes of the blood–brain barrier: permeability changes in neuroinflammation. Prog Neurobiol, 68: 311–23.

Pittock, SJ, Mayr, WT, McClelland RL. 2004. Change in MS-related disability in a population- based cohort: a 10- year follow–up study. Neurology; 62: 51-59.

Porras-Betancourt, M; Nuñez-Orozco, L; Plascencia-Alvarez, NI; Quiñones-Aguilar, S & Sauri-Suarez, S. 2007. Esclerosis Multiple. Rev Mex Neurosc 8: 57-66.

Prat A, Antel J. 2005. Pathogenesis of multiple sclerosis.Curr Opin Neurol , 18: 225-30.

Rauer, S; Euler, B; Reindl,M & Berger TH. 2006. Antimyelin antibodies and the risk of relapse in patients with a primary demyelinating event. J Neurol Neurosurg Psychiatry, 77: 739–42.

Redzic, ZB, Preston, JE, Duncan, JA, Chdobski, A & Szmydynger Chdobsk, J. 2005. The choroid plexus- cerebrospinal fluid system from development to ageing. Curr Top Dev Biol, 71: 1-52.

Reese, TS & Karnowosky, MJ 1967. Fine structural localization of a blood-brain barrier to exogenous peroxidase. J Cell Biol 34: 207-17.

Reiber H, Ungefehr ST, Jacobi CHR. 1998. The intrathecal, polyspecific and oligoclonal immune response in multiple sclerosis. Mult Scler; 4: 111–17.

Rivest S. 2009. Regulation of innate immune responses in the brain. Nat. Rev. Immunol, 9: 429-39.

Robinson-Agramonte MA. 2010. Asimilación del método de focalización isoeléctrica en agarosa y aplicación del ELISA al estudio de la respuesta de anticuerpos en el sistema nervioso central de personas con esclerosis múltiple. Revista CENIC Ciencias Biológicas, 21: 206-07.

Robinson-Agramonte M, Reiber H, Cabrera-Gomez JA, Galvizu R. 2007. Intrathecal polyspecific immune response to neurotropic viruses inmultiple sclerosis: a comparative report from Cuban patients. Acta Neurol Scand, 115: 312–18.

Robinson-Agramonte M, Reiber H, Dorta-Contreras AJ,Herna´ndez-Dıaz E. 2001. Respuesta inmune intratecal oligoclonaly poliespecı´fica en la esclerosis múltiple. Rev Neurol; 33: 809–11.

Rock R. B, Gekker G, Hu S et al. 2004. Role ofmicroglia in central nervous system infections. Clinical Microbiology Reviews, 17: 942–64.

Rose, WJ & Carlson, GN. 2007. Pathogenesis of multiple sclerosis. Continuum Lifelong Learning Neurol , 13: 35-62.

Roussel V, Yi F, Jauberteau MO, et al. 2000. Prevalence and clinical significance of anti-phospholipid antibodies in multiple sclerosis: a study of 89 patients. J Autoimmun; 14: 259–65.

Sarchielli P, Greco L, Floridi A, et al. 2003. Excitatory amino acids and multiple sclerosis: evidence from cerebrospinal fluid. Arch Neurol; 60: 1082–88.

Semra YK, Seidi OA, Sharief MK. 2002. Heightened intrathecal release of axonal cytoskeletal proteins in multiple sclerosis is associated with progressive disease and clinical disability. J Neuroimmunol, 122: 132-39.

Serafini B, Severa M, Columba-Cabezas S, Rosicarelli B, Veroni C, Chiappetta G, et al. 2010. Epstein-Barr virus latent infection and BAFF expression in B-cells in the multiple sclerosis brain: implications for viral persistence and intrathecal B-cell activation. J Neuropath Exp Neurol; 69: 677–93.

Seyfert, S & Faultish, A. 2003. Is the blood-CSF barrier alterated in disease? Acta Neurol Scand, 108: 252-56.

Shi Y, Feng Y, Kang J, et al. 2007. Critical regulation of CD4+ T cell survival and autoimmunity by beta-arrestin-1. Nat Immunol; 8: 817–24.

Silber, E; Semra, YK; Gregson, NA & Sharief MK. 2002. Patients with progressive multiple sclerosis have elevated antibodies to neurofilament subunit. Neurology 58: 1372-78.

Smith T, Groom A, Zhu B, et al. 2000. Autoimmune encephalomyelitis ameliorated byAMPA antagonists. Nat Med; 6: 62–66.

Sobel, RA. 1998. The extracellular matrix in multiple sclerosis lesions.J Neuropathol Exp Neurol, 57: 205–17

Sospedra, M &. Martin, R. 2009. MRI criteria in MS patients with negative and positive oligoclonal bands: equal fulfillment of Barkhof's criteria but different lesion patterns. J Neurol, 256: 1121-25.

Steinman L. 2007. A brief history of TH17, the first major revision in the TH1/TH2 hypothesis of T cell-mediated tissue damage. Nature Medicine, 13: 139–45.

Sternberg Z, Chadha K, Lieberman A et al. 2008. Quercetin and interferon-β modulate immune response(s) in peripheral blood mononuclear cells isolated from multiple sclerosis patients. Journal of Neuroimmunology, 205: 142–47.

Stockinger & Veldhoen M. 2007. Differentiation and function of Th17 T cells. Curr Op Immunol,19: 281–86.

Chung Y. & Dong C. 2009. Don't leave home without it: the IL- 23 visa to TH-17 cells. Nat Immunol, 10: 236–38.

Stromnes I. M., Cerretti L.M, Liggitt D., Harris R.A. & Goverman J. M. 2008. Differential regulation of central nervous system autoimmunity by TH1 and TH17 cells. Nature Medicine, 14: 337–42.

Stys PK, Lipton SA. 2007. White matter NMDA receptors: an unexpected new therapeutic target? Trends Pharmacol Sci; 28: 561–66.

Taplin CE, Barker JM. 2008. Autoantibodies in type 1 diabetes. Autoimmunity; 41: 11–18.

Tester A.M., Cox J. H., Connor A. R. et al, 2007. LPS responsiveness and neutrophil chemotaxis in vivo require PMN MMP-8 activity. PLoS ONE, 2: article e312.

Theiss C, Napirei M, Meller K. 2005. Impairment of anterograde and retrograde neurofilament transport after anti-kinesin and anti-dynein antibody microinjection in chicken dorsal root ganglia. Eur J Cell Biol 84: 29–43.

Torkildsen, O; Vedeler, CA; Nyland, HI; Myhr KM. 2006. FcγR and multiple sclerosis: an overview. Acta Neurol Scand ,113: 61–63.

Vercellino M, Merola A, Piacentino C, et al. 2007. Altered glutamate reuptake in relapsing-remitting and secondary progressive multiple sclerosis cortex: correlation with microglia infiltration, demyelination, and neuronal and synaptic damage. J Neuropathol Exp Neurol; 66: 732–39.

Villar, LM; Sádaba,MC;Roldán, E; Masjuan, J; González, P; Villarrubia, N; et al. 2005. Intrathecal synthesis of oligoclonal IgM against myelin lipids predicts an aggressive disease course in MS. J Clin Invest,115 :187-90.

Vojdani A & Lambert J. 2011a The Role of Th17 inNeuroimmuneDisorders: Target for CAM Therapy. Part II Hindawi Publishing Corporation Evidence-Based Complementary and Alternative Medicine Volume 1-7.

Vojdani A & Lambert; J. 2011.The Role of Th17 inNeuroimmuneDisorders: Target for CAM Therapy. Part I Hindawi Publishing Corporation Evidence-Based Complementary and Alternative Medicine Volume 1-8.

Vyshkina T & Kalman B. 2008. Autoantibodies and neurodegeneration in multiple sclerosis. Lab Invest, 1-12.

Wallstrom E, Diener P, Ljungdahl A, et al. 1996. Memantine abrogates neurological deficits, but not CNS inflammation, in Lewis rat experimental autoimmune encephalomyelitis. J Neurol Sci; 137: 89–96.

Weinstock-Guttman B; Ramanathan M; Lincoff N; Napoli SQ; Sharma J; et al. 2006. Study of Mitoxantrone for the Treatment of Recurrent Neuromyelitis Optica Devic Disease. Arch Neurol, 63: 957-63.

Wilson C. B, Rowell E. & Sekimata M. 2009. Epigenetic control of T-helper-cell differentiation. Nat Rev Immunol, 9: 91–105.

Winer JB. 2001. Guillain Barre syndrome. Mol Pathol; 54: 381–85.

Wingerchuck, D & Kantarci O. 2006. Epidemiology and natural history of multiple sclerosis: new insights. Curr Opin Neurol, 19: 248-54.

Zaffaroni M. 2003. Biological indicators of the neurodegenerative phase of multiple sclerosis. Neurol Sci; 24 (Suppl 5): S279–S282.

Zheng et al. 2007. Interleukin-22, a TH17 cytokine, mediates IL-23-induced dermal inflammation and acanthosis. Nature, 445 (7128): 648–51.

9

The CNS Innate Immune System and the Emerging Roles of the Neuroimmune Regulators (NIRegs) in Response to Infection, Neoplasia and Neurodegeneration

J. W. Neal[2], M. Denizot[1], J. J. Hoarau[1] and P. Gasque[1]

[1]*GRI, Immunopathology and Infectious Disease Research Grouping (IRG, GRI),*
University of La Reunion,
[2]*Neuropathology Laboratory, Dept. of Histopathology, Cardiff University Medical School,*
[1]*Reunion Island*
[2]*UK*

1. Introduction

The mammalian CNS relies upon the ancient, innate immune system, to provide defence against attack by pathogens (virus, bacteria, fungi and parasites) and the clearance of both neurotoxic proteins and apoptotic cells. The main function(s) of the CNS innate immune system can be summarised as the detection of "non self"(pathogens) and " altered self " (neurotoxic proteins and apoptotic cells), with their subsequent clearance, designed to facilitate tissue repair and rapid return to normal function. The failure to express an effective protective response to detect and remove a pathogen (non –self) prolongs the innate immune response and this is associated with autoimmunity, chronic inflammatory diseases (Multiple sclerosis) and neuro degeneration (Alzheimer's and Prion disease) (Hauwel et al., 2005 Griffiths et al., 2009). The failure to detect and clear apoptotic cells results in their accumulation and subsequent release of neurotoxic proteins and enzymes, contributing to excessive tissue damage (Griffiths et al., 2009).

2. The blood brain barrier and immuno privilege

Insects, have a brain lymph barrier, whereas, the vertebrate blood brain barrier (BBB) evolved 50-100 million years before the appearance of the adaptive immune system (Abbot 1995; Lowenstein 2002). For this reason, the CNS immune response against pathogens relies upon the ancient and highly conserved innate immune system that first appeared in limited form in the Agnatha, 500 million years ago and almost 100 million years before the emergence of the systemic adaptive immune system in bony fish. (Lowenstein 2002). The vertebrate type BBB, was therefore present, long before the adaptive immune system and this barrier provide some immunoregulatory control of the CNS response to pathogens (Abbot 1995; Lowenstein 2002).

Other protective physical barriers, are the choroid plexus between the systemic circulation and ventricular CSF (cerebro spinal fluid) and the specialized, ciliated ependymal (glia) layer, that lines ventricles containing the CSF(Martino et al., 2001). Both these epithelial layers express highly conserved receptors that are able to detect pathogens in the CSF and regulate intra CSF inflammation (McMenamin., 1999; Laflamme and Rivest 2001; Canova et al., 2006; Rivest 2009).

The presence of a BBB composed of endothelial cells linked by tight junctions and surrounded by astrocyte foot processes (Pachter et al., 2003) contributed to the development of homeostatic systems to preserve CNS electrolyte and hydrostatic pressure gradients (Abott 1995). To some extent, this also prevented infiltration into the brain by systemic cells (lymphocytes, myeloid related cells) of the more recent adaptive immune system and provided some evidence of immuno regulatory function. Once the vertebrate BBB had developed, the brain relied upon the resident glia and neurons (also perivascular cells and choroid plexus) to deliver the CNS immune response against pathogen invasion (Lowenstein 2002).

To reflect this function, the resident glial cells have been termed" amateur "innate immune cells, in contrast with the" professional" innate immune system cells such as macrophages, dendritic cells and natural killer cells (Hauwel et al., 2005).

3. The CNS innate immune response involves detection of " non self" and clearance of dangerous pathogens, neurotoxic proteins and apoptotic cells

The cells responsible for delivering the CNS innate immune response are microglia, astrocytes, endothelial cells, ependymal cells and to a lesser extent neurons (Rivest 2009). Of great importance, is the capacity of these cells to discriminate between" non –self"defined by pathogens and "altered self " (apoptotic cells and dangerous proteins)from "self " (host cells) (Takeuchi et al., 2010; Elward and Gasque 2003). This discrimination relies upon the expression by microglia and the other glia of ancient, highly conserved, pattern recognition receptors PRR (TLR, RLR, NRL) that are localized upon the cell membrane, within endosomes and also released in soluble form (Jane way 1992; Kawai and Akira 2010).

PRR, are able to detect unique, pathogen associated molecular patterns or PAMPs as represented by bacterial cell wall constituents, such as lipopolysaccharide (LPS). (Medzithov and Janeway 200). This property of the PRR is important for the danger theory as proposed by Matzinger; that while the immune system distinguishes between "self "and "non –self", it also must discriminate dangerous from non -dangerous signals (Matzinger 1994). Endogenous molecules such as S-100 proteins (Foell et al., 2007) and high mobility box group I (HMBG1) (Bianchi 2007; Castiglioni et al., 2011) are released during non -apoptotic cell injury and initiate host tissue inflammation: they are regarded as either "alarmins" or "danger signals "and are identified by the PRR of the innate immune system, because they express, damage associated molecular patterns or DAMPs (Klune et al., 2008; Biannchi 2007).

Apoptotic cells express a range of "altered self "molecules on their surface, so called apoptotic cell associated molecular patterns or ACAMPs (Elward and Gasque 2003; Gregory and Devitt 2004; Griffiths et al., 2009). The detection of " altered self" by PRR as defined by DAMPS and ACAMPs, results in the activation of signalling pathways composed of intra cellular adaptor proteins regulating the expression of pro inflammatory cytokines such as the interferons (INFα/β), interleukins (IL) and tumour necrosis factor (TNFα) (Griffiths et al 2009).

Scavenger receptors (SR), Mannose macrophage receptor (MMR), CD14, CD36, CD91(α2 macroglobulin or LRP low density lipoprotein receptor) and phosphatidylserine recepotor (PRS) are present on the host cell membrane or intracellular endosomes. These receptors are multifunctional because they detect PAMPS, ACAMPs and DAMPs to initiate engulfment and phagocytosis of pathogens or apoptotic cells (Stahl and Ezekowitz., 1998. Fadok et al., 2000 and b, Hanayama et al., 2002; Gregory and Devitt 2004; Mukhopadhyay et al., 2004.)

The resident cells of the CNS express two of the three complement pathways(CP) the classical and alternative, but not the lectin activated pathway (Gasque P et al., 2000; Morgan and Gasque 1996). The first complement component, C1q, functions as a PRR, a property shared with a wide range of other C lectins including, mannan binding protein (MBL) and the pentraxins; all these molecules are able to function as both opsonins and PRR capable of detecting PAMPS and ACAMPs. (Tenner AJ 1999; Lu et al., 2002; Thielens et al 2002; Ogden et al., 2005).

After binding to either an apoptotic cell (by detecting ACAMPS) or bacteria (through PAMPS), the opsonins provide a signal on a phagocytic cell that enhances phagcoytosis, either through activation of the complement C pathway or facilitating binding to a PRR such as the β2 integrin, CR3/CR4, receptors (Ehlers et al., 2000; Gasque et al 2000; Gasque 2004). Phagocytosis of opsonized pathogens, neurotoxic proteins and apoptotic cells by microglia and macrophages will promote a reduction in local inflammation (non -phlogistic response) stimulating the recruitment of stem cells from a distance niche and assisting tissue repair (Griffiths et al., 2009).

4. Regulatory pathways prevent an uncontrolled innate immune response; the Neuro immuno-regulatory molecules (NIRegs)

The uncontrolled activation of the innate immune response results in the production of neurotoxic factors and unregulated inflammatory cytokine release. These two factors contribute to any indiscriminate bystander damage and the amplification of underlying disease state. For this reason, the innate immune response must be regulated in order to prevent bystander neuron loss and an uncontrolled inflammatory response. There is now evidence of a group of neuro immuno regulatory (NIRegs) molecules, that by analogy are similar to T reg lymphocytes (Griffiths al., 2007; Hoarau et al., 2011). These T cells are responsible for regulating /controlling the innate immune response and for shaping the resident cells towards a protective phenotype. Several NIRegs, CD47 and CD 200, are capable of acting as "don't eat me "signals allowing host cells to evade detection and phagocytosis by microglia and macrophages (Elward and Gasque 2003; Barclay et al., 2002; Brown and Frazier., 2001; Hoek et al., 2000). The Siglecs, a family of lectins, also detect cells expressing "don't eat me" signals in the form of sialic acid containing molecules (Crocker and Varki 2005). Pathogens do not generally express sialic acid residues and the absence of sialic acids provides a " non -self " signal, sometimes referred to as an "eat me signal "and this is detected by lectins, including Siglecs, and complement proteins.

The CP is also strictly regulated by a series of complement regulatory proteins CRP (FH, CD55, CD46) preventing inappropriate activation and host destruction (Elward et al., 2005; Griffiths et al., 2009; Zipfel et al., 2009). Furthermore, components of the CP including C3a, are also capable of recruiting stem cells into areas of tissue damage and increasing growth factor expression, both facilitating tissue repair (Griffiths et al., 2010).

5. Toll like receptors (TLRs) are PRR with multiple roles in infection including pathogen detection and inflammatory response

The TLR are an ancient, highly conserved family of PRR, which belong to the type-1 trans membrane receptors. They are characterized by a cytosolic C-terminal signalling domain – Toll/interleukin -1receptor (TIR) required for intracellular signal transduction and terminal LRR(leucine rich repeats) domain that mediates the recognition of PAMPs (Kawai and Akira 2010). This family of PRR are vital for the detection of PAMPs, including cell wall lipoproteins and nucleic acids, derived from bacteria, viruses, parasites and fungi (Iwaski and Medhitov 2010).

TLR 4, or heterodimers TLR2-TLR1, TLR2-TLR6 and TLR5 (but notTLR3) binds to a ligand such as a PAMP or DAMP, the complex is internailized within the endosome and this triggers intracellular transduction pathways by recruiting the TIR interaction domain that forms multimers with, a number of adaptor proteins such as myeloid differentiation primary response protein, My D88, My D88 adaptor like (Mal, also TIR domain containing adaptor protein, TIRAP), TIR domain containing adaptor inducing IFN-γ(TRIF) and TRIF – related adaptor molecule TRAM. Activation of TLR by PAMPS recruits one of the above adaptor molecules and activates the My D 88 dependent pathway with NF- kB activation. An alternative signalling pathway following TLR binding to a ligand involves the activation of the TRIF –dependent pathway, with the induction of the type I interferon (anti -virus) response, with the expression of IFNβ and inflammatory cytokines (Netea et al., 2004 Creagh and O Neill 2006).

Mice deficient in the individual TRL negative regulatory proteins, such as zinc finger proteins, autophagy related molecules and ubiquitin are unable to regulate the inflammatory response subsequent to TLR ligand binding. This uncontrolled inflammatory response results in multi organ inflammation such as, chronic inflammatory bowel disease and auto immune arthritis. Conversly, MyD 88 deficiency reduces inflammation (Kwai and Akira 2010 for detailed discussion).

A detailed review of the intra cellular signalling pathways linked to TLR activation by viral nucleic acids, bacterial lipo proteins and other ligands, with subsequent inflammatory cytokine synthesis is outside the scope of this review, but see Takeuchi and Akira 2007; Iwaski and Medhitov 2010; Kawai and Akira 2010)

5.1 TLR act in combination with other PRRs and not always alone

Interestingly, TLR2, forms hetero dimers with TLR-1 and this combination is able to detect Gram negative bacteria, whereas the heterodimer TLR-2-TLR-6 combination recognizes Gram positive organisms. Further cooperation between TLR -4 and the SR co -receptors, CD14 and CD36, together with the C lectin receptor, dendritic cell –specific intercellular molecule -3 grabbing non –integrin (DC –SIGN), detects glucuronoxylmannans found on the cell wall of fungi (Kumar et al 2010).

5.2 TLR distribution in the CNS

Ten functional TLRs have been identified in humans, of these, nine are conserved in both humans and mice. In the human and mouse CNS, TLR 3, , TLR 7 and TLR 8 are located on the cell surface of neurons (Bisibi et al., 2002; Prehaud et al., 2005; Jackson et al., 2006), microglia (Alexopoulou et al., 2001; Olson et al., 2004; Jack 2005), astrocytes (Bsibi et al., 2001; Bisibi et al 2006 Farina et al., 2005; Rivieccio et al., 2006; Carpentier et al., 2007) ependyma and oligodendrocytes (Bsibi 2002). TLR 7 and 8 on microglia (Olson et al., 2004), astrocytes (Buchiet al., 2008) neurons (Ma et al., 2006), TLR 9 on microglia (Mc Kimme et al., 2006). Cells of the meninges, choroid plexus and circum ventricular organs are all exposed to the systemic circulation and express TLR 2 and TLR 4 (Lafalamme and Rivest 2001; Bowman et al., 2003; Laflamme et al., 2003;) see table1

TLR, 3 TLR7, TLR8 and TLR 9 are distributed within intracellular organelles, endoplasmic reticulum, lysosomes and endolysosomes so they are strategically placed to detect intra cytoplasmic viral nucleic acids, both RNA and DNA (Griffin 2003; Kumar et al., 2011). Conversly, TLR2, TLR5 and TLR 6, are present on the cell surface and detect various bacterial components (Kumar et al., 2011; Iwasaki and Medzhitov 2010)

TLRs11-13 have been described in neurons, astrocytes, ependymal and endothelial cells(Mishra er al., 2008). see table 1

5.3 TLRs; Innate immune response to bacterial infection

TLRs are expressed by glial and choroid plexus cells following bacterial infection (Bowman et al., 2003 Carpentier et al., 2008). TLR- 4 forms a complex with MD2 on the host cell surface and they provide the main Lipopolysaccharide (LPS), binding site. Further interaction between LPS binding protein with CD14, a glycophosphatidylinositol protein (GPI) with leucine repeat protein, delivers LPS to the TLR4-MD2 complex, this is internalized into endosomes and through the My88 protein intracellular signalling pathway eventually results in cytokine expression. TLR4 also detects virus envelope proteins and *Streptococcus pneumoniae* pneumolysin (Kwai and Akira 2010. Akira and Uematas., 2006).

TLR2, is able to detect a wide range of bacterial wall PAMPS, including peptidoglycan, Mycobacteria (lipoarabinomannan mycobcateria), fungal (zymosan), haemagluttin on influenza virus, together with mucin molecules from *Trypanosoma cruzi*. The glucans are a main constituent of the fungal cell wall and in association with dectins -1(a C type – lectin)are detected by the TLR2 receptor and internalized to produce a protective inflammatory response (Netea et al., 2004). TLR2 is not able to detect viral nucleic acids.

TLR5 and TLR9 detect a different range of bacterial constituents; TLR5 recognizes the flagellin protein expressed by flagellated bacteria, whereas TLR9, detects bacterial and viral DNA, especially CpG DNA motifs, that are rarely found in mammalian cells (Kawai and Akira 2010). (see table 1). TRL 11, recognizes bacteria found in the genitourinary tract as well as a profilin, a molecule expressed by *Toxoplasmosis gondii* (Yarovinsky et al., 2005), and also neurocysticercosis (Mishra er al 2008).

5.4 TLR; virus detection and the anti virus response

TLR3 detects double stranded (ds) RNA formed during replication of RNAand DNA viruses (Alexopoulou et al., 2001; Wang T et al., 2004; Daffis et al., 2008) the viral nucleic acid binds to N and C terminal sites on the TLR3 ectodomain activating the TRIF and NF- kB dependent pathways to produce an interferon type 1 anti- virus (IFN type -1) response (Paul et al., 2007)

Conversly, TLR7 and TLR 9 detect single stranded viral (ss)RNA and DNA respectively, and signal through the adaptor protein (MyD88) to initiate intracellular signalling by activating transcription factors NF-kB and the interferon regulatory factors (IRFs).

IRFs are translocated to the host cell nucleus where they regulate inflammatory cytokine synthesis and stimulate IFN type I interferon synthesis(IFNα/β expression) resulting in a protective response in adjacent cells, uninfected with a virus (Katze et al., 2002; Paul et al 2007). IFNα/βbinds to the IFN surface receptor (IFNAR) on an uninfected host cell leading to the activation of Janus kinases (JAK) with phosphorylation of transcription factors Signal Transducer and Activation of Signal (STAT1 and STAT2). These two proteins enter the host nucleus to drive the expression of IFN stimulated genes (ISGs)to intiate the anti virus host response.

Many of the emerging RNA viruses responsible for encephalitis express viral proteins that inhibit the host's innate anti -virus response by inhibiting specific steps in the pathway for IFN α/β synthesis, namely the ISGs and several anti -virus proteins blocking the hosts anti virus response (Type 1 interferon) (Griffin 2003; Paul et al., 2007) Examples of viruses and their individual proteins that block the host's IFN expression include, West Nile Fever (Envelope protein E), Influenza (Non Structual protein -1), Ebola (VP 24, VP35) Rabies (Rabies virus phosphoprotein), Enterovirus (structural protein 3C).

5.5 TLR detection of DAMPs in the absence of infection promotes inflammation

Necrotic cells release a range of endogenous proteins such as, heat shock proteins (HSP), S - 100, High mobility group box 1 Interleukin (HMGB1), ATP and mitochondrial proteins that are all regarded as DAMPS, because they can initiate an inflammatory response. (Roth et al., 2003; Lotze et al 2005; Krysko et al., 2010).

Several PRR including TLR-3, TLR-7 and TLR-9 function as sensors of tissue necrosis (Cavassani et al., 2008; Marshak- Rothstein and Rifkin 2007). Chromatin –DNA and ribonucleoprotein complexes all of which contain "self"nucleotides that activate the intracellular PRRs, TLR 7and TLR 9, resulting in an autoimmune disease(Tian et al 2010). Self nucleic acids are usually unable to activate the innate immune system, but after degradation by serum nucleases they are detected by TLRs in endolysosomes resulting in a further inflammatory response (Cavassani et al., 2008) In Systemic lupus erythematosus SLE, (a chronic inflammatory multi-organ disease charachterized by antibody production against self antigens such as DNA). On this basis SLE is regarded as a typical autoimmune disease because serum auto antibodies bind to " self" nucleic acids and are internalized by FcγR IIIa receptors on DC. These complexes are detected by TLR7 and 9, leading to interferon type I response and persistent autoimmune inflammation (Marshak- Rothstein and Rifkin 2007).

HMBG1 is an important DAMP, because it can bind to self DNA and pathogens. The receptor for activated glycation endproducts (RAGE) is also a PRR, and binds with HMBG1 to form a complex. This is delivered to endosomes containing TLR9, activating both DC and

The CNS Innate Immune System and the Emerging Roles of the Neuroimmune Regulators (NIRegs)
in Response to Infection, Neoplasia and Neurodegeneration

183

B lymphocytes, with an up regulation of inflammatory cytokines (Tian et al., 2007). The regulation of HMGBI is clearly an important factor contributing to reducing DAMP initiated inflammation. One regulator of this interaction is Thrombomodulin (CD141); it is expressed by microglia and has been shown to bind to HMBG before it can form a complex with RAGE, to prevent this complex being detected by TLR and promoting an inflammatory response. (Abeyama et al 2005).

Heat shock proteins (HSP) and S-100, are important DAMPs and also interact with TLR 2-4 /CD91 and the RAGE receptor. This complex also signals through the NF-kB pathway to activate proinflammatory cytokine expression (Foell et al., 2007; Yu et al., 2006). The regulation of DAMP initiated inflammation is not well understood; however two macrophage (and possibly microglial) related lectins, MINCL and Clec9A, both bind to ribonucleoproteins, SAP 130, released by necrotic cells preventing DAMPS binding to TLR, with a down regulation of cytokine expression (Sancho et al 2009).

6. Non-TLR PRRs in pathogen detection

6.1 RIG like receptor; RIG -1 and MDA5 receptors detect intracellular viral nucleic acids and initiate interferon synthesis

Retinoic acid inducible agent -1 and melanoma differentiation associated gene 5 (MDA5) are both RIG-1 –like receptors (RLRs) , are helicases and signal through the adaptor molecule IPS-1 (Yoneyama et al., 2004; Kato et al 2006; Kwaki and Akiar 2010). They are expressed by microglia and astrocytes, and are located in the cytosol (Miranada et al., 2009). RLRs detect mainly virus RNA, both short and long ds and ss RNA (. Fur et al., 2008; Yoshida et al., 2007) RIG-1 detects short double stranded RNA; negative sense single strand, Influenza A and Ebola viruses and positive sense single strand RNA, Japanese encephalitis and Hepatitis C (Yoneyama et al., 2004; Fuijita et al 2007., Mohamadzadeh et al., 2007) whereas, MDA-5 detects cytoplasmic positive sense RNA, for example Poliovirus. (Griffin 2003; Kato et al 2008)

6.2 RiG-1 and MDA-5 anti virus response

RIG-1 and MDA-5 contain caspase recruitment domains (CARDS) essential for down stream signalling and an intermediate DEeD/H-box RNA Helicase domain, essential for ligand binding and recognition. (Parisien et al., 2003) The interaction between the RIG-1 and MDA-5 with nucleic acid from a pathogen activates the CARD containing adaptor (IPS-1) known as Cardif, MAVS and VISA, resulting in the up regulation of interleukins and a range of anti -virus proteins (Kumar et al 2010: Kato 2006) promoting the IFN type I response, capable of inhibiting viral replication(Paul et al 2007). See table 1.

6.3 ND LR receptors; roles in the innate response against infection

The NDLR (nucleotide –binding domain leucine rich repeat) are a group of highly conserved proteins found in diverse species, including sea urchins and humans. They (twenty two have been identified in humans and thirty four in mice) are a family of intracellular cytoplasmic PRR that represent sensors for detecting Gram negative and Gram positive bacteria, mycobacteria and DAMPs (Karaparakis et al 2007: ; Ting et al., 2010; Kumar et al., 2011).

These receptors are characterized by an N -terminal effector domain caspase recruitment domain (CARD), a centrally located nucleoside binding domain NACHT (or NOD) domain for nucleotide binding and a C terminal of leucine rich (LRR) mediating PAMP ligand recognition, e. g peptioglycan and flagellin in the bacterial cell wall (Sterka and Marriott 2006: Kaparakis et al., 2007 Proell et al 2008).

The actual process wherby an NLR detects either a PAMP or DAMP, is not understood. However, the C terminal LRR region recognizes PAMPS, but the crucial step in NLR activation is the oligomerization of NACHT domain and this permits binding to a series of intracellular adaptor proteins and eventually the intiation of IFN synthesis as the inflammatory response. (Proel2008)Further information about potential homo and heterotypical interactions between NLR s is needed to determine whether or not different combinations of NLRS demonstrate functional differences. Mutations in the genes encoding individual NLR have been linked to several chronic inflammatory disorders (such as Crohn's disease and asthma) underlying the potential importance of NLR in human disease (Tinget al 2010).

The expression of the NLR in the CNS is not clearly defined, although NOD 2 is expressed by monocytes, microglia and astrocytes (Chauhan et al; 2009)

NOD1 and 2 are cytosol proteins, they are able to detect major components of bacteria cell walls, g –D glutamyl –meso –diaminopimelic acid (iE- DAP) present in numerous organisms including Listeria Bacillus subtilis, Shigella Flexneri, Campylobacter jejuni and, Helicobacter pylori; NOD-2 detects murmayl dipepetide from Salmonella Typhimurium, Mycobacteria tuberculosis, Listeria monocytogenes, Saphylococcus aureus and Neiseeria menigitidis (Sterka et al., 2006) Kumar et al 2011). Uncontrolled NOD-2 activation can, however, result in demyelinization, representing the detrimental effects of unregulated activation of the innate immune system against pathogen invasion. (Proell et al., 2008).

NLR3, is a key component of NLR- 3 inflammosome (NLR 3, ASC and procaspase -1) because it is able to detect a wide range of PAMPs including viruses (adeno and influenzaviruses), bacteria (Staphylococcus aureus) and fungi (Candida albicans) (Osawa et al., 2010) and various DAMPs (HSP and BCL-2)(Schroder 2010). Of interest, is the association between a mutation in the nucleotide –binding oligomerization domain gene 2(NOD2) and Crohn's disease, an inflammatory bowel disease (Rehaume et al; ., 2010; Ting et al., 2010).

The explanation for the role of NOD2 in some forms of bowel inflammation (Crohn's disease) provides several insights into the more general immuno regulatory roles for NOD - 2. Firstly, as an activator of the transcription factor NF-kB, to increase cytokine synthesis, or as a negative regulator of the host TLR response to pathogens, thirdly, a capacity to increase host defence by up regulating the expression of small molecular weight (18-45 amino acids) molecules called the α defensins in Paneth cells. The defensins assist with the intracellular lysis of phagocytosed bacteria, therfore regulating the severity of inflammation in the intestine wall (Rehaume et al., 2010).

The precise mechanism by which intra cellular sensing of PAMPs, such as bacterial peptidoglycan derived molecules, meso –diaminopimelic acid and muramyl dipeptide is carried out is as yet, not known (Ting et al 2010). Once a PAMP or DAMP is detected by the NLR this activates the inflammasome pathway (a complex composed of NLR, the adaptor

The CNS Innate Immune System and the Emerging Roles of the Neuroimmune Regulators (NIRegs)
in Response to Infection, Neoplasia and Neurodegeneration

185

ASC (apoptotic speck-containing protein) with a CARD and procaspase -1 increasing the expression of proinflammatory cytokines IL-β and IL-18. (Royet et al., 2007; Hoarau et al., 2011).

The involvement of NLR in virus infection requires the mitochondrial located anti virus signalling protein, MAVS (also Cardif, IPS-1, VISA), that is responsible for type I interferon response. An NLR protein family member, NLRX1, regulates the interferon type 1 response by inhibiting the interaction between RIG-1 and MAVS, whereas NOD 2, also inhibits RNA virus production through its interaction with the anti- viral protein, 2-5 oligodenylate synthase type 2 (OAS2) (Ting et al 2010). see table 1.

7. Scavenger Receptors (SR) detect pathogens, apoptotic cells and endogenous proteins; vital components of the innate immune response

7.1 CD14, CD36 and SCARB

CD14 is expressed by microglia and is both a membrane anchored glycophosphatidylinositol protein (GPI) and soluble PRR. It has a co-operative interaction with TLR- 4 to facilitate bacterial LPS detection and it interacts with apoptotic lymphocytes, via the intercellular adhesion molecule(ICAM-3) to facilitate their phagocytosis (Gregory 2000). Clearance of apoptotic cells by CD14, depends upon detection of ACAMPS and this is also an anti -inflammatory response, reducing tissue damage, because the soluble form CD14 switches off activated T cells (Pender 2001).

7.2 Scavenger receptors class A (SRAI, SRABI/II) and class B, CD36

The best characterised SR is CD36, a multifunctional receptor, expressed by microglia and astrocytes (Husemann etal., 2002). It is able to bind to phosphatidyl (PS) and oxidized low density lipoprotein, both present on apoptotic cells (as ACAMPs) as well as neurotoxic proteins such as Aβ4 (Ren et al., 1995; Coraci et al., 2002). Macrophage, CD36, co-operates with the vitronectin receptor αvβ3 (CD51/CD61) to increase phagocytosis, because this complex recognizes the protein thrombospondin (TSP) located on the surface of apoptotic cells. (Lamy et al 2007: Fadok et al., 1998).

A further receptor, Scavenger receptor B, SCARB (Lysosomal integral membrane protein II or CD36b like-2) is expressed by many different tissues and has also been identified as a receptor for the enterovirus EV71and coxsackie virus A16, although only EV71 is responsible for encephalitis. SCARB is expressed in most tissues, so it not possible to explain the neurotophic effect of EV71 as the result of this virus binding this new receptor. (Yamayoshi et al, 2009).

7.3 CD91; a multi functional PRR

The α2 macroglobulin LRP receptor-related or the lipoprotein low density lipoprotein receptor (CD91) is expressed by microglia and neurons (Marzolo et al., 2000), and functions as an entry receptor for both bacteria and viruses. HIV-1 utilizes CD91 as a docking receptor to enter the CNS via endocytosis; the toxin of the bacterium Pseudomonas is taken up by CD91 (Herz et al., 2001). Despite this evidence, the contribution made by this SR in defending against neuro infection is not yet clarified; CD91 is also able to bind toAβ4 amyloid and apoptotic cells (Marzolo et al., 2000). As the result of apoptosis, calreticulin, a soluble protein located on the endoplasmic reticulum migrates to the cell surface and becomes a potentially important ligand for phagocyte receptors, including mannan binding lectin (MBL), the first complement proteinC1q and the CD91 complex. (Ogden et al., 2001; Gardai et al., 2005)

7.4 TREM -2; a new scavenger receptor

Triggering receptor expressed by myeloid cells (TREM-2) and is an SR expressed on monocyte derived dendritic cells, osteoclasts and microglia (Takahashiet al., 2007). The TREM-2 receptor is expressed by microglia in conjunction with the receptor DAP-12 that shares many features with Draper, an ancient phagocytic receptor found in *Drosphila*. The microglial, DAP-12 receptor and Draper, both contain ITAM (immuno receptor tyrosine based activation motifs) and stimulation of this signalling pathway increases microglial phagocytosis and pro inflammatory cytokine expression. (Linnaetz et al., 2010). In vitro, microglia expressing TREM -2 demonstrated increased phagocytosis of membrane fragments from apoptotic neurons. This effect was also reproduced in experimental autoimmune encephalomyelitis(EAE)following the intravenous administration of TREM-2 in bone marrow precursor cells and was accompanied by a down regulation of tumour necrosis factor (TNFα). A loss of function mutation in both TREM-2 and Draper proteins are associated with a chronic neurodegenerative disease, Nasu-Hakola, characterized by the failure to clear neurotoxic proteins, representing a contributory factor in this form of early onset dementia (Colonna M et al., 2003). The TREM -2 mediated apoptotic response was inhibited by inflammatory signals activating the ITIM (immuno receptor tyrosine based inhibitory motifs) leading to the recruitment src homology 2 (SH) domains of syk protein kinases, preventing phagocytosis and down regulating both the microglial inflammatory and anti -pathogen responses.

7.5 Lectins as PRR in the innate immune response to infection and injury

The lectins are a range of carbohydrate binding proteins and glycoproteins, either homo or hetero oligomers of non -covalently bound, polypeptide units and carbohydrate recognition domains (CRD) that bind to a sugar molecule in a Ca 2+ dependent manner (Cambi et al., 2005). One important role for the lectins is to establish tolerance between bacteria living inside the host through molecular mimicry. Bacteria display surface lectin molecules similar to those present on host cells so bacterial lectins are detected as " self " by the host immune system, allowing them to remain in the gut with mutual benefit to both host and bacteria.

The innate immune response also includes the C- type lectins (acting as PRRs) to detect PAMPS (Endo et al., 2006; Geijten beek et al., 2009). The most important families of lectins are the Pentraxins (extracellular), the Macrophage mannose receptor (MMR) located on the endoplasmic reticulum)(Stahl and Ezowitz 1998), the non classical C-type lectins, dectins 1and 2, expressed by microglia (Brown G et al., 2006) Siglecs (cell membrane)(Crocker and Varki, 2001) and the newly identified C –type lectin member 4E (Clec4) (Sancho et al., 2009). The galectins, expressed by cerebral blood vessels, are an increasingly important family of lectins, functioning as a PRR to detect both intracranial l PAMPs and DAMPs (Sato et al., 2009; Vasa, 2009).

7.6 MMR and DC-SIGN are PRR for "non self", complex carbohydrates

Glia, express trans membrane C- type lectins (Burundi et al., 1999) namely MMR (microglia, astrocytes and peri vascular cells) (Linehan et al., 1999) and DC- SIGN receptor that recognizes "self "intercellular adhesion glycoproteins ICAM. (van Kooyk et al., 2003). The DC-SIGN receptor is expressed by peri vascular cells and a population of dendritic cells, both associated with cerebral blood vessels (Mukhtar et al., 2002; Schwartz et al., 2002; Greter., 2005). MMR and DC- SIGN function as PRRs binding to and internalising viruses by endocytosis, promoting their degradation and antigen presentation to T cells in association with MHC (Stahl et al 1998; van Kooyk et al., 2003).

Both, MMR and DC-SIGN, also recognize "non self" molecules containing a high mannose content (functioning as PAMPs), as found on enveloped viruses. Both MMR and DC-SIGN receptors provide a pathway for a virus to enter the CNS (le Cabec et al., 2005) and this is the case for Dengue (Miller et al 2008), HIV, Ebola and Marburg (both ss RNA Filo viruses), West Nile Fever virus (WNFV), Influenza A, all target MMR (Upham et al 2010.). Whereas, WNV and Ebola virus target the DC- SIGN receptor (Alvarez et al., 2002; Schwartz et al., 2002; Mohameazah et al., 2007)

7.7 Pentraxins

The pentraxins are highly conserved proteins with a cyclic multimeric structure and include the acute phase reactant C protein (CRP) and serum amyloid protein (SAP). Microglia and neurons express CRP and SAP, both of which are capable of opsonising apoptotic cells with subsequent binding to the collectin, C1q, the first C pathway protein to stimulate phagocytosis. (Elward and Gasque 2003; Nauta et al 2003). CRP recognizes apoptotic cells through binding to phosphorylcholine found in oxidized lipids which are regarded as ACAMPs (Chang et al., 2002). Pentraxins, as opsonins, also initiate phagocytosis of apoptotic cells as they are capable of binding directly to microglial Ig (FcγR) receptors and C1q (Chang et al 2002: Nauta et al., 2003) Despite this evidence, the contribution of the pentraxins to the removal of apoptotic cells from the CNS in neurodegenerative and inflammatory disease is yet to be defined.

7.8 Galectins are lectins and PRR with multiple roles

Most galectins are non – glycosylated, soluble proteins, distributed in most mammalian tissues, including the innate and adaptive immune systems (Sato et al., 2010: Vasta 2010). Glactins(previously known as S- type lectins) are expressed by cerebral vessel wall endothelium (Joubert et al., 1998). They are also examples of PRR capable of binding to viruses, bacteria (*Streptococcus pneumonia, Neisseria meningitides, Haemophilus influenza* and fungi *Candida albicans,* the protozoan *Trypanosoma cruzi* and parasite *Toxoplasmosis gondii.* Glactins are able to prevent Nipah virus entry in to endothelial cells by preventing virus fusion with ephrin B2 and B3 receptors on endothelial cell surface (Lo et al., 2010; Garner et al., 2010) However, this protective function of glactein is exploited by the HIV -1 virus, because it binds to glactin -1 and enters host cells. Organs that represent reservoirs for HIV-1 infection express abundant glactin –1 on their cell surface, confirming glactins are " non self" detecting PRR. (Sato 2009).

7.9 Defense collagens or collectins (MBL and SPA)

These are soluble molecules expressed by the liver, lungs and astrocytes (Kuraya et al., 2003; Wagner et al 2003)and include mannose binding lectin (MBL) and Lung surfactant protein A (SPA). Both these collectins are capable of recognizing carbohydrate patterns containing large numbers of mannose and fucose molecules characterized as PAMPs, and found in the cell wall of bacteria and viruses (non self), but not expressed by mammalian cells (Tenner AJ 1999; Elward Gasque 2003). The globular carboxyl C terminal of the defence collagen acts as PRR recognizes PAMPs and potentially ACAMPs, whereas the N -terminal domain links defence collagen to a receptor on phagocytic cells e. g microglia. MBL binds to Ebola and Marburg envelope gylco proteins, preventing these viruses gaining "subversive "entry to the host cell through the DC -SIGN receptor (Ji et al 2005). SPA and MBL are capable of binding to apoptotic cells and neutrophils, functioning as a bridging molecules, between the apoptotic cell and the phagocyte receptor CD91 (Vandivier et al., 2002).

7.10 Siglecs detect sialic residues as markers of "self"

Siglecs (sialic acid -binding immunoglobulin like lectins) are a subgroup of the Ig super family, type 1 membrane proteins with an amino terminal V -set immunoglobulin domain; they represent a family of receptors that detect sialylated glycoproteins and glycolipids (Crocker and Varki 2001 Crocker etal., 2007). Two group of Siglecs can be identified; Siglecs common to mammals Siglec -1(sialoahesin, CD169) (Delputte et al., 2011), Siglec 2 (CD22), myelin associated siglec 4 and those Siglecs related to the CD33 family including siglec -10, 11 and 16 (Lock et al., 2009 Mott et al., 2004). Most siglecs, are present on haemopoietic tissue however, sialoadhesin is expressed only on macrophages as a specific adhesion molecule, whereas siglec -11 is expressed by microglia (Angata et al., 2002). The CD33 family of siglecs are expressed on most mammalian cells, with each siglec having a unique specificity for a sialylated ligands (sialic acid), so there is room for overlapping functions within the family of Siglec receptors (Cao and Crocker 2010). Their main function is the detection of "self " indicated by sialic acid residues and the suppression of inappropriate microglial directed host cell phagocytosis.

7.11 Complement system provides first line defence against pathogens PAMPS, DAMPs and ACAMPs

The C system is an extremely ancient component of the innate immune system. It is thought to have evolved 300 million years ago, as part of the coagulation protein pathway. The complement system comprises of three pathways, the classical, alternative and lectin activated pathways. (Sjoberg et al., 2008; Gasque 2004; Gasque et al., 2000)

The first component of the classical C pathway, C1q, has a multimeric structure, that represents a PRR and is expressed by astrocytes and neurons (Gasque et al., 2000). C1q is able to detect a variety of pathogens, apoptotic cells and neurotoxic misfolded proteins (mutant Prions, fibrillary amyloid), antigen -antibody complexes and DNA (Nauata et al 2002; Korb et al., 1997). The identity of the C1q receptor is not well defined, but candidates include, CD93, expressed by microglia or C1qRp (Dean et al 2000 Webster et al., 2002. ; Elward and Gasque 2003).

The CNS Innate Immune System and the Emerging Roles of the Neuroimmune Regulators (NIRegs)
in Response to Infection, Neoplasia and Neurodegeneration

189

The activation of the classical C pathway generates two anaphylotoxins (C3a, C5a) responsible for recruiting inflammatory cells into areas of tissue injury, as welll as opsonins (iC3b and C3) and the cytolytic membrane activation complex (MAC). With regards to pathogens such as bacteria and fungi, the opsonins (C3b and iC3b) coat the pathogen making it a more attractive target for microglia expressing the β2 integrin (CR3 /CR4)receptors (Akiyma and Mc Geer 1990: Ehlers 2000; Reichart et al., 2003). Apoptotic cells contain activated DNA and this enables C1q to directly bind to apoptotic cells, activating the classical C pathway with the generation of opsonins C3b and iC3b, again providing targets for phagocytosis by CR3 and CR4 to reduce host cell damage (Mevorach et al., 1998; Korb et al., 1997). There is also evidence that the Ficolins (lectins) bind to ACAMPs expressed by apoptotic cells, activate complement and generate the opsonin C3, facilitating phagocytosis (Matsushita., 2010)

8. Neurodegeneration; The detection and clearance of Pathogen protein associated molecular patterns (PPAMPS) and innate immune system activation

Neurodegeneration produces neuronal loss and is characterized by intra and extra neuronal accumulation of dangerous(neurotoxic) intrinsic proteins (fibrillary amyloid, mutant prions, α–synuclein, mutant tau) classified as PPAMPs(pathogen protein associated molecular patterns) regarded as a sub type of DAMPS. PPAMPs are detected by a range of PRRs with resulting proinflammatory cytokine expression (Wyss-Coray and Mucke 2002). During chronic CNS inflammation, the accumulation of endogenous protein aggregates is perceived by the innate immune system as "stranger" or "danger" signals (DAMPs). In AD, it has been suggested that a variety of glial related PRR (CD14, TLR, CD36, CD91) with opsonins(C 1q, iC3b, C3) derived from C activation contribute to the removal of Aβ4amyloid fibrils (Coraci et al., 2002: Elkhoury et al., 2003; Fassbender et al., 2004; Alarcon et al 2005: Tahara et al., 2006; Landreth et al., 2009)The SR, CD36, facilitates the assembly of a heteromeric complex composed of CD36, TLR4 and TLR6 following binding to Aβ 4 (Stewart et al., 2010).

Aβ fibrils can activate microglia and astrocytes through TLR4 (together with CD14 and MD2 in microglia), leading to the activation of downstream inflammatory response genes (Reed - Geaghan et al., 2009; Walter et al., 2007; Chen et al., 2006: Lehnardt et al., 2003, Bamberger et al., 2003). This explanation is consistent with mice carrying a nonfunctional TLR4 crossed with a mouse model of AD (APP/PS1 double transgenic mice) having a lower level of inflammatory cytokines than wild type animals (Walter et al., 2007; Jin et al., 2008). A TLR4 polymorphism was shown to be associated with protection against late-onset AD in an Italian population, suggesting that theTLR4–mediated innate immune inflammation could influence AD pathology (Minorettiet al., 2006). TLR2 also may be a sensor for fibrillar Aβ (Chen K et al., 2006; Jana et al 2008). Blocking TLR2 signaling with antibody or by knockdown of the receptor gene *in vitro* suggested that TLR2 stimulation by Aβ promotes neurotoxic inflammation. However, mice lacking TLR2 crossed with APP/PS1 transgenic AD mice were reported to show a delay in Aβ deposition and improved behavior on memory tests (Richard et al., 2008) These apparently contradictory functions of TLR could be due to differences in the cell types as well as signaling pathways that are engaged by the amyloid peptides and/or fibrils. (Tahara et al., 2006)

NOD-like receptors (NLRs) are also involved in Aβ-induced inflammatory response. In AD, Aβ oligomers and fibrils induce lysosomal damage and trigger NALP3, a member of the NLR family that is expressed in microglia (Halle et al., 2008) NALPs activate downstream signaling proteins, such as ASC and this will lead to caspase 1 activation and increased processing of proinflammatory mediators like IL-1β and IL-18.

Fibrillary amyloid and aggregated forms of mutant prion protein are opsonized by complement components (C1q, C3) to promote clearance by macrophages and microglia CR3/CR4(Tenner 2001: Kovacs et al., 2004). In AD as the result of C1q binding to fibrillary Aβ4, the C pathway is activated increasing C3 and C5 as part of the protective response promoting clearance of the amyloid plaque (Mc Geer et al., 1989; Jian et al., 1994; Eikelenboom et al., 2002); inhibition of the complement cascade increased amyloid plaque burden (Wyss Coray and Mucke., 2002). However, in the context of acute inflammation, microglia and astrocytes express complement and it is plausible C activation on myelin/neuronal debris contributes to secondary brain injury. The formation of the MAC and non-specific binding to host cells would cause bystander damage.

In Huntington's disease the expression of C1q, C3, iC3b and C4 is increased on microglia and astrocytes, C activation is also present in experimental models of ischaemia (van Beek et al., 2000; van Beek et al., 2001: Singhrao et al., 1999). Interestingly, administration of a C1q inhibitor C1-INH, resulted in neuron protection after experimental ischaemia, but its protective effect was interpreted as independent of C1q activation of the complement pathway (De Simoni et al., 2004).

A further sensing system for Aβ, is provided by RAGE (receptor for advanced glycation endproducts) a PRR and trans membrane receptor of the immunoglobulin super family RAGE is expressed on the surface of microglia, astrocytes, vascular endothelial cells, and particularly on neurons (Fang F et al 2010). Several reports suggest that Aβ peptide as well as Aβ oligomers bind to RAGE and contributing to the activation of microglia and the production of proinflammatory mediator (Yan et al., 2006). RAGE is also suggested to play an important role in the clearance of Aβ4 and to be involved in cellular processing and signaling (Origlia et al, 2008; Takuma et al 2009). The role of the SRs, CD36, CD14 and particularly CD91, in AD is ambiguous; studies indicate that CD91 has the capacity to influence both the production and the clearance of Aβ. CD91 is a receptor for APP, apoE, and α2M, which all have been genetically linked to AD (. Bu, 2006). Clearance of Aβ complexed to these ligands could contribute to a reduction in amyloid plaque burden (Herz et al., 2001).

8.1 Phagocytosis of apoptotic cells (altered self) reduces local inflammation (the non phlogistic response)

Apoptotic cells result from the consquences of infection, ischaemic infarction and neurodegeneration; they express a range of apoptotic cell associated molecular patterns or ACAMPs on their surface. In general phagocytosis of apoptotic cells reduces local tissue inflammation, as the so called "non pholgistic response", providing some degree of local immunoregulation. (Chan et al., 2001: Chang et al., 2001; Magus et al., 2002; Griffith set al., 2009. The result of clearing apoptotic cells reduces local inflammation (non phlogistic response) and this is in contrast to the increase inflammatory response, following attempted clearance of pathogens (phlogistic response). The clearance of apoptotic cells by CD14 is anti-inflammatory (non phlogistic) as it binds to and switches off T cells (Gold1991), releases

The CNS Innate Immune System and the Emerging Roles of the Neuroimmune Regulators (NIRegs)
in Response to Infection, Neoplasia and Neurodegeneration

191

the anti-inflammatory cytokines TGFβ and prostaglandin E2, together with growth factors such as Vascular endothelial growth factor (VEGF), all reducing local inflammation and promoting tissue repair (Griffiths., 2009 et al, Golpon HA et al., 2004, Huynh et al., 2002, Voll R et al., 1997)

ACAMPs include nucleic acids and sugars, the best characterized ACAMPS are, phosphatidyl serine (PS) and calreticulin (Fadok et al., 2000: Hoffman et al 2001; Gardai et al., 2005; Gardai et al., 2006).

Glia and macrophages express PRRs that recognize ACAMPS, including the PS receptor (PSR), CD14 (in conjunction with ICAM), LRP, CD36, the soluble bridging molecules milk - fat gobulin (MFG -EGF 8), growth arrest –specific gene 6, and TREM-2 (Prieto et al., 1999, Gregory 2000; Hanayama et al., 2002; Leonardi –Essman et al., 2005 Gardaiet al., 2006). Thrombospondin, a protein expressed by glia, acts as a bridging molecule between an as yet undefined ligand on the apoptotic cell and CD36, to promote phagocytic clearance (Lamy et al., 2007). PS on apoptotic cells and IgM both bind to C1q to activate C pathway and opsonin (C3b iC3b) synthesis, to provide targets for CR3 and CR4 (Kim et al., 2002).

Animals deficient in C1q accumulate apoptotic cells, resulting in glomerulonephritis and an (SLE)- like disease, because the accumulated DNA and RNA both function as DAMPs and trigger autoimmune inflammation (Botto et al 1998). Activated microglial and Kolmer cells in the choroid plexus (Singhrao et al., 1999) express C3R /CR4 and both detect C1q, C3b, C3b as well as MBL, underlining the importance of glia for removing apoptotic cells opsonised with C from the CSF (Mevorach et al., 1998; Reichart et al., 2003). The lectins, Ficolins and MBL, are capable of interacting with ACAMPs such as calcireticulin, to initiate clearance of apoptotic cells (Ogden et al., 2001).

Phagocytes involved in apoptotic cell clearance also express, the T cell immunoglobulin domain mucin domain protein 4 receptor (TIM4) and the TAM receptors (Tyro2, Axland Mer) which bind to Gas 6 both are expressed by neurons (Lemke and Rothlin 2008). These receptors regulate the effects of TLR mediated response by inducing the expression of Suppressor of Cytokine Signalling proteins (SOCS 1 and 3), a family of intracellular inducible proteins, that inhibit cytokine synthesis. (Baker et al., 2009).

8.2 Neuroimmunoregulatory molecules (NIRegs) regulate the innate immune response and prevents inappropriate activation

One basic property of the NIRegs is their expression by host cells, but neither by pathogens nor by apoptotic cells. NIRegs interact with either macrophages or microglia to provide immuno regulation, promoting a reduction in the severity of inflammation and facilitating tissue repair (Hoarau et al., 2011).

Examples of NIRegs, include CD200 and CD47; these two molecules both represent "don't eat me" signals cells, to prevent un warranted phagocytosis, whereas the Siglecs detect sialic acid (a "don't eat me" signal) on host cells resulting in immuno regulation and inhibition of microglial activation. CRProteins modulate complement activation whereas, the the CD24/siglec 10 pathway inhibits DAMPs initiated inflammatory response (Chen et al., 2009). see table 2, for a summary of the current NIreg s.

8.3 Complement regulatory proteins (CRP) as NIRegs

To avoid self-destruction, host cells employ a range of regulatory molecules, including the CRP, which inhibit assembly of either the C3-cleaving enzymes or the formation of the membrane attack complex (MAC) on host cell surface. As pathogens lack these inhibitors, activation of the complement cascade can proceed and results in lysis or phagocytosis of microbial intruders. (Zipfle and Skerka 2009). However, animals deficient in CRP are also likely to experience severe inflammation, because unregulated activation of the C system will generate C3a and C5a, both anaphylatoxins(chemotaxis of macrophages and neutrophils) with uncontrolled activation of MAC.

Similarly, as "self" cells progress to "altered self" (apoptotic cells), there is a down-regulation of complement inhibitors (including CRP) at the cell surface including a low sialic acid content and the loss of the CRP, FH(Crocker and Verki 2001). The loss of CRP based membrane inhibitors, such as CD46, can lead to moderate and limited opsinonisation of apoptotic cells with the complement proteins (C3b, iC3b) with the promotion of phagocytosis by CR3/CR4. (Elward et al., 2005)

The soluble C1 inhibitor (C1-INH), C4b-binding protein (C4bp), factor H (fH), factor I (fI), S protein (Sp) and clusterin are all CRP, expressed by glia and neurons (Gasque 2004). C4bp is an important NIReg, because it is able to inhibit the DAMP effect of DNA released from necrotic cells and has been detected upon amyloid plaques in AD, potentially limiting C activation (Torouw et al., 2007; Torouw et al., 2005).

The other CRP are expressed on the cell membrane and include two trans membrane proteins CR1, membrane cofactor protein (MCP, CD46) and two GPI-anchored proteins, Decay Accelerating Factor (DAF, CD55) and CD59 (see comprehensive review Zipel and Skerka., 2009). Moreover, since CD55 is a ligand for CD97 on macrophages it is tantalizing to speculate that CD55-CD97 interactions could play an important role regulating phagocytosis (Hamann et al., 1996).

FH, CD55 and CD59, fulfill the criteria for an NIReg given that they are broadly expressed and extremely important in the control of complement activation on self-cells. Neurons also express NIRegs in the form of the CRP, Factor H. This CRP is able to reduce axonal degeneration (self injury) in a MOG induced EAE model, as the result of inhibiting C pathway activation. (Griffiths et al., 2009)

8.4 Siglecs are an emerging NIReg

The Siglecs, are expressed by monocytes, microglia and macrophages; they have a potentially important immuno regulatory function in the CNS (Linnartz et al., 2010) The absence of sialic acid expression on micro-organsims or apoptotic cells is detected by siglecs as a signal of "missing self "and this promotes phagocytosis (Crocker and Virki 2001). To emphasize the importance of sialic acid residues as a signal of "self", over twenty, pathogens have evolved the capacity to synthesize or capture sialic acids, providing molecular mimics of host ("self ") and thus avoiding detection by their host (Jones et al., 2003). This possibility is supported by evidence showing Group B Streptocci with siayalted surface molecules bind to neutrophils expressing siglec 9, with reduction in their killing response aiding the survival of bacteria (CaoCrocker 2010).

The CD33 related sub-family of Siglecs (includes human Siglec 10, Siglec 11, Siglec 16) and the CD22 related Siglecs, both signal through cytosolic ITIM (immuno receptor tyrosine based inhibitory motifs) that provide inhibitory regulation of receptor pathways (Crocker and Varki 2003; Lemke and Rothlin 2008). This association strengths the potential NIReg regulatory role for both CD33 and CD22 siglecs on the basis of their capacity to detect sialylated glycans (α-2, 6 α-2, 3 and α-2, 8 linked sialic acids) representing markers of" self "on host cells.

The interaction between CD22 and B cells results in a phosphorylation of ITIMS with the recruitment of the Src homology 2 domain –containing protein tyrosine phophatases(SHP-1 and SHP-2 proteins) with a down regulation of inflammatory signalling. (Crocker 2007).

Cortical neurons express high levels of CD 22 and on ligation with microglial CD45 it reduced LPS induced microglial expression of TNF-α acting as a negative regulator of microglial cytokine release (Mott et al., 2004). Siglec 11, expressing microglia have a reduced neurotoxic capacity and fail to phagocytose apoptotic material in micro glial- neuron co culture experiments. (Wang et al., 2010: Toguchi et al 2009).

CD33 related Siglecs inhibit cell proliferation, negatively regulate TLR, increase apoptosis and reduce IFN production, again through ITIM signalling pathways (Cao and Crocker 2010). The absence of sialic acid in the cell wall of a pathogen will prevent the interaction with CD22, CD33, resulting in the failure to promote an ITIM related inhibitory response with an increased host " protective " inflammatory response (Crocker 2010). The presence of sialic acid residues defines host cell as "self" and initiates an inhibitory signal to down regulate any inflammatory response and prevent inappropriate phagocytosis of host cells. A further immunoregulatory role for Siglecs is their inhibitory response to TLR signalling activated by DAMPs.

8.5 CD24/siglec 10; an NIReg pathway that regulates DAMPS and reduces tissue injury

The successful resolution of pathogen invasion of the CNS requires the detection of PAMPs and also DAMPs released by tissue injury. HMBG, S100 and HSP are all examples of a DAMPand released from cells after injury. The innate immune system can be activated by DAMPs as a consequence of being detected by a RAGE and TLRs and triggering the TLR – MyD88 –NFkB pathway (Liu et al., 2009). Of interest, is the relatively low level inflammatory response elicted by DAMPs, raising the possibility that DAMPS are capable of regulating the inflammatory response.

One pathway, capable of imunoregulating DAMPS involves, CD24, a heat stable antigen and GPI anchored protein, that binds to HMBG, reducing the pro inflammatory properties of this DAMP. Two lines of evidence support the regulatory role of CD24; individuals with polymorphisms of CD24 appear to at risk of developing so called autoimmune disease involving inflammation and when T cells are introduced into CD24 deficient mice, they undergo rapid proliferation. Furthermore CD24, is expressed in the developing CNS and by stem cells; although not fully characterized, it is known to regulate cell proliferation and neuritic outgrowth (Kleene et al., 2001: Shewan et al., 1996).

CD24 detect s DAMPs, but not PAMPS and the CD24- DAMP complex binds to the Siglec 10, which has an ITIM motif and recruits SHP-1 SHP-2 and SHIP complexes. The presence of

Siglec 10- SHIP-1 compex inhibits the DAMP-TLR /NLR based activation of the NF-kB pathway, reducing DAMP activated inflammatory cytokine expression. PAMP activation of the TLR –MyD88 –Nf-kB pathway remains intact and inflammatory cytokines are synthesised. This proposed pathway, based upon CD24 binding to DAMPS, but not PAMPS, allows the host to regulate endogenous protein activation of inflammation following infection and neuro degeneration, adding a further protective pathway to reduce the severity of tissue injury.

Mice deficient in the human homologue of siglec 10 have an increased proinflammatory response to pathogens (Chen et al., 2009). Further evidence, that the CD24/siglec 10 interaction presents an NIReg pathway is the inhibition of the inflammatory response initiated by the DAMPS, HSP 70 and HSP90 (Liu et al., 2009). The CD24 /Siglec 10 pathway represent an NIReg pathway capable of regulating endogenous DAMPs released during injury, neurodegeneration and infection. (Liu et al 2009; Hoarau et al., 20011)

8.6 CD200-200R an NIReg pathway for evasion of phagocytosis

CD200, is a well defined member of the NIRegs family it is expressed by reactive astrocytes; its counter receptor, C200R is expressed by microglia and perivascular macrophages (Barclay et al., 2002; Broderick et al., 2002 Lyons et al., 2007). The interaction between CD200 and CD200R results in down regulation of microglial phagcocytosis, preventing "self" attack (Barclay et al., 2002: Hoek et al., 2000). CD200 is a 41-47kD surface molecule and a member of the immunoglobulin Ig supergene family, characterized by two IgSF domains (Barclay et al., 2002; Wright et al., 2001). It is a highly conserved and found in invertebrates and vertebrates; like many of the glycoproteins containing this molecular arrangement they are involved with regulation of the immune system.

In the brain CD200, is expressed by microglia, cerebellar and retinal neurons, together with vascular endothelium. (Broderick et al., 2002). The counter receptor to CD200, CD200R, also contains two IgSF domains and is expressed by myeloid cells and brain microglia (Koning et al., 2009; Koning et al., 2007). In CD200 deficient mice, the number of activated microglia and macrophages were more numerous after an experimental lesion, as compared to wild type animals, providing evidence that the CD200/CD200R interaction is related to regulation of microglial activation and regulation of local inflammation (Hoek et al., 2000). This interpretation is supported by experiments in CD200 -/-mice inoculated with myelin oligodendrocyte glycoprotein MOG peptide to induce EAE. In these experiments the severity of the EAE was increased owing to the loss of CD200 regulation of microglial activity (Hoeket al., 2000). The contribution made by the CD200 (astrocytes)-CD200R (microglia) interaction on microglia in MS and AD remains to be established, although evidence for a dysregulation of CD200-CD200R pathway as a contributory factor to increase the severity of inflammation in MS has been proposed (Koning et al., 2009).

8.7 CD47-C172 an NIReg pathway as a marker of " self" or "don't eat me".

CD47, is expressed by astrocytes, neurons, macrophages and endothelium. The interaction between CD47 with the counter receptor CD172a, down regulates microglial activity, complement activation and cytokine expression, overall reducing the severity of the inflammatory response (deVries et al., 2002 Reinholdet al., 1995)

CD47 has five trans membrane regions with alternatively spliced isoforms of CD47 having a tissue specific expression, form 2 is present in bone marrow, whereas form 4 is highly expressed in brain (Reinhold et al., 1995). CD47, has two counter receptors; CD172a is expressed by myeloid cells, microglia and neurons a plasma membrane protein with three Ig domains in its extracellular component (Brown et al., 2001) and thrombospondin TSP (Lamy et al., 2007).

The interaction between CD47 with CD172a, recruits tyrosine phosphotases SHP-1 and SHP-2, with down regulation of macrophage phagocytosis, complement activation and cytokine synthesis including (Vernon –Wilson et al 2001: Brown et al., 2001: Oldenborg et al., 2001: Seiffertet al., 2001. The protective activity of CD47 could also be extended to its beneficial role in supporting neural development and promoting clearance of amyloid fibrils, albeit by mechanisms that remain ill-characterized (Bamberger et al., 2003).

The interaction between CD47 and CD172a has been shown to reduce neutrophil migration across endothelium and blocking CD47 induced expression of inflammatory cytokines by dendritic cells. CD47 is capable of inducing apoptosis in both T cells and cells deficient in CD47 i. e. loss of "self" identity, these cells are subsequently cleared rapidly from the systemic circulation by the spleen. (Oldenborg et al., 2001). The interaction between CD47 and thrombospondin promotes apoptosis of activated T cells, therefore, reducing inflammation by terminating T cell activation (Lamy et al., 2007: Sarati et al., 2008).

Hence, CD47, represents an important "don't eat me signal", preventing inappropriate phagocytosis of host cells (Elward and Gasque 2003). Apoptotic cells rapidly loose CD47, reducing its ability to bind and phosphorylate CD172a to recruit inhibitory signals and increasing their clearance through phagocytosis. The presence of CD47 on neurons and T cells is capable of promoting apoptosis through the CD95/Fas and caspase independent pathways (Manna et al., 2005). In MS, CD47, but not CD172a expression, is reduced at the edge of a chronic plaque, contributing to the loss of immuno regulation of microglia in this chronic inflammatory disease(Koning et al 2009).

The finding that viable cells are readily ingested if 'don't eat me signals' are disrupted raises the intriguing possibility that recognition and removal by phagocytosis is a default process that is actively prevented by inhibitory ligands on viable cells. Whether or not the CD47-CD172a pathway is capable of regulating microglial activity in disease remains to be determined. (Hoarau et al., 2011)

9. Emerging NIRegs; semaphorins and suppressor of cytokine signalling proteins (SOCS)

9.1 Semaphorins and microglia represent a potential pathway to regulate the host inflammatory response

The semaphorins are a diverse group of highly conserved trans membrane and extra cellular proteins with an extra cellular, 500 amino acid cysteine rich, semaphorine domains. Semaphorins bind to a diverse range of receptors; in the brain, plexins and neuropilins whereas in the immune system, the C -type lectin, CD72 is expressed mainly by T cells, but also on DC and macrophages. The functional importance of the semaphorins was initially directed towards control of axon growth, but it is now apparent these molecules are important immuno regulators in the CNS (Takegahara et al., 2005).

The interaction between Sema 4D (originally CD100), a trans membrane semaphorine, and the immune system CD72 results in an increased expression of cytokines by B cells, because Sema 4D turns off the inhibitory ITIM associated pathway (Suzuki et al., 2008). In the CNS microglia are activated by Sema 4D binding to plexin B1, rather than the CD72 molecule that is also expressed by microglia (Okuno et al; 2009)

Interestingly, plexin B1 and Sema 4D deficient mice are resistant to EAE induced by MOG derived peptide, because of the failure to generate MOG –specific T cells, emphasising the importance of functional Sema 4D for T cell activation and differentiation within the CNS (Takegahara et al., 2005). Antibodies raised against Sema 4D reduced inflammation during EAE, this was explained as the result of blocking T cells expressing Sema 4D interacting with microglial plexin to promote expression of pro inflammatory cytokines (Okuno et al., 2009).

In contrast to the other NIReg pathways, Sema 4D, increases the host inflammatory response by upregulating the level of cytokine expression and microglial activation. The regulation provided by Sema4D ensures the host inflammatory response is appropoiate to counter the effects of pathogens and neurtoxic proteins. Conversly inhibition of the SEMA 4D-plexin pathway represents a potential new target to suppress and regulate neuro inflammation.

9.2 Suppressor of cytokine signalling proteins (SOCS)

SOCS, are a family of eight intracellular, cytokine inducible proteins, expressed by CNS cells (microglia, astrocytes and neurons) that inhibit IFN signalling in CNS cells (Baker etal., 2010). Through activation of STAT transcription factors the C terminal of the SOCS binds to and inhibits phosphorylated tyrosine residues on Janus kinases (JAK), in addition the of the N terminus contains a kinase inhibitory region, and this also inhibits INF synthesis and blocks the NF-kB pathway. In the brain, SOCS1 and 3 are induced by a variety of inflammatory cytokines including INFγand LPS. Overall, SOCS 1and 3 are examples of NIRegs because they block the JAK/STAT pathway regulating glial and neuron inflammatory cytokine synthesis.

SOCS1 and SOCS3 have potentially important clinical applications. Administration of SOCS-1 to experimental animals prevents EAE by inhibiting JAK-2 mediated phosphorylation reducing the expression of inflammatory cytokines IL-2, IL -5 and TNFα raising the possibility that SOCS-1 is a potential therapeutic agent to treat inflammatory mediated demyelination (Baker et al 2010)Furthermore, the level of SOCS 3 exppressed by T cells in relapsed MS was less than in remission and this correlated with STAT levels, such that reduced SOCS allowed STAT to rise increasing inflammatory cytokine levels and increasing the likelihood of relapse. (Baker et al 2009 for review of clinical studies involving SOCS)

9.3 Loss of immuno surveillance, NIRegs and CNS neoplasia

Glioblastoma (GBM), is the most common primary brain tumour in adults, it is highly aggressive and infiltrates throughout the brain. These tumours have developed the capacity to escape immune surveillance by suppressing the host anti -glioma response. Failure to promote an anti glioma response is associated with an accumulation of immunosuppressive, CD4-Fox P3+ regulatory T cells, both within and surrounding the tumour (Sonabend et al.,

The CNS Innate Immune System and the Emerging Roles of the Neuroimmune Regulators (NIRegs)
in Response to Infection, Neoplasia and Neurodegeneration

197

2008). Glioma stem cells and macrophages are also capable of inducing immuno supression in host microglia, because they express the anti -inflammatory cytokines TGF-1β MIC-1macrophage inhibitory factor and also inhibit microglial phagocytosis (Wu et al., 2010; Hussain et al., 2006). A pivotal role in this apparent loss of anti- glioma response is the inhibition of the JAK/STAT signalling pathway in glioma cells with resulting cell proliferation, inhibition of both host cell inflammatory response and tumour immuno surveillance (Brantley et al., 2008). The inhibition of STAT signalling pathway in GBM is thought to result from an over expression of the NIReg, SOCS -1that inhibits STAT and function as an immuno-modulatory molecule by blocking IFNβ and CD40, with the down regulation of both MHC I and II expression in GBM. However, the function role of the other SOCS proteins (SCOCS- 3) in GBM remains to be clarified; in vitro SOCS -3 increases the IL-10 mediated anti-inflammatory response and radio resistance, but therapeutic inhibition of STATalso promotes microglial recognition of glioma cells (Baker et al., 2009).

Glioma cells express a limited range of TLR and application of various ligands including LPS and Poly I; C did not have any therapeutic effect, probably due to the failure to stimulate intra tumour Antigen Presenting Cells. (Grauner et al., 2008. However, the injection of the TLR9 ligand, CpG, an oligonucleotide, resulted in effective anti glioma response with inhibition of local Tregs, together with an T effector cell mediated anti -glioma respons. TLR9 is not present in host cells surrounding the glioma, providing an explanation for the apparent failure of host cell to produce an effective T cell response (Grauner et al., 2008). The intra tumour injection of ligands such as CpG to selectively stimulate host expression of TLR is of potential therapeutic importance.

One further protective strategy employed by gliomas to evade imuno surveillance is the expression of C regulator proteins. Activation of C pathway is potentially able to lyse tumour cells, but several glioma cells lines have been shown to express complement regulators CD59, CD55, CD46 and FH on their cell surface, preventing C attack and generation of lytic MAC(Maenpaa A et al., 1996, Junnikkala S et al., 2000). One possible therapeutic route is infact, the use of surface CD46, this Creg is very similar to the adenovirus receptors (adenovirus serotype 3) and provides a target to deliver an adenovirus containing anti- glioma therapy. (Ulasov et al 2006)

Outside the CNS, squamous cell carcinoma of the skin, leukaemias and myeloma cells up regulate surface expression of the NIReg, CD200, and this inhibits local immune detection promoting metastatic potential. After spreading to local lymph nodes, metastatic tumour cells that are CD200+ interact with local CD200R+ myeloid drived cells such as macrophages and potentially microglia, enhancing their survival, conversely loss of CD200 reduces metastatic tumour survival. The expression of CD200 is a property of the primary tumour and this expression did not vary according the type of tissue infiltrated by metastatic tumour (Stumpova et al., 2010).

10. Conclusion

The host inflammatory reaction is required to counter the detrimental effects of pathogen invasion (encephalitis and meningitis) and the accumulation of amyloid, mutant prions (neurodegenerative disease). One consequence of the host's protective inflammatory reaction is an inevitable amount of associated tissue injury. The detrimental effects of tissue injury have to be to be balanced against the, consequences of not removing a pathogen (or clearing neurotoxic proteins), usually this leads to peristent inflammation preventing any tissue repair. This balance between protective and destructive consquences is the so called "double edged sword"effect, that accompanies brain inflammation (Wyss- Coray and Mucke 2002). The role of the NIRegs is to modulate the level of the protective inflammatory response, in order to provide the "appropriate amount " of inflammation to allow the efficent clearance of pathogens and neurotoxic proteins from the brain.

The immune response against "non self" (pathogens, neurotoxic protiens) must be critically regulated in order to provide conditions of tissue repair without excessive destruction of "self "or host cells. Self (host) must be distinguish from " non –self "as defined by, pathogens PAMPs, apoptotic cells ACAMPs and "danger proteins" (HMGB1, HSP and S100) classified as (DAMPs). Non self (PAMPS, DAMPS), is detected by a range of intracellular and trans membrane PRR (TLR, RIG, NDLR,) whereas the scavenger receptors CD14, CD36, C lectins and TREM-2 provide a clerance pathway for apoptotic cells and neurotoxic proteins. Activation of the complement pathway by pathogens and neurotoxic proteins (Fibrillary Amyloid and mutant prion protein) results in MAC formation and anaphylotoxins C3a and C5a, all promoting inflammation and tissue destruction. The C pathway also assists the SR clear apoptotic cells through opsonins C3 and C4 localization on the surface of apoptotic cells.

To prevent excessive host tissue destruction, (NIRegs) must control the proinflammatory response and efficiently clear apoptotic cells (non-phlogistic response), before they are able to release neurotoxic enzymes to increase host tissue destruction. NIRegs, provide cell surface signals (CD200, CD47, sialic acid, CD46,) to identify "self " and through interaction with counter receptors (CD200R, CD172a, FH, Siglecs, CD24 –Siglec,) utilizing ITAM /ITIM pathways, inhibit microglial activation and phagocytosis of host cells. The C pathway is regulated by a series of CRP also regarded as NIRegs, because they reduce C activation and excessive host tissue destruction. The inhibiton of CRPs on tumour cells could provide a mechanism to increase host anti -tumour cell lysis as well as providing receptors for the delivery of viruses carrying anti glioma reagents. One emerging pathway controls, microglial activation as the result of T cells expressing Sema 4D; inhibiton of this pathway resulted in a down regulation of the severity of inflammation in MOG induced EAE. Similarly, the contribution made by the SOCS family of intracellular proteins to regulating the innate immune response in a diverse range of neuroinflammatory conditions requires clarification.

The therapeutic benefit of NIRegs is apparent, but to date, there is only limited evidence for their influence in clinical examples of neuro-degneration and neuro-inflammation. CD200-CD200R, CD47 and SOCS have been detected in MS tissue providing evidence for dys regulation of the host inflammatory response. There is some experimental evidence to show PAMPS and DAMPs can be distinguished by the host and DAMP initiated inflammation is regulated by the emerging NIReg, CD24/Siglec, pathway. The cellular localization and functional importance for each of the NIRegs is summarised in table 2.

It is highly likely the NIRegs provide a range of potentially important therapeutic reagents that selectively regulate the host immune response and promote tissue repair in a variety of brain infections (viral and bacterial), neurodegerative diseases and neoplasia. The opportunity presented by the NIRegs as the means to selectively regulate the CNS immune response to a wide range of pathogens and neurotoxic proteins should be exploited as a matter of some importance.

Pattern Recognition Receptor PRR	Ligand detected	PRR and CNS cell expression	Function	Host Innate immune response
TLR2	Bacterial cell wall peptidoglycan Zymosan (Fungi) Haemagluttin (Measles virus)	Microglia Astrocytes Choroid plexus	Form hetero dimres with TLR-1 to detect Gram neg ative bacteria Co operates with Dectin -1to detect fungi	Microglia increased pro inflammatory cytokines Phagocytosis
TLR3	ds RNA	Neurons microglia astrocytes oligodendroglia	West Nile Virus Detect necrosis and danger signals (HMGB, HSP)	Microglial IFNβ TNFα IL-6 Systemic cytokines and BBB receptor
TLR4	Bacteria Lipopolysacahride LPS	Microglia, astrocytes ependyma Choroid plexus	Cooperates with CD36, CD14 and DC-SIGN to detect fungi and *Streptococcus pneumonia*	Microglia and astrocyte inflammatory cytokines phagocytosis of apoptotic cells
TLR 5	Flagellin, bacterial protein	Macrophage		
TLR7	ssRNA	Microglia, astrocytes ependyma, neurons	Influenza A Detect necrosis and "danger signal "HMGB, HSP	Astrocytes increased TNFα IFNβ MCP-1
TLR8	ssRNA	Neurons	RNA viruses	Astrocytes increased TNF α, IFNβ, MCP-1
TLR9	CpG DNA	Microglia, astrocytes	Detect necrosis and "danger signals" HMBG-1	Microglia express TNFα, IL-12, NO HMBG-1 /RAGE detected by TLR-9
TLR11	Profilin, bacterial protein	Genitourinary Neurons	Detects Toxoplasmosis Neurocysticerosis	Inflammatory cytokines
RIG-1	Short dsRNA	Microglia, astrocytes	Japanese encephalitis virus Influenza A, Ebola virus	Astrocytes express IFNβ, IL-6, IL-8 RANTES
MDA-5	Long dsRNA	Microglia astrocytes	?Nipah virus, polio virus,	Microglia express IFNβ
NOD like	Bacterial cell wall		*Listeria bacillius Shigella*	

Receptors NOD-1 and NOD-2		?Microglia, astrocytes	*Flexneri Helicobacter pylori Mycobacterium tuberculosis*	
NLR -3 (NLP-3)	Bacterial cell wall peptidglycan peptidoglycan and virus proteins	? in CNS	Bacteria Viruses Crohn's disease	Inflammasome(NLR ASC, procaspase -1) is engaged to produce inflammatory cytokines

Table 1. Shows the individual ligands detected by TLR and Non- TLR (R LR MDA and NLR), Pattern Recognition Receptors PRR in the CNS. The cellular distribution of each of these receptors in the CNS is provided together with their contribution to host CNS innate immune system in response to pathogens(PAMPS and danger signals (DAMPS).

Neuroimmuoregulatory (NIReg)	NIReg-receptor/ligand	Cell –cell interaction	Mechanism of immune regulation	Human disease
CD200 Astrocyte	CD200R microglia	Astrocyte – microglia	Reduce phagocytosis	Alzheimer's (AD) Multiple sclerosis (MS)
CD47 Astrocyte Endothelium neuron	CD172a myeloid cells microglia	Astrocyte – microglia	Reduce phagocytosis and cytokine expression	Multiple sclerosis
Complement regulators FH, CD46, CD55, CD59 C4bp CD46 (MCP) CD55(DAF)	Sialic acid Complement proteins	Astrocytes Microglia Neurons	Reduce C activation	Neurodegenerative disease AD Huntington's disease Inhibits complement regulation of glioma lysis
Siglecs CD33 family Siglec 10 Siglec 11	Sialic acid Detect absence of sialic acids " non self"	NK cells Microglia	Reduces inflammation ITIM pathway	Bacterial infection; bacteria mimic sialic acids to become " self "
CD24 -Siglec 10 pathway	DAMPs HMGB-1	microglia stem cells	Binds with SHP -1, this complex inhibits DAMPS activation of NF-kB	Reduces DAMP associated inflammation Polymorphisms in CD24 associated with autoimmune disease
Suppressor of cytokine synthesis SOCS1 SOCS3	Inhibits IFN and IL cytokine stimulation of cytokine expression	Microglia astrocytes neurons	Blocks JAK/STAT cytokine pathway	Glioblastoma SOCS increased SOCS reduced in relapsed MS

Thrombomodulin CD141	HMBG1/ DAMPS	Microglia	Blocks HMBG binding to RAGE and TLR activation	
Semaphorin SEMA4	CD72 on T cells Plexin B1 on microglia	T cell with microglia	Blocks ITIM increases cytokine expression	Sema4D deficiency reduced EAE severity

Table 2. The potential of NIRegs and their cellular localization, ligands and mechanism whereby they produce immuno regulation. In the final column there is information relating to their contribution to infection, neurodegeneration and neuro inflammation as well as neoplasia, in the human CNS.

11. References

Abbot, NJ. Morphology of non mammalian glial cells; functional implications. Chapter 4. in Neuroglia ed Kettleman H, Ransom BR. Oxford University Press 1995

Abeyama, K, D. M Stren, Y Ito, K Kawahara, Y. Yoshimoto, M. Tanka, T. Uchmura, N. Ida, Y. Yamakazi, S. Ymada, Y. Yamamoto, H. Yamamoto, S, Iino, N Taniguchi I. Maruyama. 2005. The terminal domain of thrombomodulin sequesters high mobility group B-1 protein, a novel anit inflammatory mechanism. J Clin. Invest. 115: 1267-1274.

Akira, S, S. Uematsu, O. Takeuchi. 2006. Pathogen recognition and innate immunity. Cell 124: 783-801.

Akiyma, H, Mc Geer. 1990. Brain microglia constitutively express beta -2 integrins. J Neuroimmunology. ; 39: 81-93.

Alexopoulou, L., A. C. Holt, R. Medzhitov, and R. A. Flavell. 2001. Recognition of double-stranded RNA and activation of NF-kappaB by Toll- like receptor 3. Nature 413: 732-738. 39.

Alarcon R, C. Fuenzalida, M. Santibanez, and R von Bernardi. 2005. Expression of scavenger receptors in glial cells. Comparing the adhesion of astrocytes and microglia from neonatal rats to surface bound beta amyloid. J Biol Chem. ; 280: 30406- 30415.

Alvarez, C., , F. Lasala, J. Carrillo, O. Munz, A. L. Corbi and R. Delgado. 2002. C Type le ctins DC In-SIGN and L-SIGN mediate cellular entry y Ebola virus in *cis* and *trans*. J Virol 76 (13); 6841-6844.

Angata, T., S. C. Kerr, D. R. Greaves, N. M. Varki, P. R. Crocker, and A. Varki. 2002. Cloning and characterization of human Siglec-11. A recently evolved signaling that can interact with SHP-1 and SHP-2 and is expressed by tissue macrophages, including brain microglia. J Biol Chem 277: 24466-24474.

Babcock, A. A., M. Wirenfeldt, T. Holm, H. H. Nielsen, L. Dissing-Olesen, H. Toft-Hansen, J. M. Millward, R. Landmann, S. Rivest, B. Finsen, and T. Owens. 2006. Toll-like receptor 2 signaling in response to brain injury: an innate bridge to neuroinflammation. J Neurosci 26: 12826-12837

Baker, B. J. L. Nowoslawski -Akhtar and E. N. Benveniste. 2009. SOCS1 and SOCS3 in the control of CNS immunity. TIMS 30 (8): 392-400

Bamberger, M. E., M. E. Harris, D. R. McDonald, J. Husemann, and G. E. Landreth. 2003. A cell surface receptor complex for fibrillar beta-amyloid mediates microglial activation. J Neurosci 23: 2665-2674.

Barclay, A. N., G. J. Wright, G. Brooke, and M. H. Brown. 2002. CD200 and membrane protein E interactions in the control of myeloid cells. Trends in Immunology 23: 285-290.

Bianchi, M. E, 2007. DAMPSs, PAMPS and alarmins: all we need to know about danger. Journ Leukocyte Biology 81: 1-5.

Botto, M, E. M. Dell, 'Angnola EM, Golay J, et al. 1998. Homozygous C1q deficiency causes glomerulonephritis associated with multiple apoptotic bodies. Nat Genetics. 19: 1956-59

Bowman, C. C., A. Rasley, S. L. Tranguch, and I. Marriott. 2003. Cultured astrocytes express toll-like receptors for bacterial products. Glia 43: 281-291.

Bsibsi, M., R. Ravid, D. Gveric, and J. M. van Noort. 2002. Broad expression of Toll-like receptors in the human central nervous system. Journal of Neuropathology and Experimental Neurology 61: 1013-1021.

Broderick, C., R. M. Hoek, J. V. Forrester, J. Liversidge, J. Sedgwick, A. D. Dick. 2002. Constitutive retinal expression of CD200 regulates resident microglial and activation state of inflammatory cells during experimental autoimmune uveoretinitis Am J Path 1612: 1669-1677.

Brown, E. J., and W. A. Frazier. 2001. Integrin-associated protein (CD47) and its ligands. 11: 130-135.

Brown, G. 2006 Dectin -1 a signaling non TLR pattern recognition receptor. Nature Rev Immunol 6: 33-43.

Bsibsi, M., C. Persoon-Deen, R. W. Verwer, S. Meeuwsen, R. Ravid, and J. M. Van Noort. 2006. Toll-like receptor 3 on adult human astrocytes triggers production of neuron protective mediators. Glia 53: 688-695.

Brantley, E. C, and E. N. Benveniste, 2008. Signal transducer and activator of transcription - 3: a molecular hub for signaling pathways in gliomas. Mol Cancer Res: 6(5): 675-684

Bu, G., J. Cam, and C. Zerbinatti. 2006. LRP in amyloid-beta production and metabolism. Ann N Y Acad. Sci. 1086: 35-53.

Burudi, E. M, P. D Stahl and A. Regnier-Vigouroux. 1999. Identification and functional characterization of the mannose receptor in astrocytes. Glia 25: 44-55.

Butchi, N. B., S. Pourciau, M. Du, T. W. Morgan, and K. E. Peterson. 2008. Analysis of the neuroinflammatory response to TLR7 stimulation in the brain: comparison of multiple TLR7 and/or TLR8 agonists. J Immunol 180: 7604-7612.

Cambi, A., M. Koopman, C. G Figdor. 2005. C type lectins detect pathogens. Cell Microbiol 7(4): 481-488.

Cameron, J. S., L. Alexopoulou, J. A. Sloane, A. B. DiBernardo, Y. Ma, B. Kosaras, R. Flavell, S. M. Strittmatter, J. Volpe, R. Sidman, and T. Vartanian. 2007. Toll-like receptor 3 is a potent negative regulator of axonal growth in mammals. J Neurosci 27: 13033-13041.

The CNS Innate Immune System and the Emerging Roles of the Neuroimmune Regulators (NIRegs)
in Response to Infection, Neoplasia and Neurodegeneration

203

Canova, C., J. W. Neal, and P. Gasque. 2006. Expression of innate immune complement regulators on brain epithelial cells during human bacterial meningitis. J Neuroinflammation 3: 22.

Cao, H, and P. R. Crocker. 2010. Evolution of CD33 –related siglecs: regulating host immune functions and escaping pathogen exploitation. Immunology 132: 18-26.

Carpentier, P. A., W. S. Begolka, J. K. Olson, A. Elhofy, W. J. Karpus, and S. D. Miller. 2005. Differential activation of astrocytes by innate and adaptive immune stimuli. Glia 49: 360-374.

Carpentier, P. A., D. S. Duncan, and S. D. Miller. 2008. Glial toll-like receptor signaling in central nervous system infection and autoimmunity.

Carpentier, P. A., B. R. Williams, and S. D. Miller. 2007. Distinct roles of protein kinase R and toll-like receptor 3 in the activation of astrocytes by viral stimuli. Glia 55: 239-252.

Castiglioni, A, V Canti, P. Rovere-Queriniand, A. A, Manfredi. 2011. High mobility box 1(HGBM1) as a master regulator of innate immunity. Cell Tis Res 343: 189-199.

Cavassani, K. A., M. Ishii, H. Wen, M. A. Schaller, P. M. Lincoln, N. W. Lukacs, C. M. Hogaboam, and S. L. Kunkel. 2008. TLR3 is an endogenous sensor of tissue necrosis during acute inflammatory events. J Exp Med 205: 2609-2621.

Chan A, T. Magus, and R Gold R. 2001. Phagocytosis of apoptotic inflammatory cells by microglia and modulation by different cytokines; mechanism for removal of apoptotic cells in the inflamed nervous system. Glia; 33: 87-95.

Chang G, N. M. Barbaro, R. O Pieper. 2002. Phosphatidylserine- dependent phagocytosis of cells by normal human microglia, astrocytes and glioma cells. Neuro oncol 2002; 3: 174-183.

Chauhan, V. S., D. G. Sterka, Jr., S. R. Furr, A. B. Young, and I. Marriott. 2009. NOD2 plays an important role in the inflammatory responses of microglia and astrocytes to bacterial CNS pathogens. Glia 57: 414-423.

Chen, GY, J Tang P, L Zheng, Y Liu. 2009. CD24 and siglec 10 selectively repress tissue damage- induced immune responses. Science 323: 1722-1725.

Chen, K., P. Iribarren, J. Hu, J. Chen, W. Gong, E. H. Cho, S. Lockett, N. M. Dunlop, and J. M. Wang. 2006. Activation of Toll-like receptor 2 on microglia promotes cell uptake of Alzheimer disease-associated amyloid beta peptide. J Biol Chem 281: 3651-3659.

Colonna, M, . 2003. TREMs in the immune system and beyond. Nat Rev Immunol 6: 445-453.

Coraci, I. S, H. J., Berman, J. W, Hulette, C. Dufour, J. H. Campanella, G. K, Luster, AD, Silverstein, J. B. El Khoury. 2002. CD36, a Class B Scavenger Receptor, is expressed on Microglia in Alzheimer's disease brains and can mediate production of reactive oxygen species in response to beta-amyloid fibrils. Am J Pathol 160: 101-112.

Creagh, E. M, L. A. J O'NEIL. 2006. TLRs, NLRs and RLRs; a trinity of pathogen sensors that cooperate in innate immunity. Trends in Immunology 277: 352-357.

Crocker, P. R., A. Varki. 2001. Siglecs, sialic acids and innate immunity Trends in Immunology 22 6: 337-342.

Crocker, P. R, J. C. Paulson and A. Varki. 2007. Siglecsand their roles in the immune system. Nature reviews in Immunol; 7 255-266

Daffis, S., M. A. Samuel, M. S. Suthar, M. Gale, Jr., and M. S. Diamond. 2008. Toll-like receptor 3 has a protective role against West Nile virus infection. J Virol 82: 10349-10358.

Dean, Y D, McGreal EP, Akatsu H, et al. Molecular and cellular properties of the rat AA4 antigen, a C type lectin -like receptor with structural homolgy to thrombomodulin. J Biol Chem 2000; 275: 34382 -34392

Delputte, P. L, H. Van Gorp, H. W. Favoreel, I. Hoebeke, I. Delrule, H. Dewerchin, , F Verdnock, B. Verhasselt, E. Cox, H. J. Nauwynck. 2011 Porcine Siaoladhesin (CD 169/Siglec -1) is an endocytic receptor that allows targeted delivery of toxins and antigens to macrophages PLos ONE 6: e1682

De Simoni, M. G., E. Rossi, C. Storini, S. Pizzimenti, C. Echart, and L. Bergamaschini. 2004. The powerful neuron protective action of C1-inhibitor on brain ischemia-reperfusion injury does not require C1q. Am J Pathol 164: 1857-1863.

de Vries, H. E., J. J. Hendriks, H. Honing, C. R. De Lavalette, S. M. van der Pol, E. Hooijberg, C. D. Dijkstra, and T. K. van den Berg. 2002. Signal-regulatory protein alpha-CD47 interactions are required for the transmigration of monocytes across cerebral endothelium. J Immunol 168: 5832-5839.

Ehlers, M. R. 2000. CR3: a general purpose adhesion-recognition receptor essential for innate immunity. Microbes Infect 2: 289-294.

Eikelenboom, P., C. Bate, W. A. Van Gool, J. J. Hoozemans, J. M. Rozemuller, R. Veerhuis, and A. Williams. 2002. Neuroinflammation in Alzheimer's disease and prion disease. Glia 40: 232-239.

El Khoury, J. B., K. J. Moore, T. K. Means, J. Leung, K. Terada, M. Toft, M. W. Freeman, and A. D. Luster. 2003. CD36 mediates the innate host response to beta-amyloid. J Exp Med 197: 1657-1666.

Elward, K., and P. Gasque. 2003. "Eat me" and "don't eat me" signals govern the innate immune response and tissue repair in the CNS: emphasis on the critical role of the complement system. Mol Immunol 40: 85-94.

Elward, K., M. Griffiths, M. Mizuno, C. L. Harris, J. W. Neal, B. P. Morgan, and P. Gasque. 2005. CD46 plays a key role in tailoring innate immune recognition of apoptotic and necrotic cells. J Biol Chem 280: 36342-36354.

Endo, Y, M., Takahashi, T. Fujita. 2006. Lectin complement system and pattern recognition. Immunobiology 211(4): 283-293.

Fadok, V. A, B. D. L. Rose, D. M, Pearson, A. B Ezekewitz, P. M. Henson. 2000. A receptor for phosphatidylserine specific clearance of apoptotic cells. Nature 405: 85-90.

Fadok, V. A, W. M. Bratton, P. M. Henson PM. 1998. CD36 is required for phagocytosis of apoptotic cells by human macrophages that use either a phosphatidylserine receptor or the vitronectin receptor (alpha v beta 3). J Immunol 161: 6350-6357.

Fang F, L. F. Lue, S. Yan, H. Xu, J. S. Luddy, D. Chen, D. GWalkr D. M. Stern, S. Yan, A. N. Schmidt, J. X. Chen and S. S. Yan. 2010. RAGE- dependent signaling in microglia contributes to neuroinflammation, A beta accumulation, and impaired learning memory in a mouse model of Alzheimer's disease Faseb 4: 1043-105

The CNS Innate Immune System and the Emerging Roles of the Neuroimmune Regulators (NIRegs)
in Response to Infection, Neoplasia and Neurodegeneration

205

Farina, C., M. Krumbholz, T. Giese, G. Hartmann, F. Aloisi, and E. Meinl. 2005. Preferential expression and function of Toll-like receptor 3 in human astrocytes. J Neuroimmunol 159: 12-19.

Fassbender, K., S. Walter, S. Kuhl, R. Landmann, K. Ishii, T. Bertsch, A. K. Stalder, F. Muehlhauser, Y. Liu, A. J. Ulmer, S. Rivest, A. Lentschat, E. Gulbins, M. Jucker, M. Staufenbiel, K. Brechtel, J. Walter, G. Multhaup, B. Penke, Y. Adachi, T. Hartmann, and K. Beyreuther. 2004. The LPS receptor (CD14) links innate immunity with Alzheimer's disease. Faseb J 18: 203-205.

Foell, D., H. Wittkowski, T. Vogl, and J. Roth. 2007. S100 proteins expressed in phagocytes: a novel group of damage-associated molecular pattern molecules. J Leukoc Biol 81: 28-37.

Fujita, T., K. Onoguchi, K. Onomoto, R. Hirai, and M. Yoneyama. 2007. Triggering antiviral response by RIG-I-related RNA helicases. Biochimie 89: 754-760.

Furr, S. R, V. S. Chauhan, D. Sterka Jr, V. Grdzelishvilli and I Marriot. 2008. Characterization of retinoic acid-inducible gene-I expression in primary murine glia following exposure to vesicular stomatitis virus. J Neurovirol; : 1-11.

Gardai, S, D. L. Bratton, C. AOgden, P. M. Henson. 2006. Recognition ligands on apoptotic cells; a perspective. J Leukco Biol 2006; 79: 896-903

Gardai, S. J., K. A. McPhillips, S. C. Frasch, W. J. Janssen, A. Starefeldt, J. E. Murphy-Ullrich, D. L. Bratton, P. A. Oldenborg, M. Michalak, and P. M. Henson. 2005. Cell-surface calreticulin initiates clearance of viable or apoptotic cells through trans-activation of LRP on the phagocyte. Cell 123: 321-334.

Garner, O. B, HC Aguilar JA, Fulcher, EL, Levroney R, Harrison, L. L. Wright, V Robinson, Aspericueta, M Panico, SM Hasalam, HR Morris A Dell, B. Lee and L. G. Baum 2010. Endothelial galectin -1 binds to specific glycans on nipah virus fusion protein and inhibits maturation mobility and functions to block syncytia formation. PloS Pathog; 15; 6 e10000993

Gasque, P. 2004. Complement: a unique innate immune sensor for danger signals. Mol Immunol 41: 1089-1098.

Gasque, P., Y. D. Dean, E. P. McGreal, J. VanBeek, and B. P. Morgan. 2000. Complement components of the innate immune system in health and disease in the CNS. Immunopharmacology 49: 171-186. 56.

Geijtenbeek, T. B., and S. I. Gringhuis. 2009. Signalling through C-type lectin receptors: shaping immune responses. Nat Rev Immunol 9: 465-47

Golpon, H,A.,V.A.Fadok.,LTaraseviciene. –Stewart 2004 Life after corpse engulfment, phagocytosis of apoptotic cells leads to VEGF secretionand cell growth Faseb 18; 1716-1718

Gregory, C. D. 2000. CD14 dependent clearance of apoptotic cells: relevance to the immune system. Current Opinions in Immunology 12: 27-34.

Gregory, C. D., and A. Devitt. 2004. The macrophage and the apoptotic cell: an innate immune interaction viewed simplistically? Immunology 113: 1-14.

Greter, M, Heppner FL, Lemos MP, Odermatt BM, Goebels N, Laufer T, et al. 2005 Dendritic cells permit immune invasion of the CNS in an animal model of multiple sclerosis. Nature Medicine; 11: 328-334

Griffin, D. E. 2003. Immune responses to RNA-virus infections ofthe CNS. Nat Rev Immunol 3: 493-502.

Griffiths, M. R, , J. W. Neal, P. Gasque. 2007. Innate immunity and protective neuroninflammation new emphasis on the role of neuroimmune regulatory proteins. Int Rev Neurobiol 82: 29-55

Griffiths, M. R., P. Gasque, and J. W. Neal. 2009. The multiple roles of the innate immune system in the regulation of apoptosis and inflammation in the brain. J Neuropathol Exp Neurol 68: 217-226.

Griffiths, M. R, J. W. Neal, M. Fontaine, T. Das, P. Gasque. 2009. Complement factor H, a marker of self protects against experimental autoimmune encephalomyelitis. J Immunol. 182: 4368-4377.

Grauer, OM, JW Molling, E. Bennink, L. W. J Toonen, R. M. P Sutmuller, S. Nierkens and G. J, Adema, 2008. TLR Ligands in the local treatment of established murine gliomas. JI 181: 6720-6729.

Halle, A., V. Hornung, G. C. Petzold, C. R. Stewart, B. G. Monks, T. Reinheckel, K. A. Fitzgerald, E. Latz, K. J. Moore, and D. T. Golenbock. 2008. The NALP3 inflammasome is involved in the innate immune response to amyloid-beta. Nat Immunol 9: 857-865.

Hanayama, R., M. Tanaka, K. Miwa, A. Shinohara, A. Iwamatsu, and S. Nagata. 2002. Identification of a factor that links apoptotic cells to phagocytes. Nature 417: 182-187.

Hamann, J., B. Vogel, G. M. van Schijndel, and R. A. van Lier. 1996. The seven-span transmembrane receptor CD97 has a cellular ligand (CD55, DAF). J Exp Med 184: 1185-1189.

Hauwel, M., E. Furon, C. Canova, M. R. Griffiths, J. W. Neal, and P. Gasque. 2005. Innate (inherent) control of brain infection, brain inflammation and brain repair: the role of microglia, astrocytes, "protective" glial stem cells and stromal ependymal cells. Brain Res Brain Res Rev 48: 220-233.

Helmy, K. Y., K. J. Katschke, Jr., N. N. Gorgani, N. M. Kljavin, J. M. Elliott, L. Diehl, S. J. Scales, N. Ghilardi, and M. van Lookeren Campagne. 2006. CRIg: a macrophage complement receptor required for phagocytosis of circulating pathogens. Cell 124: 915-927

Herz, J., and D. K. Strickland. 2001. LRP: a multifunctional scavenger and signaling receptor. J Clin Invest 108: 779-784.

Hoek RM, R. S., Murphy CA, Wright GJ, Goddard R, Zurawski SM, Blom B, Homola ME, Streit WJ, Brown MH, Barclay AN, Sedgwick JD. 2000. Down-regulation of the Macrophage Lineage Through Interaction with OX2 (CD200). Science 290: 1768.

Hoffman PR de Cathelineau AN Ogden CA et al, et al 2001. Phosphatidyl serine(PS) inducesPS receptor mediated macropinocytosis and promoted clearance of apoptotic cells. J Cell Biol; 155: 649-660

Hoarau, J. J, . Krejbich-Troto, M. C. Jaffar –Bandjee, T. Das, V. Thon-Hon, S. Kumar J. W. Neal, P. Gasque. 2011 The natural healing properties of innate immune receptors and neuroimmune regulatory proteins (NIRegs) in the CNS. CNS Drug Targets 10(1): 25-43

The CNS Innate Immune System and the Emerging Roles of the Neuroimmune Regulators (NIRegs)
in Response to Infection, Neoplasia and Neurodegeneration

207

Husemann, J., J. D. Loike, R. Anankov, M. Febbraio, and S. C. Silverstein. 2002. Scavenger receptors in neurobiology and neuropathology: their role on microglia and other cells of the nervous system. Glia 40: 195-205.

Hussain, S. F, D. Yeng, D. Suki, K. Aldape, A. B Heimberger. 2006. The role of human glioma infiltrating microglia/macrophages in mediating antitumour –immune resonse. Neuro Oncol 8 (3) 261-279

Iwasski A, Medzhitov 2010 Regulation of adaptive immunity by the innate system Science 327: 291-295.

Jack, C. S., N. Arbour, J. Manusow, V. Montgrain, M. Blain, E. McCrea, A. ShapiJack and J. P. Antel. 2005. TLR signaling tailors innate immune responses in human microglia and astrocytes. J Immunol 175: 4320-4330.

Jackson, A. C., J. P. Rossiter, and M. Lafon. 2006. Expression of Toll-like receptor 3 in the human cerebellar cortex in rabies, herpes simplex encephalitis, and other neurological diseases. J Neurovirol 12: 229-234.

Jana, M., C. A. Palencia, and K. Pahan. 2008. Fibrillar amyloid-beta peptides activate microglia via TLR2: implications for Alzheimer's disease. J Immunol 181: 7254-7262.

Janeway, Jr, CA 1992 The immune system evolved to discriminate infectious nonself from non infectious self. Immunol Today; 13: 11-16.

Ji- X, Gg. Olinger, S. Aris, Y. Chen, H. Gewurz, and G. T. Spear. 2005 Mannose binding lectin binds to Ebola and Marburg envelope glycoproteins resulting in blocking of virus interaction with DC-SIGN and complement –mediated virus neutralization. J Gen Virol; 86: 2535-2542.

Jin, J. J., H. D. Kim, J. A. Maxwell, L. Li, and K. Fukuchi. 2008. Toll-like receptor 4-dependent upregulation of cytokines in a transgenic mouse model of Alzheimer's disease. J Neuroinflammation 5: 23.

Jones, C., M. Virji, and P. R. Crocker. 2003. Recognition of sialylated meningococcal lipopolysaccharide by siglecs expressed on myeloid cells leads to enhanced bacterial uptake. Mol Microbiol 49: 1213-1225.

Joubert ,RS Kuchler,J. Zanetta P. Bladier ,D V Avellana-Adalid V M Caron M, Doinel C , CVincedon –galactoside binding lectin in. 1989. Immunohistochemical localization of a rat central nervous system 1. Light –and electron microscopical studies on developing cerebral cortex and corpus callosum. Dev Neuroci 1989 11: 397-413.

Karaparakis, M, D. J, Philpott, and R. L. Ferrero. 2007 Mammalian NLR proteins; discriminating foe from friend. Immuno Cell Biol 85(6): 495-502.

Kato, H, O. Takeguchi and S. Sato et al Differential roles of MDA5 and RIG-1 helicases in the recognition of RNA viruses. Nature: 441: 101-105.

Katze, M. G., Y. He, and M. Gale, Jr. 2002. Viruses and interferon: a fight for supremacy. Nat Rev Immunol 2: 675-687.

Kawai, T, S. Akira. 2010. The role of pattern – recognition receptors in innate immunity Update on Toll-like receptors. Nat Immunol 11: 373-384.

Kim, S. J, D. Gershov, X. Ma, N. Brot, and K. B. Elkon. 2002. I PLA -2 activation during apoptosis promotes the exposure of membrane lysophosphatidylcholine leading to binding by natural immunoglobulin M antibodies and complement activation. J Exp Med; 196: 655-665.

Kleene, R, H. Yang, M. Kutscheand, M. Schachner. 2001The neural recognition molecule is a sialic binding lectin for CD24, which induces promotion and inhibition of neurite outgrowth. J Biol Chem 276: 21656-21663.

Klune, J. R, R. Dhupar, J. Cardinal, T. R Billiar and A. Tsung. 2008. HMGB-1: Endogenous Danger signalling. Mol Med 14: 476-484

Koning N, D. F. Swab, R. M Hoek, I. Huitinga. 2009. Distribution of the immune inhibitory molecules CD200 and CD200Rin the normal central nervous system and multiple scelrosis lesions suggests neuron-glia and glia glia interactions. J Neuropath Exp Neurol 68(2): 159-167

Koning, N., L. Bo, R. Hoek, . 2007. Down regulation of macrophage inhibitory molecules in Multiple sclerosis lesions. Ann Neurol; 62: 504 -514

van Kooyk, Y. and, T. B. H Geijenbeek. 2003. DC-SIGN: escape mechanism for pathogens. Nature Rev Immunol 3: 697-709

Korb, L. C., and J. M. Ahearn. 1997. C1q binds directly and specifically to surface blebs of apoptotic human keratinocytes: complement deficiency and systemic lupus erythematosus revisited. J Immunol 158: 4525-4528.

Kovacs, G. G., P. Gasque, T. Strobel, E. Lindeck-Pozza, M. Strohschneider, J. W. Ironside, H. Budka, and M. Guentchev. 2004. Complement activation in human prion disease. Neurobiol Dis 15: 21-28.

Krysko, D. V, P Agostinis, O. Krysko, A. D. Garg C. Bachert, B. N Lanbrecht and P. Vanenabeele. 2011. Emerging role of damage-associated molecular patterns derived from mitochondria in inflammation. Trends in Immunol 32: 157-164.

Kumar, H, Kawai T and S Akira 2011 Pathogen Recognition by The Innate Immune system. International reviews of Immunology 30: 16-42

Kuraya, M., M. Matsushita, Y Endo, etal. 2003Expression of H-ficoline / Hahkata antigen mannose, binding lectin associated serine protease (MASP-1) and MASP3 by human glioma cell line T98G. Int Immunol; 15: 109-117

Laflamme, N., and S. Rivest. 2001. Toll-like receptor 4: the missing link of the cerebral innate immune response triggered by circulating gram-negative bacterial cell wall components. Faseb J 15: 155-163.

Laflamme, N., G. Soucy, and S. Rivest. 2001. Circulating cell wall components derived from gram-negative, not gram-positive, bacteria cause a profound induction of the gene-encoding Toll-like receptor 2 in the CNS. J Neurochem 79: 648-657.

Laflamme, N., H. Echchannaoui, R. Landmann, and S. Rivest. 2003. Cooperation between toll-like receptor 2 and 4 in the brain of mice challenged with cell wall components derived from gram-negative and gram-positive bacteria. Eur J Immunol 33: 1127-1138.

le Cabec, . V, L. J. Emorine, I. Toesca, C. Cougoule, I. Maridonneau-Parini. 2005. The human macrophage mannose receptor is not a professional phagocytic receptor. 77: 934-943

The CNS Innate Immune System and the Emerging Roles of the Neuroimmune Regulators (NIRegs)
in Response to Infection, Neoplasia and Neurodegeneration

209

Leonardi-Essmann, F., M. Emig, Y. Kitamura, R. Spanagel, and P. J. Gebicke-Haerter. 2005. Fractalkine-up regulated milk-fat globule EGF factor-8 protein in cultured rat microglia. J Neuroimmunol 160: 92-101

Lamy L, Foussat A, Brown EJ, et al. Interactions between CD47 and thrombospondin reduce inflammation. J Immunol 2007; 178: 5930 -5939

Landreth, G. E., and E. G. Reed-Geaghan. 2009. Toll-like receptors in Alzheimer's disease. Curr Top Microbiol Immunol 336: 137-153

Lehnardt, S., L. Massillon, P. Follett, F. E. Jensen, R. Ratan, P. A. Rosenberg, J. J. Volpe, and T. Vartanian. 2003. Activation of innate immunity in the CNS triggers neurodegeneration through a Toll-like receptor 4-dependent pathway. Proc Natl Acad Sci U S A 100: 8514-8519.

Lemke, G, . C. V Rothlin. Immunobiology of the TAM receptor. 2008. Nat Rev Immunol 8(5)327-336.

Linehan, SA, L. Martinez –Pomares, P. G Stahl, and S. Gordon. 1999. Mannose receptor and its putative ligand in normal murine lymphoid and non lymphoid organs; In situ expression of mannose receptor by selected macrophages, endothelial cells perivascular microglia and mesangial cells, but not dendritic cells. J Exp Med 1999; 189: 1961-1972.

Linnartz, B., Y Wang, and H Neumann. 2010. Microglial Immuno receptor Tyrosine –Based activation and Inhibition motif signalling in Neuro inflammtion. International Journal of Alzheimer's disease 10. 4061/2010/587463.

Liu, Y, GY, Chen and P Zheng. 2009. CD24-siglec G/10 discriminates danger from pathogen associated molecular patterns. Trends in Immunol 12: 557-561.

Lo MK, MillerD, Aljofan M, Mungall BA, Rollin PE, Bellini WJ PE Rota 2010 Characterization of the antiviral and inflammatory responses against Nipah virus in endothelial cells and neurons. Virology; 404(1): 78-88

Lock, K., J. Zhang, J. Lu, S. H. Lee, and P. R. Crocker. 2004. Expression of CD33-related siglecs on human mononuclear phagocytes, monocyte-derived dendritic cells and plasmacytoid dendritic cells. Immunobiology 209: 199-207.

Lotze, M. T., and K. J. Tracey. 2005. High-mobility group box 1 protein (HMGB1): nuclear weapon in the immune arsenal. Nat Rev Immunol 5: 331-342.

Lowenstein, PR 2002 Immunology of viral-vector-mediated gene transfer into the brain: an evolutionary developmental perspective. Trends in Immunology 23: 23-3012.

Lyons A, EJ Downer SCrotty, YM Nolan: KHMills MA Lynch 2007 CD200 ligand receptor interaction modulates microglial activation in vivo and in vitro: a role for IL-4. J Neurosci 27: 830-8313

Lu, J., C. Teh, U. Kishore, and K. B. Reid. 2002. Collectins and ficolins: sugar pattern recognition molecules of the mammalian innate immune system. Biochim Biophys Acta 1572: 387-400.

Ma, Y., J. Li, I. Chiu, Y. Wang, J. A. Sloane, J. Lu, B. Kosaras, R. L. Sidman, J. J. Volpe, and T. Vartanian. 2006. Toll-like receptor 8 functions as a negative regulator of neurite outgrowth and inducer of neuronal apoptosis. J Cell Biol 175: 209-215.

Magnus. T. C, O. Grauer, K. V. Toyka, RGold. 2001. Microglial phagocytosis of apoptotic inflammatory T cells leads to down regulation of microglial immune activation. J Immunol; 167; 5004-10.

Martino, G., R. Furlan, G. Comi, and L. Adorini. 2001. The ependymal route to the CNS: an emerging gene-therapy approach for MS. Trends Immunol 22: 483-490.

McGeer, P. L., H. Akiyama, S. Itagaki, and E. G. McGeer. 1989. Activation of the classical complement pathway in brain tissue of Alzheimer patients. Neurosci Lett 107: 341-346.

McKimmie, C. S., D. Roy, T. Forster, and J. K. Fazakerley. 2006. Innate immune response gene expression profiles of N9 microglia are pathogen-type specific. J Neuroimmunol 175: 128-141.

McMenamin, PG Distribution and Phenotype of dendritic cells and resident tissue macrophages in the dura mater. J Comp Neurol 1999; 405: 553-562.

Manna P, J. Dimitry P. E. Oldenborg, W. A. Frazier. 2005. CD 47 augments Fas /CD95 mediated Apoptosis. J Biol Chem; 280: 29637-29644.

Marshak –Rothstein, A and I. R. Rifkin. 2007. Immunologically active autoantigens: the roll of toll like recepotrs in the development of chronic inflammatory disease Ann Rev Immunol 25; 419-441

Marzolo MP, R. von Berhardi, N. C. Inestrosa. 2001. Mannose receptor is present in a functional state in rat microglial cells. J Neuroscience Res 2001; 58: 387-395.

Matushita, M 2009 Ficolins: complement –activating lectins involved in Innate Immunity J Innate Immunity; 2: 24-32

Matzinger, P. 2007. Friendly and dangerous signals: is the tissue in control? Nat Immunol 8: 11-13.

Medzhitov R, and CA Janeway. 2000. Innate immune recognition mechanisms and pathways. Immuno Rev; 173: 89-9.

Mevorach, D, J. O Mascraenhas, D. Gershov and K. B, Elkon. 1998. Complement dependant clearance of apoptotic cells by human macrophages. J Exp Med; 188: 2313-2320.

Miller, J. L., B. J deWet, L. Martinez-Pomares, C. M. Radcliffe, R. W. Dwek, and S Gordon. 2008. The mannose receptor mediates dengue virus infection of macropahges. PlosPathog 4: e17.

Minoretti, P., C. Gazzaruso, C. D. Vito, E. Emanuele, M. Bianchi, E. Coen, M. Reino, and D. Geroldi. 2006. Effect of the functional toll-like receptor 4 Asp299Gly polymorphism on susceptibility to late-onset Alzheimer's disease. Neurosci Lett 391: 147-149.

Miranda, J., K. Yaddanapudi, M. Hornig, and W. I. Lipkin. 2009. Astrocytes recognize intracellular polyinosinic-polycytidylic acid via MDA-5. Faseb J 23: 1064-1071.

Mishra, B. B., U. M. Gundra, J. M. Teale. 2008. Expression and distribution of Toll –like receptors 11-13 in the brain during murine neurocysticercosis. J Neuroinflammation 12: 5 53

Mohamadzadeh, M., L Chen, Schmaljohn AL. 2007. How Ebola and Marburg viruses battle the immune system. Nature Reviews in Immunology; 7: 556-567.

Morgan, B. P., and P. Gasque. 1996. Expression of complement in the brain: role in health and disease. Immunol Today 17: 461-466.

Mott, R. T., G. Ait-Ghezala, T. Town, T. Mori, M. Vendrame, J. Zeng, J. Ehrhart J Mullan and
   J. Tan 2004 Neuronal expression of CD22: novel mechanism for inhibiting
   microglial proinflammatory cytokine production. Glia 4: 369-379.

Mukhopadhyay, S., and S. Gordon. 2004. The role of scavenger receptors in pathogen
   recognition and innate immunity. Immunobiology 209: 39-49.

Mukhtar M., S. Harley, P. Chen M, BouHamdan, C. Patel, E. Acheampong, R. J. Pomerantz.
   2002. Primary isolated human brain microvascular endothelial cells express diverse
   HIV/SIV associated chemokine co receptors and DC-SGN and L-SIGN. Virology:
   297(1): 78-88.

Nauta, A. J, M. Daha, R. van Kooten, A. Roos. 2003. Recognition and clearance of apoptotic
   cells; a role for complement and pentraxins. Trends in Immunol; 24: 148-15425.

Netea, M. G, C. van der Graaf, J. W. M. Van der Meer, B. J. Kulberg. 2004. Toll like receptors
   and the host defence against microbial pathogens; bringing specificity to the innate
   –immune system. J Leuk Biol 75: 749-755

Ogden, CA, A. de Cathelineau P. R. D, Hoffman, B. Bratton, B. Ghebrehiwet, V. A. Fadok, P.
   M. Henson. 2001. C1q and mannose binding lectin engagement of cell surface
   calreticulin and CD91 initiates micropinocytosis and uptake of apoptotic cells. J
   Exp Med; 194: 78-795.

Okuno, T., Y. Nakatsuji, M. Moriya, H. Takamatsu, S Nijima, N Takegahara, T. Toyofuku,
   Ynakagawa, S. Kang, R. H. Friedel, S Sakoda, H Kikutani, and A. Kumangooh.
   2010. Roles of Sema 4-D Plexin –B1 interactions in the central nervous system for
   pathogenesis of Experimental Autoimmune Encephalomyelitis. J Immunol 3: 1499-
   1506.

Oldenborg, P. A., H. D. Gresham, and F. P. Lindberg. 2001. CD47-signal regulatory protein
   alpha (SIRPalpha) regulates Fcgamma and complement receptor-mediated
   phagocytosis. J Exp Med 193: 855-862.

Olson, J. K., and S. D. Miller. 2004. Microglia initiate central nervous system innate and
   adaptive immune responses through multiple TLRs. J Immunol 173: 3916-3924.

Origlia, N., M. Righi, S. Capsoni, A. Cattaneo, F. Fang, D. M. Stern, J. X. Chen, A. M.
   Schmidt, O. Arancio, S. D. Yan, and L. Domenici. 2008. Receptor for advanced
   glycation end product-dependent activation of p38 mitogen-activated protein
   kinase contributes to amyloid-beta-mediated cortical synaptic dysfunction. J
   Neurosci 28: 3521-3530.

Osawa, R., K. L. Williams, and N. Singh. 2011. The inflammasome regulatory pathway and
   infections: Role in patho physiology and clinical implications. J Infection 62; 119-
   129

Pachter, J. S, H. de Vries and Z. Fabry. 2003. The Blood brain barrier and its Role in the
   central nervous system. J Neuropath Exp Neurol 62: 593-604

Parisien JP, Bamming D, Komuo A. 2009et al A shared interface mediates paramyxovirus
   interference with antiviral RNA helicases MDA5 and LGP2. J Virol 2009; (14): 7252-
   7260

Paul, S., C. Ricour, C. Sommereyns, F. Sorgeloos, and T. Michiels. 2007. Type I interferon
   response in the central nervous system. Biochimie 89: 770-778.

Pender, MP, and Rist MJ Apoptosis of inflammatory cells in immune control of the nervous system; role of glia. Glia 2001; 36: 137- 144.

Prehaud, C., F. Megret, M. Lafage, and M. Lafon. 2005. Virus infection switches TLR-3-positive human neurons to become strong producers of beta interferon. J Virol 79: 12893-12904.

Prieto, A. L., J. L. Weber, S. Tracy, M. J. Heeb, and C. Lai. 1999. Gas6, a ligand for the receptor protein-tyrosine kinase Tyro-3, is widely expressed in the central nervous system. Brain Res 816: 646-661.

Proell, M, SJ Riedl, JH Fritz, AM Rojas, and R Schwarzenbacher. 2008. The Nod –Like Receptor (NLR) family: a tale of similarities and differences. PLos ONE 3 e2119.

Reed-Geaghan, E. G., J. C. Savage, A. G. Hise, and G. E. Landreth. 2009. CD14 and toll-like receptors 2 and 4 are required for fibrillar A{beta}-stimulated microglial activation. J Neurosci 29: 11982-11992.

Reichert, F., and S. Rotshenker. 2003 Complement -receptor 3and scavenger -receptor-AI/ myelin phagocytosis in microglia and macrophages Neurobiology of disease; 12; 65-72

Rehaume, L. M, T. Jouault, M. Chamaillard. 2010. Lessons from the inflammasome: a molecular sentry linking Candida and Crohn's disease. Trends in Immunology; 2 171-176.

Reinhold, M. I., F. P. Lindberg, D. Plas, S. Reynolds, M. G. Peters, and E. J. Brown. 1995. In vivo expression of alternatively spliced forms of integrin-associated protein (CD47). J Cell Sci 108 (Pt 11): 3419-3425.

Ren tein R L, J Allen, et al. CD36 gene transfer confers capacity for phagocytosis of cells undergoing apoptosis. J Exp Med 1995; 181: 1857 1872

Richard, K. L., M. Filali, P. Prefontaine, and S. Rivest. 2008. Toll-like receptor 2 acts as a natural innate immune receptor to clear amyloid beta 1-42 and delay the cognitive decline in a mouse model of Alzheimer's disease. J Neurosci 28: 5784-5793.

Rivest. S, Regulation of innate of immune responses in the brain 2009. Nature Rev in Immunol 9: 429-439

Rivieccio, M. A., H. S. Suh, Y. Zhao, M. L. Zhao, K. C. Chin, S. C. Lee, and C. F. Brosnan. 2006. TLR3 ligation activates an antiviral response in human fetal astrocytes: a role for viperin/cig5. J Immunol 177: 4735-4741.

Roth, J., T. Vogl, C. Sorg, and C. Sunderkotter. 2003. Phagocyte-specific S100 proteins: a novel group of proinflammatory molecules. Trends Immunol 24: 155-158.

Royet, J., and R. Dziarski. 2007. Peptidoglycan recognition proteins: pleiotropic sensors and effectors of antimicrobial defenses. Nat Rev Microbiol 5: 264-277.

Sancho, D, O. PJoffre, N. C Rogers, D. Martinez, P. Hernanz-Falcon, I. Rosewell E. Reis and C Sousa. 2009. Identification of a dendritic cell receptor that couples sensing of necrosis to immunity. Nature. 458: 899-903.

Sarati M, G. Fontin, M. Raymond and S. Susin. 2008. CD47 in the immune response: role of thrombospondin and SIRP alpha reveres signaling. Curr Drug Targets ; 9: 842-850.

Sato S., C. St –Pierre, P. Bhaumik, and J. Nieminen. 2009. Galectins in innate immunity: dual functionof host soluble beta galactoside-binding lectins as damage associated

The CNS Innate Immune System and the Emerging Roles of the Neuroimmune Regulators (NIRegs)
in Response to Infection, Neoplasia and Neurodegeneration

213

molecular patterns(DAMPs) and as receptors for pathogen associated molecular patterns (PAMPs). Imunol Review 230: 172-187.

Schwartz, A. J, X. Alvarez, A. A Lackner. 2002. Distribution and immunophenotype of DC-SIGN -expressing cells in SIV infected and uninfected macaques. AIDS research and Human retroviruses. 2002; 18 (14): 1021-1029

Seiffert, M., P. Brossart, C. Cant, M. Cella, M. Colonna, W. Brugger, L. Kanz, A. Ullrich, and H. J. Buhring. 2001. Signal-regulatory protein alpha (SIRP alpha) but not SIRPbeta is involved in T-cell activation, binds to CD47 with high affinity, and is expressed on immature CD34(+)CD38(-) hematopoietic cells. Blood 97: 2741-2749.

Shewan D V Calaora PNielsen, Cohen, G Rougon, and H Moreau. 1996. mCD24, a glycoprotein transiently expressed by neurons is an inhibitor of neurite growth J Neurosci 16(8): 2624-2634

Singhrao, S. K, J. W Neal., Gasque P, and Newman G. R. 1999. Increased Complement Biosynthesis By Microglia and Complement Activation on Neurons in Huntington's disease. Experimental Neurology 159: 362-376

Singhrao, S. K, J. W. Neal, N. K. Rushmere, B. P Morgan, P. Gasque et al. 1999 Differential expression of individual complement regulators in the brain and choroid plexus. Lab Invests 10: 1247-1259

Sjoberg, A. P, L. A Trouw, A. M Bloom. 2009. Complement activation and inhibition: a delicate balance. Trends in Immunology 30 (92): 83-90.

Schroder, , K., and J. Tschopp. 2010. The inflammasomes. Cell 140: 821-832.

Stahl, P. D, and R. E. Ezekowitz. 1998 The mannose receptor is a pattern recognition receptor involved in host defence. Curr Opin Immunol 10: 50-55.

Stewart, C. R., L. M Stuart, K. Wilkinson, J. M. van Gils, J. Deng, A. Halle, K. J. Rayner, L. Boyer, R. Zhong, W. A. Frazier, A, Lacy –Hulbert, J, El Khoury, D. T. Golenbock, KJ More. 2010. CD36 ligands promote sterile inflammation through assembly of a Toll –like receptor 4and 6 heterodimer. Nat Immunol 12: 155-161.

Sonabend, A. M., C. E Rolle, and M. S Lesniak. 2008. The role of regulatory T cells in malignant gliomas. Anticancer Res 28(2B) 1143-1150.

Sterka, D., Jr., and I. Marriott. 2006. Characterization of nucleotide-binding oligomerization domain (NOD) protein expression in primary murine microglia. J Neuroimmunol 179: 65-75.

Sterka, D., Jr., D. M. Rati, and I. Marriott. 2006. Functional expression of NOD2, a novel pattern recognition receptor for bacterial motifs, in primary murine astrocytes. Glia 53: 322-330.

Stumpova, M., D Ratner, E. B Desciak, Y. D Eliezri and DM Owens. 2010. The immunosuppressive surface ligand CD200 augments the metastatic capcity of Squamous cell carcinomas. Cancer Res. 70: 2962-2972.

Suzuki, K., A. Kumanogoh, H. Kikutani. 2008. Semaphorins and their receptors on immune cell interaction. Nature Immunology: 9 17-27.

Tahara, K., H. D. Kim, J. J. Jin, J. A. Maxwell, L. Li, and K. Fukuchi. 2006. Role of toll-like receptor signaling in A beta uptake and clearance. Brain 129: 3006-3019.

Takahashi, K, C, . D. P. Rochford and H, Neumann. Clearance of apoptotic neurons without inflammation by microglial triggering receptor expressed on myeloid cells -2. J Exp Med 2005; 201: 647-657.

Takegahara, N, A. Kumanogoh, H Kikutani. 2005 Semaphorins: a new class of immunoregulatory molecules Proc. Trans. R Soc B 360: 1673-1168

Takeuchi, O., and S. Akira. Pattern recognition receptors and inflammation. Cell 140: 805-820.

Tenner, A. J. 1999. Membrane Receptors for soluble defense collagens. Current Opinion in Immunology 11: 34-41.

Tenner, A. J. 2001. Complement in Alzheimer's disease: opportunities for modulating protective and pathogenic events. Neurobiol Aging 22: 849-861.

Thielens, N. M, P. Tacnet –Delormeand, G. J. Arlaud. 2002. Interaction of C1q and mannan – binding lectin with viruses. Immunology 205: 563-574

Tian, J, A. M. Avalos, S. Y. Mao, B. Chen, , K Senthil, H. Wu, P Parroche, S Drabic, D Golenbock, C. Sirois, J. Hua, L. L. An, L Audoly GLeRosa ABierhaus, P. Naworth, A. Marshak –Rothstein, M. K. Crow, K Fitzgerald E. Latz, P. A Kiener, and A J Coyle. 2007. Toll like receptor 9 –dependent activation by DNA- containing immune coplexes is mediated by HMGB1 and RAGE. Nature Immunol 8: 487-49. .

Ting, J. P. Y, J. A, Duncan, Y. Lei. 2010 How the Non inflammasome NLRS function in the innate immune system. Science 327: 286-290.

Toguchi, M., D. Gonnzalez, S. Furukawa, S. Inagaki. 2009. Involvement of Sema-4D in the control of microglial activation. Neurochem Int 55: 573-580.

Trouw L, A. Bengtssona, K. A, Gelderman, B Dahlback, G. Sturfelt, A. M. Blom 2007. C4b - binding protein and factor H compensate for the loss of membrane bound complement inhibitors to protect apoptotic cells against excessive complement attack. J Biol Chem; 282: 28540-28548

Trouw L, Nielsen HM, Minthon LE Londos, G Landburg Rverhuis, S Janciauskiene, AM Blom, 2008C4b- binding protein in Alzheimer's disease: binding to Abeta 1-42 and to dead cells. Mol Immunol 2008; 45: 3649-3660

Upham JP, Pickett D, Anders T, Reading C. Macrophage receptors for Influenza A virus: role for the macrophage galactose-type lectin and mannose receptor in viral entry. J Virol 2010; 84(3): 3730-3737

Van Beek, J., O. Nicole, C. Ali, A. Ischenko, E. T. MacKenzie, A. Buisson, and M. Fontaine. 2001. Complement anaphylatoxin C3a is selectively protective against NMDA-induced neuronal cell death. Neuroreport 12: 289-293.

Van Beek, J., M. Bernaudin, E. Petit, P. Gasque, A. Nouvelot, E. T. MacKenzie, and M. Fontaine. 2000. Expression of receptors for complement anaphylatoxins C3a and C5a following permanent focal cerebral ischemia in the mouse. Exp Neurol 161: 373-382.

van Kooyk, and T. B. H. Geijenbeek. DC-SIGN escape mechanism for pathogens Nat Review Immunol 2003; 3: 697-709.

Vandivier, RW, Ogden CA, Fadok VA, P. R. Hofmann, Brown, M. Botto, M. J. Walport J. H. Fisher, . PM. Henson, K. E. Greene. 2002. Role of surfactant proteins A, D and

The CNS Innate Immune System and the Emerging Roles of the Neuroimmune Regulators (NIRegs)
in Response to Infection, Neoplasia and Neurodegeneration

215

C1qin the clearance of apoptotic cells in vivo and in vitro: calcireticulin and CD91 as a common collectin receptor complex. J Immunol; 169: 3978-3986

Vasta, G. Roles of galectins in infection. Nature Reviews in Microbiology; 7: 424-438.

Vernon-Wilson, E. F., W. J. Kee, A. C. Willis, A. N. Barclay, D. L. Simmons and M. H. Brown. 2000. CD47 is a ligand for rat macrophage membrane signal regulatory protein SIRP (OX41) and human SIRPalpha 1. Eur J Immunol 30: 2130-2137.

Voll R, Herrmann, Roth EA. 1997 Immunosuppresive effects of apoptotic cells Nature; 390: 350-351

Wagner, S., Lynch, NJ, Walter W, etal. 2003 Differential expression of the murine mannose-binding lectins A and C in lymphoid and nonlymphoid organs and tissues. J Immunol; 170: 1462-1465.

Walter, S., M. Letiembre, Y. Liu, H. Heine, B. Penke, W. Hao, B. Bode, N. Manietta, J. Walter, W. Schulz-Schuffer, and K. Fassbender. 2007. Role of the toll-like receptor 4 in neuroinflammation in Alzheimer's disease. Cell Physiol Biochem 20: 947-956.

Wang, J., I. and L. Campbell. 2002. Cytokine signaling in the brain: putting a SOCS in it? *J Neurosci Res* 67: 423-427.

Wang, T., T. Town, L. Alexopoulou, J. F. Anderson, E. Fikrig, and R. A. Flavell. 2004. Toll-like receptor 3 mediates West Nile virus entry into the brain causing lethal encephalitis. Nat Med 10: 1366-1373.

Wang, Y, H. Neumann. 2010. Alleviation of neurotoxicity by microglial human Siglec- 11. J Neurosci 30 (9) 3482 -4388.

Webster, S, D, , M. D Galavan, E. Ferran, W. Garzon –Rodriguez, C. G. Glabe, A. J. Tenner Antibody –mediated phagocytosis of the amyloid beta peptide in microglia is differentially modulated by microglia. J Immunol; 12: 7496-74503.

Wu, A, J. Wei, L. Y. Wong, Y. Wang, W. Priebe, W. Qiao, R. Sawaya and A. B Heimbergerg. 2010 Glioma cancer stem cells induce immunosuppressive macrophages /microglia. Neuro Oncol. 12: 113-1125

Wright, G. J., M. Jones, M. J. Puklavec, M. H. Brown, and A. N. Barclay. 2001. The unusual distribution of the neuronal/lymphoid cell surface CD200 (OX2) glycoprotein is conserved in humans. 102: 173-179.

Wyss-Coray, T., and L. Mucke. 2002. Inflammation in neurodegenerative disease. A double-edged sword. Neuron 35: 419-432.

Yagami, T., K. Ueda, K. Asakura, N. Okamura, T. Sakaeda, G. Sakaguchi, N. Itoh, Y. Hashimoto, T. Nakano, and M. Fujimoto. 2003. Effect of Gas6 on secretory phospholipase A(2)-IIA-induced apoptosis in cortical neurons. Brain Res 985: 142-149.

Yamayoshi, S, Y. Yamashita, J. Li, N. Hanagata, TMinowa, T, Takemura, 2009. Scavenger receptor B2 is a cellular receptor for enterovirus 71. Nat Med; 15: 798-801

Yan, S. D, A. Bierhaus, P. P. Naworth, D. M. Stern. 2009. RAGE and Alzheimer's disease: a progression factor for amyloid induced cellular perturbation ?J. Alzheimers Dis 16: 833-843

Yoneyama, M., M. Kikuchi, T. Natsukawa, N. Shinobu, T. Imaizumi, M.

Miyagishi, K. Taira, S. Akira, and T. Fujita. 2004. The RNA helicase RIG-I has an essential function in double-stranded RNA-induced innate antiviral responses. Nat Immunol 5: 730-737.

Yarovinsky, F., D. Zhang, J. F. Andersen, G. L. Bannenberg, C. N. Sheran, M. S. Hayden, S Hieiny, F. S Sutterwala, R. A. Flavell, S. Ghosh, A. Sher. 2005 TRL-11 activation of dendritic cells by a protozoan profilin-like protein. Science 308: 1626-1629.

Yoshida, H., T. Imaizumi, S. J. Lee, K. Tanji, H. Sakaki, T. Matsumiya, A. Ishikawa, K. Taima, E. Yuzawa, F. Mori, K. Wakabayashi, H. Kimura, and K, Satoh. 2007. Retinoicacid-inducible gene-I mediates RANTES/CCL5 expression in U373MG human astrocytoma cells stimulated with double-stranded RN A. Neurosci Res 58: 199-206.

Yu, MH, Wang, A Ding, DT Golenbock, E Latz, CJ Cura, MJ Fenton, K Tracey and H Yang. 2006. HMGB1 signals through toll like receptor (TLR) 4 and TLR 2. Shock 2: 174-179.

Zipfel, P. F., and C. Skerka. 2009. Complement regulators and inhibitory proteins. Nat Rev Immunol 9: 729-740.

10

Regulatory B Cells - Implications in Autoimmune and Allergic Disorders

Susanne Sattler[1]*, Luciën E.P.M. van der Vlugt[2], Leonie Hussaarts[2],
Hermelijn H. Smits[2] and Fang-Ping Huang[1]
[1]Imperial College London,
[2]Leiden University Medical Center,
[1]UK
[2]The Netherlands

1. Introduction

B lymphocytes represent a major component of the immune system and their best understood effector functions are antibody production, presentation of antigens to T cells and the modulation of immune responses via cytokine production. Although most of these functions serve to amplify immune responses, B cells have also been demonstrated to downregulate inflammatory reactions and induce tolerance. As such, regulatory B (Breg) cells have been implicated in various inflammatory conditions. There is evidence for Breg cell deficiencies in human autoimmune diseases and various adoptive transfer experiments in mouse models of autoimmune and allergic conditions indicate that Breg cells are capable of suppressing disease development. In this review we endeavour to give an overview of the current knowledge about regulatory B cell immunobiology and their implications in autoimmune and allergic disorders.

2. Regulatory B cells

B cells with regulatory capacity have become the focus of intense investigations in recent years. However, the general concept that B cells might have the ability to induce tolerance, was introduced already in the 1970s by Katz et al., who demonstrated that depletion of B cells from splenocytes abolished their ability to inhibit an inflammatory reaction in a delayed type hypersensitivity (DTH) model (Katz, Parker et al. 1974; Mauri and Ehrenstein 2008). More than 20 years later, Janeway and co-workers were the first to demonstrate a role of B cells in protection from autoimmunity, showing that B cell-deficient mice failed to undergo spontaneous remission from experimental autoimmune encephalomyelitis (EAE) (Wolf, Dittel et al. 1996). The term 'regulatory B cells' was introduced shortly afterwards, by Mizoguchi and Bhan, who identified an IL-10 producing B cell subset in gut-associated lymphoid tissues (GALT) with upregulated CD1d expression, which suppressed progression of intestinal inflammation by downregulating inflammatory cascades (Mizoguchi, Mizoguchi et al. 2002). Breg cells are now considered a key regulatory cell type

---

* SS and LvdV contributed equally to this work

capable of suppressing effector functions of various target cells including T cells, dendritic cells (DC) and macrophages, and can even convert effector T cells into regulatory T cells (Tian, Zekzer et al. 2001; Matsushita, Horikawa et al. 2010; Ronet, Hauyon-La Torre et al. 2010; Wong, Puaux et al. 2010).

2.1 Breg cell populations in mice and humans

Although the existence of a regulatory subset of B cells is generally accepted, there is still some controversy concerning their origin and relationship to other B cell populations (Vitale, Mion et al. 2010). In mice, B cells are classified according to their developmental origin, into B1 and B2 cells. B1 lymphocytes are considered an innate type of lymphocytes and appear early in life. They produce antibodies with a limited diversity to common pathogens and can respond quickly and independently of T cells. B2 lymphocytes on the other hand are further subdivided into marginal zone (MZ) and follicular B cells in the spleen and circulating B cells in the peripheral blood, each with very specific characteristics and functions (Hardy and Hayakawa 2001). Regulatory B cells or their precursors seem to be able to arise from different subpopulations of both B1 and B2 cells. As shown in Table 1, several Breg cell populations with varying surface phenotypes have been identified in various mouse model systems as well as in different human disease conditions. Some regulatory B cell populations have also been shown to be induced in diverse disease settings and in response to many different exogenous and endogenous stimuli. Toll-like receptor (TLR) signalling via TLR-2, 4 and 9 as well as B cell receptor (BCR) signalling and co-stimulation mediated by CD40, CD80/CD86 or B-cell activating factor (BAFF) has been demonstrated to induce B cells with suppressive activity (Fillatreau, Sweenie et al. 2002; Mauri, Gray et al. 2003; Blair, Chavez-Rueda et al. 2009; Kala, Rhodes et al. 2010; Lampropoulou, Calderon-Gomez et al. 2010; Yang, Sun et al. 2010). One prominent type of 'natural' B cells with regulatory capacity has been isolated from naive mouse spleens and termed B10 cells by reason of their IL-10-dependent suppressive function. Phenotypically these B cells seem to be predominantly $CD1d^{hi}CD5^+$, thus they share surface markers with $CD5^+$ B1 cells ($CD21^{hi}CD23^+IgM^{hi}CD1d^{hi}Cd93^{int}$), MZ B cells ($CD1d^{hi}CD21^{hi}CD23^{lo}IgM^{hi}$) and transitional 2 (T2)-MZ precursor B cells ($CD1d^{hi}CD21^{hi}CD23^{hi}IgM^{hi}$), but do not exclusively belong to one of these B cell subpopulations (Yanaba, Bouaziz et al. 2008). The human equivalent to mouse B10 cells has been identified recently as a small population within peripheral blood $CD24^{hi}CD27^+B$ cells (Iwata, Matsushita et al. 2011). In analogy to regulatory-type T cells, which can been subdivided into Treg, Tr1 and Th3 according to their expression of FoxP3, IL-10 and transforming growth factor (TGF)-β, respectively, it has been proposed to classify human regulatory B cells into 'Breg', Br1 (B10) and Br3 (Noh and Lee 2011).

Because of the variety of Breg cell populations and inducing factors, several models have been proposed that try to explain their origin and development. The first model put forward by Mizoguchi et al. states that distinct Breg cell populations are generated from already existing B cell subsets depending on distinct activation processes (Mizoguchi and Bhan 2006). According to this hypothesis, innate type regulatory B cells are generated from MZ B cells in the spleen upon stimulation with inflammatory signals such as lipopolysaccharides (LPS) or CpG via toll-like receptors (TLR). On the other hand, acquired type regulatory B cells develop from follicular B cells following activation with CD40 ligand and/or B cell receptor (BCR) ligation with self-antigen. A second model proposed by Lampropoulou et al. states that B cells acquire suppressive function due to a hierarchical process of stepwise B

species	phenotype	initial identification	organ of origin	major effector function	disease condition
mouse	B10	(Yanaba, Bouaziz et al. 2008)	spleen	IL-10	CHS
mouse	T2 MZ	(Carter, Vasconcellos et al. 2011) (Evans, Chavez-Rueda et al. 2007)	spleen	IL-10	arthritis
mouse	MZ	(Gray, Miles et al. 2007)	spleen	IL-10	CIA
mouse	B1	(Nakashima, Hamaguchi et al. 2010)	peri-toneum	IL-10	CHS
mouse	CD1d^{hi}	(Amu, Saunders et al. 2010) (Mizoguchi, Mizoguchi et al. 2002)	spleen	IL-10	AAI, IBD anaphylaxis
mouse	CD23$^+$	(Wilson, Taylor et al. 2010)	mes. LN	?	AAI, EAE
sheep	CD21$^+$ B2	(Booth, Griebel et al. 2009)	Peyer's patches	IL-10	healthy
human	immature trans B	(Blair, Norena et al. 2010)	blood	IL-10 CD80/ CD86	SLE
human	'B10 (Br1)'	(Iwata, Matsushita et al. 2011)	blood	IL-10	healthy and autoimmune
human	CD1d^{hi}	(Correale, Farez et al. 2008)		IL-10	
human	'Br3'	(Lotz, Ranheim et al. 1994)	blood	TGF-β	CLL
human	'Breg'	(Noh, Choi et al. 2010)	blood	FoxP3	healthy

Table 1. B cell populations with regulatory phenotypes in different species. B cell populations with regulatory capacity have been identified in various different experimental settings or disease conditions in mice, humans and sheep. CHS: contact hypersensitivity, T2-MZ: transitional 2 marginal zone, CIA: collagen induced arthritis, AAI: allergic airway inflammation, IBD: inflammatory bowel disease, mes.LN: mesenteric lymphnodes, EAE: experimental autoimmune encephalomyelitis, SLE: systemic lupus erythematosus, CLL: chronic lymphocytic leukemia.

cell activation, with TLR ligands initiating the process and BCR and CD40 engagement serving to further reinforce this differentiation. According to this model, all activated B cells have the capacity to become regulatory B cells after activation (Lampropoulou, Calderon-Gomez et al. 2010). A third model, based on shared phenotypic markers between most described IL-10 producing B cell populations, claims that all different B cell populations contain distinct Breg cell precursors, which mature to IL-10 producing cells upon activation (DiLillo, Matsushita et al. 2010). Taken together, currently available information suggests, that in addition to distinct 'natural' Breg cell populations arising from specific Breg cell progenitors, members of many B cells subsets are potentially able to acquire suppressive functions as a negative feedback mechanism in response to activation.

2.2 Immunological effector functions of regulatory B cells

Regulatory B cells employ a variety of mechanisms to modulate immune responses and target many different immune cell types, such as dendritic cells (DC) (Matsushita, Horikawa et al. 2010), macrophages (Wong, Puaux et al. 2010) as well as both T helper 1 (Th1) and Th2 cells (Tian, Zekzer et al. 2001; Ronet, Hauyon-La Torre et al. 2010). Their most prominent effector function is the production of the potent immunosupressive cytokine IL-10, however different subsets also produce TGF-β (Fig. 1) or suppress target cells via cell contact-dependent mechanisms (Fig. 2).

2.2.1 Release of cytokines

As depicted in figure 1, many Breg cell functions have been demonstrated to be mediated by the release of immunosuppressive cytokines. **IL-10** is the hallmark cytokine of regulatory B cells. It has been shown to be essential for the Breg cell suppressive functions in many autoimmune models. Accordingly, the protective function of Breg cells in collagen induced arthritis (CIA), experimental autoimmune encephalomyelitis (EAE), non-obese diabetes (NOD) and inflammatory bowel disease (IBD) is abrogated if B cells are deficient in IL-10 production (Fillatreau, Sweenie et al. 2002; Dalwadi, Wei et al. 2003; Mauri, Gray et al. 2003; Hussain and Delovitch 2007; Booth, Griebel et al. 2009). B cell derived IL-10 efficiently suppresses proliferation and inflammatory cytokine production of T cells (Fillatreau, Sweenie et al. 2002; Mauri, Gray et al. 2003) and can also induce forkhead box P3 (FoxP3) positive regulatory T cells (Gray, Miles et al. 2007; Blair, Chavez-Rueda et al. 2009). Some of these effects might be indirect and due to the effects of IL-10 on innate cell types, as IL-10 is well known to inhibit antigen presentation and pro-inflammatory cytokine production by DC, monocytes and macrophages (Moore, de Waal Malefyt et al. 2001).

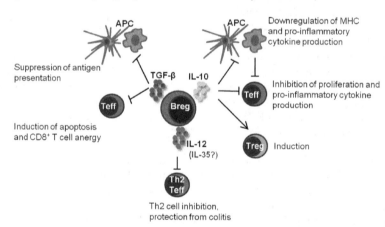

Fig. 1. Suppressive functions of Breg cells mediated by the release of cytokines. Breg cells secrete immunosuppressive cytokines causing downregulation of antigen presenting cell (APC) function, inhibition of T effector cell function and induction of regulatory T cells. Breg: regulatory B cells, Teff/reg: effector/regulatory T cells, APC: antigen presenting cells.

IL-10, **TGF-β** is the second immunosuppressive cytokine found to be secreted by some Breg cell populations to downregulate inflammatory immune responses (Tian, Zekzer et al. 2001; Parekh, Prasad et al. 2003). Similar to IL-10, TGF-β suppresses inflammatory cytokine production by T cells and inhibits the function of antigen presenting cells (APC). In addition, TGF-β induces apoptosis in target effector cells and acts as a negative regulator of mucosal immune responses (Takenoshita, Fukushima et al. 2002).

Interestingly, although not generally considered suppressive, **IL-12** production by B cells has also been demonstrated to have immunomodulatory capacity in a T cell receptor (TCR)α knockout mouse model of Th2-mediated colitis. In this model, IL-10 mediated induction of IL-12 secreting B cells is involved in protection from colitis, as IL-12p35-deficient double knockout mice as well as mice treated with anti-IL-12p40 antibodies developed a more severe colitis compared to control mice (Sugimoto, Ogawa et al. 2007).

2.2.2 Cell contact-dependent suppressive mechanisms

Independent of cytokine secretion, several B cell surface molecules have been implicated in the suppressive functions of regulatory B cells (Fig. 2). **CD1d** is not only a major phenotypic marker highly expressed on many Breg cell populations, it has also been suggested to have an active role in Breg cell-mediated suppression. CD1d is a major histocompatibility complex (MHC) class I-like molecule and is responsible for the presentation of lipid antigens to Natural Killer T (NKT) cells (Chiu, Park et al. 2002; Borg, Wun et al. 2007). Mizoguchi et al. showed that upregulation of CD1d on B cells is associated with B cell-mediated protection against intestinal mucosal inflammation (Mizoguchi, Mizoguchi et al. 2002).

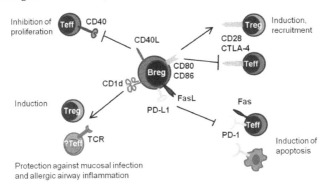

Fig. 2. Suppressive functions of Breg cells mediated by cell contact-dependent mechanisms. Breg cells express several cell surface molecules that cause inhibition of T effector cell function, induction of target cell apoptosis and induction of regulatory T cells. Breg: regulatory B cells, Teff/reg: effector/regulatory T cells, TCR: T cell receptor, PD-1: programmed death-1, PD-L1: programmed death-ligand1, FasL: Fas-Ligand, CTLA-4: cytotoxic T-lymphocyte protein 4, CD40L: CD40-Ligand.

As NKT cells had earlier been shown to be protective in mouse models of diabetes (Lehuen, Lantz et al. 1998) and colitis (Saubermann, Beck et al. 2000), it was feasible to assume that the activation of NKT cells was the underlying mechanism of protection in these models. However, as the TCRα knockout mice used in the studies by Mizoguchi et al., do not have NKT cells, the protective effect in this experimental setting has to be mediated by another CD1d responsive cell type. Amu et al. later confirmed a CD1d[high] Breg cell-dependent, but

NKT cell-independent mechanism of protection in a model of worm mediated protection from allergic airway inflammation (Amu, Saunders et al. 2010). Another group reported, that CD1d expression on APC and splenic MZ B cells was necessary for efficient generation of regulatory T cells in CD1d-reactive NKT cell-dependent tolerance in immune privileged sites such as the eye (Sonoda and Stein-Streilein 2002).

As described earlier, **CD40-CD40L** interaction seems to play an important role in the differentiation of regulatory B cells. In addition, there are reports indicating that CD40 signalling on target cells might also be involved in the suppressive mechanisms of B cells. Upon activation, B cells express CD40L on their surface (Wykes, Poudrier et al. 1998) and CD40-CD40L interaction has been shown to mediate suppression of colonic inflammation by inhibition of T cells (Bhan, Mizoguchi et al. 2000). Other costimulatory molecules involved in cell contact-dependent suppressive functions of B cells, are the B7 costimulatory receptors **CD80 and CD86**. Interaction of B7 surface receptors with their inhibitory ligands cytotoxic T-lymphocyte protein 4 (CTLA-4) or CD28 on target cells is crucial in regulating T cell activation and peripheral tolerance (Fife and Bluestone 2008). Expression of B7 molecules has been shown to be essential for recovery from EAE due to B cell-mediated generation and recruitment of regulatory T cells (Mann, Maresz et al. 2007) as well as for the suppression of colonic inflammation through inhibition of effector T cell proliferation (Bhan, Mizoguchi et al. 2000).

Moreover, evidence exists that Breg cells upregulate surface molecules like Fas ligand (FasL) and programmed death-ligand 1 (PDL-1), which upon interaction with their receptors can directly induce apoptosis in target cells. Lundy and Fox demonstrated that in a mouse model of rheumatoid arthritis, splenic CD5+ B cells express high levels of FasL and that induced T cell apoptosis indeed was due to FasL-mediated direct killing by B cells (Lundy and Fox 2009). In EAE, Bodhankar et al. showed that the well established protective effect of estrogen is mediated by B cells. The treatment, besides increasing the percentage of IL-10-producing regulatory B cells, also induced upregulation of **PD-L1** expression on B cells (Bodhankar, Wang et al. 2011). Furthermore, in murine experimental stroke, PD-L1 and PD-L2 expressing B cells were found to be protective due to their capacity to inhibit the activation of inflammatory T cells, macrophages and microglial cells through upregulation of PD-1 expression (Ren, Akiyoshi et al. 2011).

3. Regulatory B cells in autoimmune diseases

In homeostasis as well as during acute immune responses a delicate balance between activating and suppressing subsets of immune cells has to be maintained. Disrupting this balance often leads to immunodeficiencies or autoimmune diseases. In particular, the balanced ratio between effector and regulatory T cells has been demonstrated to be of crucial importance in maintaining immune homeostasis, and the role of Treg cells has been well established in autoimmune diseases (O'Connor and Anderton 2008; Yang, Tian et al. 2008; Huang and Sattler 2011). Recently, various studies have also found critical roles and possible clinical relevance of regulatory B cells in both systemic and organ-specific autoimmune diseases (Lemoine, Morva et al. 2009).

3.1 Regulatory B cells in systemic autoimmune diseases

Systemic autoimmune diseases are defined by their multi-organ involvement. Antibodies reactive to a wide variety of ubiquitous autoantigens including DNA, cell surface molecules as well as intracellular matrix proteins can cause tissue damage in various target organs. Although the underlying cause leading to systemic autoimmunity remains unclear, several genetic and environmental factors and immunological mechanisms have been implicated.

3.1.1 Systemic lupus erythematosus

Systemic lupus erythematosus (SLE) is a systemic autoimmune condition often considered the prototype of autoimmune diseases. It is mainly characterised by the presence of auto-antibodies to a variety of self antigens, particularly against nuclear components (Mills 1994). Because of the high production of pathogenic auto-antibodies, B cells are considered a major contributor to SLE pathogenesis and several therapies targeting B cells in SLE patients have been introduced (Sabahi and Anolik 2006). In addition however, there is evidence for the existence of a subset of B cells with regulatory capacity in lupus (Amano, Amano et al. 2003). Furthermore, human SLE patients have been shown to have an increased percentage of B10 and B10pro cells in peripheral blood (Iwata, Matsushita et al. 2011). However, regulatory B cells isolated from the peripheral blood of SLE patients might be functionally impaired, as they appeared to be unresponsive to CD40 stimulation, produced less IL-10 and lacked the capacity to suppress T cells (Blair, Norena et al. 2010).

Interesting insights into a possible dual role of B cells in lupus were obtained from CD19 deficient lupus-prone mice (NZB/W mice). Although, auto-antibody accumulation was significantly delayed in these mice, nephritis appeared earlier and survival was reduced compared to wild type NZB/W mice. Adoptive transfer of wild type CD1d^{hi}CD5$^+$ splenic B cells containing IL-10 producing regulatory B cells into CD19 deficient recipients significantly prolonged survival (Watanabe, Ishiura et al. 2010). Adoptive transfer of *in vitro* anti-CD40 stimulated T2 B cells into lupus-prone mice also improved renal disease and survival by an IL-10-dependent mechanism. This effect was explained by the suppression of Th1 responses and the induction of IL-10 producing and regulatory T cells. Direct *in vivo* administration of anti-CD40 also reversed established lupus disease (Blair, Chavez-Rueda et al. 2009). A possible role for innate immune signalling in the pathogenesis of SLE has been suggested previously (Lenert, Goeken et al. 2003) and TLR-9 signalling in marginal zone B cells has been demonstrated to induce higher IL-10 production in lupus-prone mice compared to controls. These high levels of B cell derived IL-10 inhibits the production of IL-12 by macrophages and DC and consequently can modulate T cell mediated inflammatory responses (Lenert, Brummel et al. 2005).

3.1.2 Rheumatoid arthritis

Rheumatoid arthritis (RA) is a common T cell-dependent chronic inflammatory disease characterised by synovial proliferation and excessive pro-inflammatory cytokine production, resulting in cartilage and bone destruction (Firestein 2003). Data available on Breg cells in human rheumatoid arthritis are limited, however similar to lupus patients, an increased percentage of B10 and B10pro cells in the peripheral blood of rheumatoid arthritis patients has been observed, indicating that regulatory B cells might play a role in this autoimmune condition too (Iwata, Matsushita et al. 2011). To date, the majority of the experimental data available on arthritis, has been obtained from the murine model of collagen-induced arthritis (CIA), which mimics the immunopathogenesis of human rheumatoid arthritis (Trentham, Townes et al. 1977). Using this model, adoptive transfer of

IL-10 producing B cells has been demonstrated by different groups to prevent the development of arthritis as well as to ameliorate already established disease (Mauri, Gray et al. 2003; Evans, Chavez-Rueda et al. 2007; Gray, Miles et al. 2007).

Mauri and co-workers were the first to show that adoptive transfer of *in vitro* anti-CD40 activated splenic B cells prevented the development of arthritis. The B cells used in these experiments were shown to produce increased amounts of IL-10 and inhibited Th1 differentiation (Mauri, Gray et al. 2003). Work by Evans et al. demonstrated that the number of endogenous IL-10 producing MZ and their precursors T2 MZP B cells were increased during the remission phase of arthritis and that adoptive transfer of T2 MZP to CIA mice prevented disease progression and alleviated established disease. Again, the underlying mechanism seemed to be the reduction of a Th1 type immune response in the presence of immunosuppressive cytokines, rather than cell contact-dependent mechanisms (Evans, Chavez-Rueda et al. 2007). Gray et al. induced IL-10 producing regulatory B cells in the spleen of CIA mice by administration of apoptotic thymocytes. Regulatory B cells induced in this manner *in vivo* as well as upon passive transfer after *in vitro* induction, were effective in protecting mice from autoimmune joint inflammation (Gray, Miles et al. 2007).

3.2 Regulatory B cells in organ-specific autoimmune diseases

In contrast to systemic autoimmune diseases, organ-specific autoimmune conditions are characterised by cell- and auto-antibody-mediated immune responses directed specifically against antigens which are only localised in a particular organ such as the pancreatic islets in type I diabetes or the central nervous system in multiple sclerosis.

3.2.1 Inflammatory bowel disease

Inflammatory Bowel Disease (IBD) refers to a group of conditions characterised by inflammation in the intestinal tract, with Crohn's disease (CD) and ulcerative colitis (UC) accounting for the majority of cases. While in CD chronic inflammation is mainly mediated by the Th1 pathway, UC is also associated with the presence of auto-antibodies, leading to the initial assumption that B cells might play a role in disease initiation (Mizoguchi, Mizoguchi et al. 1996; Bhan, Mizoguchi et al. 1999).

Studies in various mouse models of IBD demonstrating the protective roles of B cells, were among the earliest publications to document the existence and relevance of regulatory B cells. Mizoguchi et al. used a mouse model deficient in TCRα that spontaneously develops UC-like chronic colitis and demonstrated that B cells were not required to initiate disease at all, but could actually suppress colitis (Mizoguchi, Mizoguchi et al. 1997). These B cells were later shown to appear during chronic intestinal inflammation, exhibit upregulated CD1d expression and release IL-10 (Mizoguchi, Mizoguchi et al. 2002). Furthermore, adoptive transfer experiments confirmed a protective role of B cells via mechanisms like IL-10 production and induction of regulatory T cells (Bhan, Mizoguchi et al. 2000; Mizoguchi, Mizoguchi et al. 2002; Wei, Velazquez et al. 2005). Several additional studies performed by different groups using various mouse models have confirmed that B cells can regulate UC-like intestinal inflammation (Gerth, Lin et al. 2004; Hokama, Mizoguchi et al. 2004; Su, Guo et al. 2004; Sugimoto, Ogawa et al. 2007) as well as Crohn's disease-like conditions (Dalwadi, Wei et al. 2003; Wei, Velazquez et al. 2005; Ostanin, Pavlick et al. 2006).

Interestingly, B cells producing IL-12 in an IL-10-dependent manner, have also been demonstrated to be protective in a mouse model of UC-like Th2-mediated colitis (Sugimoto, Ogawa et al. 2007). In Crohn's disease-like Th1-mediated colitis, IL-12 was initially considered to be pathogenic, however a recent report suggests that IL-23 sharing the common subunit p40 (p19/p40) rather than IL-12 (p35/p40) is pro-inflammatory and the one to mediate disease (Cua, Sherlock et al. 2003; Yen, Cheung et al. 2006). Importantly, both IL-12 subunits p35 and p40 have been demonstrated to be crucial in B cell mediated attenuation of colitis (Sugimoto, Ogawa et al. 2007). However, it needs to be noted that a possible contribution of another potent suppressive cytokine sharing the p35 subunit, namely IL-35, has not been taken into account (Collison, Workman et al. 2007; Niedbala, Wei et al. 2007).

3.2.2 Multiple sclerosis

Multiple sclerosis (MS) is considered a T cell-mediated autoimmune condition that results in inflammatory lesions, demyelination and axonal damage in the central nervous system (CNS). A mouse model mimicking human MS, experimental autoimmune encephalomyelitis (EAE) has been used widely to investigate the underlying immunological mechanisms and the components of the immune system involved in disease pathogenesis (Baxter 2007). Similar to other autoimmune diseases, clonal expansion of B cells and the production of auto-antibodies, indicate that B cells contribute to the pathogenesis of MS (Colombo, Dono et al. 2000; Fraussen, Vrolix et al. 2009). However, the effects of anti-CD20-mediated B cell depletion in the EAE model depend crucially on timing, as treatment shortly after disease onset reduced disease severity, while depletion prior to disease induction or at the peak of disease did not change the disease course or even led to disease exacerbation (Matsushita, Yanaba et al. 2008). Exacerbation of disease indicates a protective role of B cells and Wolf et al. were one of the first groups to show that there might indeed be an additional protective function of B cells in EAE. They demonstrated that although the incidence and severity of disease was comparable between mice genetically deficient in mature B cells and wild type control mice, B cell deficient mice failed to undergo spontaneous recovery and developed chronic disease instead (Wolf, Dittel et al. 1996).

Several recent studies confirm these findings showing in addition that IL-10 producing B cells are responsible for this protective effect (Fillatreau, Sweenie et al. 2002; Matsushita, Fujimoto et al. 2006; Lampropoulou, Hoehlig et al. 2008). Furthermore, adoptive transfer experiments revealed a possible therapeutic potential of isolated regulatory B cells in EAE (Mann, Maresz et al. 2007; Matsushita, Yanaba et al. 2008; Rafei, Hsieh et al. 2009; Kala, Rhodes et al. 2010). Considering the extensive use of MS treatments that are dependent on B cell depletion, it seems crucial to define this dual role of B cells in the progression of disease. Lee-Chang et al. demonstrated that homeostasis of the B cell subsets is altered during the preclinical and acute phases of EAE, where the percentage of B cells with regulatory phenotype are significantly reduced (Lee-Chang, Lefranc et al. 2011), indicating again that timing is an important consideration when targeting B cells during therapy. It was also shown that B cell depletion reduced the frequency of regulatory T cells, and increased the pro-inflammatory polarising capacity of the remaining myeloid APC (Weber, Prod'homme et al. 2010).

Interestingly, in human MS patients, peripheral blood B cells produced less IL-10 in response to TLR-9 as well as CD40 and BCR stimulation compared to healthy controls (Duddy, Niino et al. 2007; Hirotani, Niino et al. 2010). This might indicate that Breg cells in human MS patients are functionally impaired, or simply exhausted due to chronic pro-inflammatory stimulation, and thereby are implicated in disease development.

3.2.3 Type 1 diabetes

Type 1 diabetes (T1D) and the spontaneous disease that develops in the corresponding mouse model (non-obese diabetic (NOD) mouse), is characterised by autoimmune destruction of the insulin-producing pancreatic β cells. Attack on β cells is primarily mediated by T cells (Anderson and Bluestone 2005), however B cells and humoral immunity also play a role, especially in disease initiation (Silveira and Grey 2006; Xiu, Wong et al. 2008). Despite the pathogenic role of B cells in disease initiation, B cells activated *in vitro* can maintain tolerance and transfer protection from disease in NOD mice (Tian, Zekzer et al. 2001; Hussain and Delovitch 2007). Transfusion of BCR-stimulated B cells reduced the incidence and delayed the onset of disease, when given repeatedly starting at a young age before disease onset. Disease protection was dependent on IL-10 and correlated with the polarisation of T cells towards a Th2 phenotype (Hussain and Delovitch 2007). In a different experimental setting, transfer of *in vitro* LPS-stimulated B cells protected NOD mice from spontaneous diabetes. As these B cells were shown to express FasL and secrete TGF-β, this effect was attributed to the triggering of apoptosis in Th1 cells and/or the inhibition of APC activity (Tian, Zekzer et al. 2001).

4. Regulatory B cells in allergic diseases

The vast majority of studies on regulatory B cells has been focused on autoimmunity models. However, recent studies indicate that Breg cells may also be instrumental in reducing T-helper 2 (Th2) skewed immune diseases, such as allergies. Allergies are dysregulated immune responses towards normally harmless allergens that result in an expansion of polarised Th2 cells, elevated immunoglobulin E (IgE) production and eosinophilia (Kay 2000). Common allergic diseases include allergic asthma, rhinitis, atopic dermatitis, and food allergies. Allergic asthma is characterised by reversible airway obstruction and airway remodelling upon exposure to inhaled aeroallergens such as house dust mite (HDM), grass pollen, or pet dander. In allergic rhinitis (hay fever), allergen exposure leads to irritation and inflammation of the nasal airways, whereas atopic dermatitis is an inflammatory, chronically relapsing, non-contagious and pruritic skin disorder. In food allergies, exposure to food products such as peanuts, fruits or milk may lead to allergic symptoms including gastrointestinal and respiratory distress, or life-threatening anaphylactic responses (Kay 2000).

Traditionally, B cells have been known for their capacity to produce antibodies, thereby contributing to humoral immunity and clearance of pathogens. During allergic disorders, B cells are driven to preferentially class-switch to IgE isotypes in the presence of local IL-4 and this forms a central element in the acute inflammatory responses to allergens. Allergen-specific IgE binds to Fc-receptors (FcR) on mast cells and basophils and subsequent exposure to the same allergen leads to degranulation and inflammation. So far, reports evaluating B cell function other than Ig(E) production in allergies are limited. Nevertheless, a few reports suggest that in allergic inflammation, like in autoimmunity, B cells can have a regulatory role (Hussaarts, van der Vlugt et al. 2011). For example, B cells isolated from OVA tolerant mice were able to dampen acute allergic airway inflammation via the TGF-β induced conversion of CD4+CD25-T cells into functionally suppressive CD4+CD25+FoxP3+ T regulatory cells (Singh, Carson et al. 2008). In addition, B cells were also shown to control experimental cockroach allergen-induced inflammation by the induction of FasL-mediated apoptosis of CD4+ T cells. In mice lacking B1a B cells, it was demonstrated that in particular the CD5+ B1a B cell population was important for protective CD4+ T cell apoptosis (Lundy, Berlin et al. 2005). Furthermore, two reports have studied the presence of human IL-10 or TGF-β producing B cells in non-IgE mediated food allergy. In response to the milk antigen, casein, the frequency of IL-10 or TGF-β producing CD5+ peripheral blood B cells increased in healthy donors whereas the frequency declined in allergic donors (Noh, Choi et al. 2010; Lee, Noh et al. 2011). In addition, our group observed less IL-10 producing B cells in response to LPS in house dust mite allergic asthma patients compared to healthy controls (Mlejnek and van der Vlugt 2012). These findings support the notion that Breg cells may form an important regulatory arm of the immune system and seem to be dysfunctional in allergic disorders.

5. Implications of pathogen-induced Breg cells in autoimmunity and allergy

The onset of hyperinflammatory disorders such as allergies and autoimmunities seems to be partly genetic, as the risk for developing disease increases when a parent or a sibling is affected (Mariani 2004; von Mutius 2009). However, the steep increase in the incidence of hyperinflammatory disorders over the last few decades in the Western world has suggested that environmental factors may also have a major impact. Fast changes in lifestyle, housing, improved hygiene and vaccinations in industrialised countries have resulted in reduced microbial exposure during early childhood (Wills-Karp, Santeliz et al. 2001; Yazdanbakhsh, Kremsner et al. 2002), which may allow for uncontrolled inflammatory responses against either innocuous or self-antigens later in life. In support of this 'hygiene' hypothesis, several epidemiological studies have pointed towards a reversed relationship between hyperinflammatory disorders and microbial exposure, such as bacterial, viral and helminth infections.

5.1 Hyperinflammatory disorders and the 'hygiene hypothesis'

Parasites are regarded to be master manipulators of the host immune system. A negative correlation between the rates of parasitic infections in developing countries and the prevalence of allergic symptoms and atopic sensitisation in children has been highlighted in a number of studies in different geographical areas (Flohr, Quinnell et al. 2009). Strikingly, long-term anti-helminth treatment resulted in increased atopic reactivity to house dust mite, supporting a direct link between helminth exposure and protection against allergic diseases (Lynch, Hagel et al. 1993; van den Biggelaar, Rodrigues et al. 2004). In addition, helminth infected MS patients showed better clinical disease outcome compared to control MS patients (Correale, Farez et al. 2008). A relationship between helminth infections and protection against hyperinflammatory disorders has also been established in various mouse models for food allergy (Nagler-Anderson 2006), asthma (Smits, Hammad et al. 2007; Amu, Saunders et al. 2010), T1D (Zaccone, Fehervari et al. 2003; Liu, Sundar et al. 2009), CIA

(Osada, Shimizu et al. 2009) and EAE (La Flamme, Ruddenklau et al. 2003; Wilson, Taylor et al. 2010). Furthermore, different cross-sectional studies show that children living in farming environments are protected from childhood asthma and atopy and this correlation has been attributed to contact with livestock (Ege, Frei et al. 2007) and hay and the consumption of raw cow's milk (Douwes, Cheng et al. 2008; Loss, Apprich et al. 2011). In farming environments, both outdoor and indoor microbial exposure are higher and more diverse compared to nonfarming environments (von Mutius, Braun-Fahrlander et al. 2000; Ege, Mayer et al. 2011). More detailed analysis of the dust composition showed that a lower risk of asthma was associated with Gram-negative bacteria and fungi of the *Eurotium* and *Penicillium* species (Ege, Frei et al. 2007; Ege, Mayer et al. 2011). Inhalation is a main route of exposure to pathogens, but ingestion of orofecal microbes (Matricardi, Rosmini et al. 1997) or colonization of certain probiotic bacteria stimulating the gut associated lymphoid tissue (GALT) may also help to avoid allergic responses or certain autoimmune conditions. A direct association between the composition of the gastrointestinal microbiome and the risk of developing allergies has been described in several studies, suggesting that *Lactobacilli* and *Bifidobacterium bifidum* have a protective effect (Bjorksten, Sepp et al. 2001; Johansson, Sjogren et al. 2011). Also in line with this data, changes in faecal microbiota were detected in autoimmune patients suffering from Crohn's disease and ulcerative colitis (Manichanh, Rigottier-Gois et al. 2006; Frank, St Amand et al. 2007).

Altogether these findings indicate that microbial exposure during early life seems to be important to prevent hyperinflammatory conditions. Various studies have indicated that the development of the regulatory arm of the immune system is instrumental for this protection, and so far have highlighted a role for Treg cells (Wohlfert and Belkaid 2008). However, there is a growing amount of evidence showing a protective role for Breg cells induced by infectious agents.

5.2 Pathogen-induced Breg cells are protective in autoimmune and allergic conditions

One of the first observations that helminths, such as *Schisostoma mansoni*, could induce suppressive B cells was made in μMT mice, which lack mature B cells. These mice show increased *S.mansoni*-induced tissue pathology compared to infected wild-type mice (Jankovic, Cheever et al. 1998). Subsequent studies with *S. mansoni* demonstrated that B cells isolated from helminth-infected mice could play a protective role in allergy, as transfer of B cells protected recipient mice against systemic fatal anaphylaxis or OVA-induced airway inflammation via the production of IL-10 (Mangan, Fallon et al. 2004; Mangan, van Rooijen et al. 2006; Amu, Saunders et al. 2010). Interestingly, these regulatory mechanisms were only active during the chronic phase of infection (Smits, Hammad et al. 2007). Similar results were obtained in *Heligosomoides polygyrus*-infected mice, where CD19+CD5-CD23hi B cells isolated from mesenteric lymph nodes of chronically infected mice were able to suppress Derp1-induced airway inflammation, although independently of IL-10 (Wilson, Taylor et al. 2010). Interestingly, *S. mansoni*-induced Breg cells also incurred protection against allergic airway inflammation via the induction of regulatory T cells (Amu, Saunders et al. 2010). However, Breg-induced immune regulation was only partially dependent on Treg cell induction as we could demonstrate in conditional FoxP3 knockout mice (van der Vlugt and Labuda 2012). In addition, B cell induced FasL-mediated apoptosis of CD4+ T cells appeared to be another mechanism used by Breg cells to control inflammation during schistosome infections (Lundy and Boros 2002). Helminth-induced Breg cells also ameliorated symptoms of several autoimmune diseases. Adoptive transfer of B cells isolated from *H. polygyrus* infected mice, dramatically reduced EAE severity in uninfected recipients (Wilson, Taylor et al. 2010) and B cells from helminth infected MS patients suppressed T cell activation *in vitro* (Correale, Farez et al. 2008). The production of B cell IL-10 and the induction of Treg cells were important in the reduction of inflammation. Treg cell induction was further shown to be dependent on expression of B7 costimulatory molecules, as B7 deficient B cells failed to efficiently recruit Treg cells into the CNS and mediate recovery from EAE clinical disease (Mann, Maresz et al. 2007). In addition to helminthic infection, bacterial exposure may also enhance the activity of Breg cells. For example, TLR signaling on B cells is required for the recovery from EAE. Interestingly, although both TLR-4 (LPS) and TLR-9 (CpG) signaling induced IL-10 expression in B cells, only LPS stimulation via TLR-2/4 was capable of inducing recovery from EAE (Lampropoulou, Hoehlig et al. 2008). Furthermore, tissue damage as a result of invading pathogens may induce apoptosis and can influence the development of Breg cells. Injection of apoptotic cells into mice has been shown to induce Breg cells and reduce inflammatory processes in a collagen-induced arthritis model (Gray, Miles et al. 2007). Overall, there is a strong case for the capacity of various pathogens to induce functional Breg cells that are protective against inflammation-driven pathology.

6. Possible therapeutic applications targeting Breg cells in autoimmune and allergic disorders

Several studies have highlighted the relevance of Breg cells in downmodulating inflammation in autoimmune and allergic disorders. In addition to the direct effects via cytokine production, Breg cells also function indirectly via the induction or recruitment of regulatory T cells and therefore may have promising therapeutic potential. However, the mechanism underlying the formation of regulatory B cells and their implications in existing therapies must be fully understood, before these pathways can be exploited for therapeutic purposes.

6.1 Pathogen-driven pathways for the induction and expansion of Breg cells

As demonstrated in figure 3, Breg cells can be induced by bacterial or parasitic infections. Therefore, the identification of the secreted or excreted pathogenic compound(s) driving Breg cell induction provides useful information for the development of therapeutic interventions. Indeed, the fact that live schistosome worms could induce IL-10 producing Breg cells from splenic B cells in an *in vitro* culture system, suggests that helminth antigens have a direct effect on B cells (Amu, Saunders et al. 2010). Helminth-related TLR ligands may be a likely candidate responsible for helminth-induced Breg cell formation, given the implication of certain TLR ligands in the induction of Breg cells in autoimmune models (as discussed above). Notably, lacto-N-fucopentaose-III (LNFPIII), a sugar found on soluble egg antigens (SEA) interacts with TLR-4 and stimulates splenic B cells to produce IL-10 (Velupillai and Harn 1994). Likewise, microfilarial extracts from *Leishmania major*, and *Brugia malayi*, which both bind to TLR-4, can induce IL-10 production by B cells (Palanivel, Posey et al. 1996). Furthermore, lyso-phosphatidylserine, a lipid derived from *S. mansoni* worms ligated TLR-2 on human monocyte-derived DC and promoted Treg cell activity (van der Kleij, Latz et al. 2002). Although it is unclear whether this TLR-2 ligating molecule has an effect on the formation of Breg cells, SEA stimulation of human B cells did result in TLR-2 mediated elevated IL-10 production (Correale and Farez 2009).

Bacterial infections such as *Helicobacter felis* induced IL-10 producing B cells via TLR-2 signalling and were also able to suppress *Helicobacter*-induced pathology via the induction of IL-10 producing T cells (Sayi, Kohler et al. 2011). Other bacterial structures, such as CpG oligonucleotides (ODN) binding to TLR-9, are also well known to be strong inducers of B cell IL-10 production (Barr, Brown et al. 2007; Bouaziz, Calbo et al. 2010). Interestingly, administration of CpG ODN to mice potently inhibited acute and established asthma, allergic rhinitis and conjunctivitis (Fonseca and Kline 2009). Additionally, human clinical trials with CpG ODN conjugated with ragweed antigen revealed that ragweed allergy subjects developed a shift in immune response from Th2 towards a dominant Th1 profile (Simons, Shikishima et al. 2004) and a decrease in clinical allergy symptoms two years after treatment (Tulic, Fiset et al. 2004). Although the role of IL-10 producing B cells was not studied in those clinical trials, a recent study in mice clearly showed that immunosuppressive IL-10 producing follicular B cells appeared after CpG treatment. These Breg cells were responsible for the reduction in late phase experimental allergic conjunctivitis (Miyazaki, Kuo et al. 2009), suggesting that the administration of CpG can also form an important therapeutic approach to induce Breg cell activity.

6.2 Induction and expansion of Breg cells by chemical drugs used in medical treatment

Clonal expansion of B cells and the production of auto-antibodies indicate that B cells contribute to the pathogenesis of several autoimmune diseases. Accordingly, B cell depletion therapy using Rituximab (anti-CD20) has shown promising effects in clinical trials (Bar-Or, Calabresi et al. 2008; Hauser, Waubant et al. 2008). However, possible implications for regulatory B cells in the treatment of human autoimmune diseases have been indicated by recent studies investigating the immunological mechanisms of drugs already used for medical treatment of human patients (Fig. 3). A very recent report shows that an antibody acting as an IL-6R antagonist (Tocilizumab), which has recently been introduced as therapy for rheumatoid arthritis, causes regulatory CD25+ B cells to increase their TGF-β expression and alter their activation status, indicating that the beneficial effects of Tocilizumab are due to an induction or expansion of regulatory B cells (Snir, Kessel et al. 2011).

Beneficial effects of several drugs used in the treatment of multiple sclerosis also seem to be mediated by regulatory B cells. Glatiramer acetate (GA) is a drug safely used in MS patients, and it has been demonstrated that the beneficial effects of GA were abrogated in B cell-deficient mice. Furthermore, adoptive transfer of B cells from GA-treated mice inhibited the proliferation of autoreactive T cells as well as the development of Th1 and Th17 cells, but promoted IL-10 production in recipient mice (Kala, Rhodes et al. 2010; Begum-Haque, Christy et al. 2011). Estrogen, a hormone drug with well established therapeutic effects on MS, was shown to depend on B cells as well. In EAE, estrogen-mediated protection from disease was associated with a general increase in the percentage of IL-10-producing regulatory B cells as well as an upregulation of PD-L1 expression on B cells, possibly leading

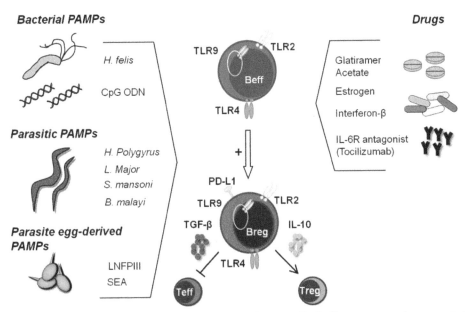

Fig. 3. Pathways for the induction and expansion of Breg cells. Different secreted or excreted (non)pathogenic compounds of bacteria, parasites or their eggs can drive Breg cell induction. These compounds have been shown to bind to TLR and thereby induce Breg cell development. Additionally, Breg cell promoting activities were found in several registered drug-based treatments for autoimmune diseases. As a consequence, Breg cells start to produce anti-inflammatory cytokines IL-10 and TGF-β, inhibit Teff cell proliferation and induce Treg cells. PAMPs: pathogen associated molecular patterns, TLR: Toll-like receptor, Breg: regulatory B cells, Teff/reg: effector/regulatory T cells, LNFPIII: lacto-N-fucopentaose-III, SEA: soluble egg antigens.

to direct target cell apoptosis (Bodhankar, Wang et al. 2011). As previous studies on B cells from human MS patients have demonstrated a defective IL-10 producing capacity (Duddy, Niino et al. 2007; Hirotani, Niino et al. 2010), upregulation of IL-10 production by B cells might be of importance in disease resolution in MS patients undergoing treatment. Indeed, a study on human patients treated with IFN-β demonstrated that their B cells showed a lower proliferative response *in vitro* than B cells from untreated patients. *In vitro* IFN-β treatment of B cells shifted their cytokine profile and induced IL-10 secretion (Ramgolam, Sha et al. 2011).

7. Concluding remarks

The underlying mechanisms leading to inflammatory conditions such as autoimmune diseases and allergies are diverse and far from being fully understood. However, it has become obvious that a balance between effector and regulatory functions of different subsets of immune cells is crucially important in the maintenance of a healthy steady-state situation.

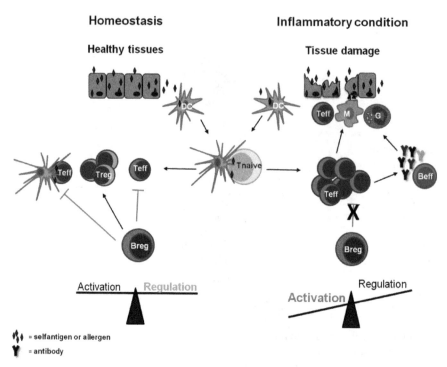

Fig. 4. Regulatory B cells in homeostasis and disease. Under normal conditions regulatory B cells control T effector cell activation and proliferation in response to harmless self antigens and allergens, and induce and activate regulatory T cells. If Breg cell mediated control fails, effector T cells can proliferate and activate antibody producing B cells as well as innate immune cell types causing tissue damage. Beff/reg: effector/regulatory B cells, Teff/reg: effector/regulatory T cells, Tnaive: naive T cells, DC: dendritic cells, M: macrophages, G: granulocytes.

Regulatory B cells are an exciting new player on the regulatory side of this constant struggle for balance. As depicted in figure 4, in the healthy immune system Breg cells help to control effector cell activation, by releasing immunosuppressive cytokines and inducing target cell apoptosis. The broad target cell range of their cytokines allows them to inhibit pro-inflammatory functions of both innate immune cells, such as DC and macrophages as well as cells of the adaptive immune system, such as effector T cells of both the Th1 and Th2 lineage. On the other hand they also amplify the regulatory arm of immune responses by inducing regulatory T cells. Impaired regulatory capacity of Breg cells might play a role in the development of inflammatory diseases. Uncontrolled effector T and B cell activation can ultimately lead to inflammation and tissue damage in various target organs. Correspondingly, several treatments demonstrated to be beneficial in autoimmune and allergic diseases seem to affect the immune system at the level of B cells by amplifying their regulatory capacity. Currently much effort is put into therapies aiming to induce regulatory T cells. However, targeting regulatory B cells instead holds the added benefit of indirectly affecting all target cell types of Breg cells, including regulatory T cells, making it a more efficient approach. Therefore, further research is needed to increase our understanding of Breg cell biology in health and disease, as targeting Breg cells for therapeutic applications holds great promise for the future treatment of autoimmune and allergic inflammatory conditions.

8. References

Amano, H., E. Amano, et al. (2003). "The Yaa mutation promoting murine lupus causes defective development of marginal zone B cells." *J Immunol* 170(5): 2293-2301.

Amu, S., S. P. Saunders, et al. (2010). "Regulatory B cells prevent and reverse allergic airway inflammation via FoxP3-positive T regulatory cells in a murine model." *J Allergy Clin Immunol* 125(5): 1114-1124 e1118.

Anderson, M. S. and J. A. Bluestone (2005). "The NOD mouse: a model of immune dysregulation." *Annu Rev Immunol* 23: 447-485.

Bar-Or, A., P. A. Calabresi, et al. (2008). "Rituximab in relapsing-remitting multiple sclerosis: a 72-week, open-label, phase I trial." *Ann Neurol* 63(3): 395-400.

Barr, T. A., S. Brown, et al. (2007). "TLR-mediated stimulation of APC: Distinct cytokine responses of B cells and dendritic cells." *Eur J Immunol* 37(11): 3040-3053.

Baxter, A. G. (2007). "The origin and application of experimental autoimmune encephalomyelitis." *Nat Rev Immunol* 7(11): 904-912.

Begum-Haque, S., M. Christy, et al. (2011). "Augmentation of regulatory B cell activity in experimental allergic encephalomyelitis by glatiramer acetate." *J Neuroimmunol* 232(1-2): 136-144.

Bhan, A. K., E. Mizoguchi, et al. (2000). "Regulatory role of mature B cells in a murine model of inflammatory bowel disease." *International Immunology* 12(5): 597-605.

Bhan, A. K., E. Mizoguchi, et al. (1999). "Colitis in transgenic and knockout animals as models of human inflammatory bowel disease." *Immunol Rev* 169: 195-207.

Bjorksten, B., E. Sepp, et al. (2001). "Allergy development and the intestinal microflora during the first year of life." *J Allergy Clin Immunol* 108(4): 516-520.

Blair, P. A., K. A. Chavez-Rueda, et al. (2009). "Selective targeting of B cells with agonistic anti-CD40 is an efficacious strategy for the generation of induced regulatory T2-like B cells and for the suppression of lupus in MRL/lpr mice." *J Immunol* 182(6): 3492-3502.

Blair, P. A., L. Y. Norena, et al. (2010). "CD19(+)CD24(hi)CD38(hi) B cells exhibit regulatory capacity in healthy individuals but are functionally impaired in systemic Lupus Erythematosus patients." *Immunity* 32(1): 129-140.

Bodhankar, S., C. Wang, et al. (2011). "Estrogen-induced protection against experimental autoimmune encephalomyelitis is abrogated in the absence of B cells." *Eur J Immunol* 41(4): 1165-1175.

Booth, J. S., P. J. Griebel, et al. (2009). "A novel regulatory B-cell population in sheep Peyer's patches spontaneously secretes IL-10 and downregulates TLR9-induced IFNalpha responses." *Mucosal Immunol* 2(3): 265-275.

Borg, N. A., K. S. Wun, et al. (2007). "CD1d-lipid-antigen recognition by the semi-invariant NKT T-cell receptor." *Nature* 448(7149): 44-49.

Bouaziz, J. D., S. Calbo, et al. (2010). "IL-10 produced by activated human B cells regulates CD4(+) T-cell activation in vitro." *Eur J Immunol* 40(10): 2686-2691.

Carter, N. A., R. Vasconcellos, et al. (2011). "Mice lacking endogenous IL-10-producing regulatory B cells develop exacerbated disease and present with an increased frequency of Th1/Th17 but a decrease in regulatory T cells." *J Immunol* 186(10): 5569-5579.

Chiu, Y. H., S. H. Park, et al. (2002). "Multiple defects in antigen presentation and T cell development by mice expressing cytoplasmic tail-truncated CD1d." *Nat Immunol* 3(1): 55-60.

Collison, L. W., C. J. Workman, et al. (2007). "The inhibitory cytokine IL-35 contributes to regulatory T-cell function." *Nature* 450(7169): 566-569.

Colombo, M., M. Dono, et al. (2000). "Accumulation of clonally related B lymphocytes in the cerebrospinal fluid of multiple sclerosis patients." *J Immunol* 164(5): 2782-2789.

Correale, J. and M. Farez (2009). "Helminth antigens modulate immune responses in cells from multiple sclerosis patients through TLR2-dependent mechanisms." *J Immunol* 183(9): 5999-6012.

Correale, J., M. Farez, et al. (2008). "Helminth infections associated with multiple sclerosis induce regulatory B cells." *Ann Neurol* 64(2): 187-199.

Cua, D. J., J. Sherlock, et al. (2003). "Interleukin-23 rather than interleukin-12 is the critical cytokine for autoimmune inflammation of the brain." *Nature* 421(6924): 744-748.

Dalwadi, H., B. Wei, et al. (2003). "B cell developmental requirement for the G alpha i2 gene." *J Immunol* 170(4): 1707-1715.

DiLillo, D. J., T. Matsushita, et al. (2010). "B10 cells and regulatory B cells balance immune responses during inflammation, autoimmunity, and cancer." *Ann N Y Acad Sci* 1183: 38-57.

Douwes, J., S. Cheng, et al. (2008). "Farm exposure in utero may protect against asthma, hay fever and eczema." *Eur Respir J* 32(3): 603-611.

Duddy, M., M. Niino, et al. (2007). "Distinct effector cytokine profiles of memory and naive human B cell subsets and implication in multiple sclerosis." *J Immunol* 178(10): 6092-6099.

Ege, M. J., R. Frei, et al. (2007). "Not all farming environments protect against the development of asthma and wheeze in children." *J Allergy Clin Immunol* 119(5): 1140-1147.

Ege, M. J., M. Mayer, et al. (2011). "Exposure to environmental microorganisms and childhood asthma." *N Engl J Med* 364(8): 701-709.

Evans, J. G., K. A. Chavez-Rueda, et al. (2007). "Novel suppressive function of transitional 2 B cells in experimental arthritis." *J Immunol* 178(12): 7868-7878.

Fife, B. T. and J. A. Bluestone (2008). "Control of peripheral T-cell tolerance and autoimmunity via the CTLA-4 and PD-1 pathways." *Immunol Rev* 224: 166-182.

Fillatreau, S., C. H. Sweenie, et al. (2002). "B cells regulate autoimmunity by provision of IL-10." *Nat Immunol* 3(10): 944-950.

Firestein, G. S. (2003). "Evolving concepts of rheumatoid arthritis." *Nature* 423(6937): 356-361.

Flohr, C., R. J. Quinnell, et al. (2009). "Do helminth parasites protect against atopy and allergic disease?" *Clin Exp Allergy* 39(1): 20-32.

Fonseca, D. E. and J. N. Kline (2009). "Use of CpG oligonucleotides in treatment of asthma and allergic disease." *Adv Drug Deliv Rev* 61(3): 256-262.

Frank, D. N., A. L. St Amand, et al. (2007). "Molecular-phylogenetic characterization of microbial community imbalances in human inflammatory bowel diseases." *Proc Natl Acad Sci U S A* 104(34): 13780-13785.

Fraussen, J., K. Vrolix, et al. (2009). "B cell characterization and reactivity analysis in multiple sclerosis." *Autoimmun Rev* 8(8): 654-658.

Gerth, A. J., L. Lin, et al. (2004). "An innate cell-mediated, murine ulcerative colitis-like syndrome in the absence of nuclear factor of activated T cells." *Gastroenterology* 126(4): 1115-1121.

Gray, M., K. Miles, et al. (2007). "Apoptotic cells protect mice from autoimmune inflammation by the induction of regulatory B cells." *Proc Natl Acad Sci U S A* 104(35): 14080-14085.

Hardy, R. R. and K. Hayakawa (2001). "B cell development pathways." *Annu Rev Immunol* 19: 595-621.

Hauser, S. L., E. Waubant, et al. (2008). "B-cell depletion with rituximab in relapsing-remitting multiple sclerosis." *N Engl J Med* 358(7): 676-688.

Hirotani, M., M. Niino, et al. (2010). "Decreased IL-10 production mediated by Toll-like receptor 9 in B cells in multiple sclerosis." *J Neuroimmunol* 221(1-2): 95-100.

Hokama, A., E. Mizoguchi, et al. (2004). "Induced reactivity of intestinal CD4(+) T cells with an epithelial cell lectin, galectin-4, contributes to exacerbation of intestinal inflammation." *Immunity* 20(6): 681-693.

Huang, F.-P. and S. Sattler (2011). "Regulatory T Cell Deficiency in Systemic Autoimmune Disorders – Causal Relationship and Underlying Immunological Mechanisms." *Autoimmune Disorders - Pathogenetic Aspects, Mavragani Clio (Ed.), ISBN 978-953-307-643-0, InTech.*

Hussaarts, L., L. E. van der Vlugt, et al. (2011). "Regulatory B-cell induction by helminths: Implications for allergic disease." *J Allergy Clin Immunol* 128(4): 733-739.

Hussain, S. and T. L. Delovitch (2007). "Intravenous transfusion of BCR-activated B cells protects NOD mice from type 1 diabetes in an IL-10-dependent manner." *J Immunol* 179(11): 7225-7232.

Iwata, Y., T. Matsushita, et al. (2011). "Characterization of a rare IL-10-competent B-cell subset in humans that parallels mouse regulatory B10 cells." *Blood* 117(2): 530-541.

Jankovic, D., A. W. Cheever, et al. (1998). "CD4+ T cell-mediated granulomatous pathology in schistosomiasis is downregulated by a B cell-dependent mechanism requiring Fc receptor signaling." *J Exp Med* 187(4): 619-629.

Johansson, M. A., Y. M. Sjogren, et al. (2011). "Early colonization with a group of Lactobacilli decreases the risk for allergy at five years of age despite allergic heredity." *PLoS One* 6(8): e23031.

Kala, M., S. N. Rhodes, et al. (2010). "B cells from glatiramer acetate-treated mice suppress experimental autoimmune encephalomyelitis." *Exp Neurol* 221(1): 136-145.

Katz, S. I., D. Parker, et al. (1974). "B-cell suppression of delayed hypersensitivity reactions." *Nature* 251(5475): 550-551.

Kay, A. B. (2000). "Overview of 'allergy and allergic diseases: with a view to the future'." *Br Med Bull* 56(4): 843-864.

La Flamme, A. C., K. Ruddenklau, et al. (2003). "Schistosomiasis decreases central nervous system inflammation and alters the progression of experimental autoimmune encephalomyelitis." *Infect Immun* 71(9): 4996-5004.

Lampropoulou, V., E. Calderon-Gomez, et al. (2010). "Suppressive functions of activated B cells in autoimmune diseases reveal the dual roles of Toll-like receptors in immunity." *Immunol Rev* 233(1): 146-161.

Lampropoulou, V., K. Hoehlig, et al. (2008). "TLR-activated B cells suppress T cell-mediated autoimmunity." *J Immunol* 180(7): 4763-4773.

Lee-Chang, C., D. Lefranc, et al. (2011). "Susceptibility to experimental autoimmune encephalomyelitis is associated with altered B-cell subsets distribution and decreased serum BAFF levels." *Immunol Lett* 135(1-2): 108-117.

Lee, J. H., J. Noh, et al. (2011). "Allergen-specific transforming growth factor-beta-producing CD19+CD5+ regulatory B-cell (Br3) responses in human late eczematous allergic reactions to cow's milk." *J Interferon Cytokine Res* 31(5): 441-449.

Lehuen, A., O. Lantz, et al. (1998). "Overexpression of natural killer T cells protects Valpha14- Jalpha281 transgenic nonobese diabetic mice against diabetes." *J Exp Med* 188(10): 1831-1839.

Lemoine, S., A. Morva, et al. (2009). "Regulatory B cells in autoimmune diseases: how do they work?" *Ann N Y Acad Sci* 1173: 260-267.

Lenert, P., R. Brummel, et al. (2005). "TLR-9 activation of marginal zone B cells in lupus mice regulates immunity through increased IL-10 production." *J Clin Immunol* 25(1): 29-40.

Lenert, P., A. Goeken, et al. (2003). "Innate immune responses in lupus-prone Palmerston North mice: differential responses to LPS and bacterial DNA/CpG oligonucleotides." *J Clin Immunol* 23(3): 202-213.

Liu, Q., K. Sundar, et al. (2009). "Helminth infection can reduce insulitis and type 1 diabetes through CD25- and IL-10-independent mechanisms." *Infect Immun* 77(12): 5347-5358.

Loss, G., S. Apprich, et al. (2011). "The protective effect of farm milk consumption on childhood asthma and atopy: The GABRIELA study." *J Allergy Clin Immunol* 128(4): 766-773 e764.

Lotz, M., E. Ranheim, et al. (1994). "Transforming growth factor beta as endogenous growth inhibitor of chronic lymphocytic leukemia B cells." *J Exp Med* 179(3): 999-1004.

Lundy, S. K., A. A. Berlin, et al. (2005). "Deficiency of regulatory B cells increases allergic airway inflammation." *Inflamm Res* 54(12): 514-521.

Lundy, S. K. and D. L. Boros (2002). "Fas ligand-expressing B-1a lymphocytes mediate CD4(+)-T-cell apoptosis during schistosomal infection: induction by interleukin 4 (IL-4) and IL-10." *Infect Immun* 70(2): 812-819.

Lundy, S. K. and D. A. Fox (2009). "Reduced Fas ligand-expressing splenic CD5+ B lymphocytes in severe collagen-induced arthritis." *Arthritis Res Ther* 11(4): R128.

Lynch, N. R., I. Hagel, et al. (1993). "Effect of anthelmintic treatment on the allergic reactivity of children in a tropical slum." *J Allergy Clin Immunol* 92(3): 404-411.

Mangan, N. E., R. E. Fallon, et al. (2004). "Helminth infection protects mice from anaphylaxis via IL-10-producing B cells." *J Immunol* 173(10): 6346-6356.

Mangan, N. E., N. van Rooijen, et al. (2006). "Helminth-modified pulmonary immune response protects mice from allergen-induced airway hyperresponsiveness." *J Immunol* 176(1): 138-147.

Manichanh, C., L. Rigottier-Gois, et al. (2006). "Reduced diversity of faecal microbiota in Crohn's disease revealed by a metagenomic approach." *Gut* 55(2): 205-211.

Mann, M. K., K. Maresz, et al. (2007). "B cell regulation of CD4+CD25+ T regulatory cells and IL-10 via B7 is essential for recovery from experimental autoimmune encephalomyelitis." *J Immunol* 178(6): 3447-3456.

Mariani, S. M. (2004). "Genes and autoimmune diseases - a complex inheritance." *MedGenMed* 6(4): 18.

Matricardi, P. M., F. Rosmini, et al. (1997). "Cross sectional retrospective study of prevalence of atopy among Italian military students with antibodies against hepatitis A virus." *BMJ* 314(7086): 999-1003.

Matsushita, T., M. Fujimoto, et al. (2006). "Inhibitory role of CD19 in the progression of experimental autoimmune encephalomyelitis by regulating cytokine response." *Am J Pathol* 168(3): 812-821.

Matsushita, T., M. Horikawa, et al. (2010). "Regulatory B cells (B10 cells) and regulatory T cells have independent roles in controlling experimental autoimmune encephalomyelitis initiation and late-phase immunopathogenesis." *J Immunol* 185(4): 2240-2252.

Matsushita, T., K. Yanaba, et al. (2008). "Regulatory B cells inhibit EAE initiation in mice while other B cells promote disease progression." *J Clin Invest* 118(10): 3420-3430.

Mauri, C. and M. R. Ehrenstein (2008). "The 'short' history of regulatory B cells." *Trends Immunol* 29(1): 34-40.

Mauri, C., D. Gray, et al. (2003). "Prevention of arthritis by interleukin 10-producing B cells." *J Exp Med* 197(4): 489-501.

Mills, J. A. (1994). "Systemic lupus erythematosus." *N Engl J Med* 330(26): 1871-1879.

Miyazaki, D., C. H. Kuo, et al. (2009). "Regulatory function of CpG-activated B cells in late-phase experimental allergic conjunctivitis." *Invest Ophthalmol Vis Sci* 50(4): 1626-1635.

Mizoguchi, A. and A. K. Bhan (2006). "A case for regulatory B cells." *J Immunol* 176(2): 705-710.

Mizoguchi, A., E. Mizoguchi, et al. (1996). "Cytokine imbalance and autoantibody production in T cell receptor-alpha mutant mice with inflammatory bowel disease." *J Exp Med* 183(3): 847-856.

Mizoguchi, A., E. Mizoguchi, et al. (1997). "Suppressive role of B cells in chronic colitis of T cell receptor alpha mutant mice." *J Exp Med* 186(10): 1749-1756.

Mizoguchi, A., E. Mizoguchi, et al. (2002). "Chronic intestinal inflammatory condition generates IL-10-producing regulatory B cell subset characterized by CD1d upregulation." *Immunity* 16(2): 219-230.

Mlejnek, E. and L.E.P.M. van der Vlugt (2012). "Impaired IL-10 expression by CD24hiCD27+ regulatory B cells in response to LPS in allergic asthmatic patients." *submitted*.

Moore, K. W., R. de Waal Malefyt, et al. (2001). "Interleukin-10 and the interleukin-10 receptor." *Annu Rev Immunol* 19: 683-765.

Nagler-Anderson, C. (2006). "Helminth-induced immunoregulation of an allergic response to food." *Chem Immunol Allergy* 90: 1-13.

Nakashima, H., Y. Hamaguchi, et al. (2010). "CD22 expression mediates the regulatory functions of peritoneal B-1a cells during the remission phase of contact hypersensitivity reactions." *J Immunol* 184(9): 4637-4645.

Niedbala, W., X. Q. Wei, et al. (2007). "IL-35 is a novel cytokine with therapeutic effects against collagen-induced arthritis through the expansion of regulatory T cells and suppression of Th17 cells." *Eur J Immunol* 37(11): 3021-3029.

Noh, G. and J. H. Lee (2011). "Regulatory B cells and allergic diseases." *Allergy Asthma Immunol Res* 3(3): 168-177.

Noh, J., W. S. Choi, et al. (2010). "Presence of Foxp3-expressing CD19(+)CD5(+) B Cells in Human Peripheral Blood Mononuclear Cells: Human CD19(+)CD5(+)Foxp3(+) Regulatory B Cell (Breg)." *Immune Netw* 10(6): 247-249.

O'Connor, R. A. and S. M. Anderton (2008). "Multi-faceted control of autoaggression: Foxp3+ regulatory T cells in murine models of organ-specific autoimmune disease." *Cell Immunol* 251(1): 8-18.

Osada, Y., S. Shimizu, et al. (2009). "Schistosoma mansoni infection reduces severity of collagen-induced arthritis via down-regulation of pro-inflammatory mediators." *Int J Parasitol* 39(4): 457-464.

Ostanin, D. V., K. P. Pavlick, et al. (2006). "T cell-induced inflammation of the small and large intestine in immunodeficient mice." *Am J Physiol Gastrointest Liver Physiol* 290(1): G109-119.

Palanivel, V., C. Posey, et al. (1996). "B-cell outgrowth and ligand-specific production of IL-10 correlate with Th2 dominance in certain parasitic diseases." *Exp Parasitol* 84(2): 168-177.

Parekh, V. V., D. V. Prasad, et al. (2003). "B cells activated by lipopolysaccharide, but not by anti-Ig and anti-CD40 antibody, induce anergy in CD8+ T cells: role of TGF-beta 1." *J Immunol* 170(12): 5897-5911.

Rafei, M., J. Hsieh, et al. (2009). "A granulocyte-macrophage colony-stimulating factor and interleukin-15 fusokine induces a regulatory B cell population with immune suppressive properties." *Nat Med* 15(9): 1038-1045.

Ramgolam, V. S., Y. Sha, et al. (2011). "B cells as a therapeutic target for IFN-beta in relapsing-remitting multiple sclerosis." *J Immunol* 186(7): 4518-4526.

Ren, X., K. Akiyoshi, et al. (2011). "Programmed Death-1 Pathway Limits Central Nervous System Inflammation and Neurologic Deficits in Murine Experimental Stroke." *Stroke.*

Ronet, C., Y. Hauyon-La Torre, et al. (2010). "Regulatory B cells shape the development of Th2 immune responses in BALB/c mice infected with Leishmania major through IL-10 production." *J Immunol* 184(2): 886-894.

Sabahi, R. and J. H. Anolik (2006). "B-cell-targeted therapy for systemic lupus erythematosus." *Drugs* 66(15): 1933-1948.

Saubermann, L. J., P. Beck, et al. (2000). "Activation of natural killer T cells by alpha-galactosylceramide in the presence of CD1d provides protection against colitis in mice." *Gastroenterology* 119(1): 119-128.

Sayi, A., E. Kohler, et al. (2011). "TLR-2-activated B cells suppress Helicobacter-induced preneoplastic gastric immunopathology by inducing T regulatory-1 cells." *J Immunol* 186(2): 878-890.

Silveira, P. A. and S. T. Grey (2006). "B cells in the spotlight: innocent bystanders or major players in the pathogenesis of type 1 diabetes." *Trends Endocrinol Metab* 17(4): 128-135.

Simons, F. E., Y. Shikishima, et al. (2004). "Selective immune redirection in humans with ragweed allergy by injecting Amb a 1 linked to immunostimulatory DNA." *J Allergy Clin Immunol* 113(6): 1144-1151.

Singh, A., W. F. t. Carson, et al. (2008). "Regulatory role of B cells in a murine model of allergic airway disease." *J Immunol* 180(11): 7318-7326.

Smits, H. H., H. Hammad, et al. (2007). "Protective effect of Schistosoma mansoni infection on allergic airway inflammation depends on the intensity and chronicity of infection." *J Allergy Clin Immunol* 120(4): 932-940.

Snir, A., A. Kessel, et al. (2011). "Anti-IL-6 receptor antibody (tocilizumab): a B cell targeting therapy." *Clin Exp Rheumatol.*

Sonoda, K. H. and J. Stein-Streilein (2002). "CD1d on antigen-transporting APC and splenic marginal zone B cells promotes NKT cell-dependent tolerance." *Eur J Immunol* 32(3): 848-857.

Su, T. T., B. Guo, et al. (2004). "Signaling in transitional type 2 B cells is critical for peripheral B-cell development." *Immunol Rev* 197: 161-178.

Sugimoto, K., A. Ogawa, et al. (2007). "Inducible IL-12-producing B cells regulate Th2-mediated intestinal inflammation." *Gastroenterology* 133(1): 124-136.

Takenoshita, S., T. Fukushima, et al. (2002). "The role of TGF-beta in digestive organ disease." *J Gastroenterol* 37(12): 991-999.

Tian, J., D. Zekzer, et al. (2001). "Lipopolysaccharide-activated B cells down-regulate Th1 immunity and prevent autoimmune diabetes in nonobese diabetic mice." *J Immunol* 167(2): 1081-1089.

Trentham, D. E., A. S. Townes, et al. (1977). "Autoimmunity to type II collagen an experimental model of arthritis." *J Exp Med* 146(3): 857-868.

Tulic, M. K., P. O. Fiset, et al. (2004). "Role of toll-like receptor 4 in protection by bacterial lipopolysaccharide in the nasal mucosa of atopic children but not adults." *Lancet* 363(9422): 1689-1697.

van den Biggelaar, A. H., L. C. Rodrigues, et al. (2004). "Long-term treatment of intestinal helminths increases mite skin-test reactivity in Gabonese schoolchildren." *J Infect Dis* 189(5): 892-900.

van der Kleij, D., E. Latz, et al. (2002). "A novel host-parasite lipid cross-talk. Schistosomal lyso-phosphatidylserine activates toll-like receptor 2 and affects immune polarization." *J Biol Chem* 277(50): 48122-48129.

van der Vlugt, L. E. P. M. and L. A. Labuda (2012). "Schistosomes induce regulatory features in human and mouse CD1dhi B cells: inhibition of allergic inflammation by IL-10 and regulatory T cells." PloS One. *Accepted.*

Velupillai, P. and D. A. Harn (1994). "Oligosaccharide-specific induction of interleukin 10 production by B220+ cells from schistosome-infected mice: a mechanism for regulation of CD4+ T-cell subsets." *Proc Natl Acad Sci U S A* 91(1): 18-22.

Vitale, G., F. Mion, et al. (2010). "Regulatory B cells: evidence, developmental origin and population diversity." *Mol Immunol* 48(1-3): 1-8.

von Mutius, E. (2009). "Gene-environment interactions in asthma." *J Allergy Clin Immunol* 123(1): 3-11; quiz 12-13.

von Mutius, E., C. Braun-Fahrlander, et al. (2000). "Exposure to endotoxin or other bacterial components might protect against the development of atopy." *Clin Exp Allergy* 30(9): 1230-1234.

Watanabe, R., N. Ishiura, et al. (2010). "Regulatory B cells (B10 cells) have a suppressive role in murine lupus: CD19 and B10 cell deficiency exacerbates systemic autoimmunity." *J Immunol* 184(9): 4801-4809.

Weber, M. S., T. Prod'homme, et al. (2010). "B-cell activation influences T-cell polarization and outcome of anti-CD20 B-cell depletion in central nervous system autoimmunity." *Ann Neurol* 68(3): 369-383.

Wei, B., P. Velazquez, et al. (2005). "Mesenteric B cells centrally inhibit CD4+ T cell colitis through interaction with regulatory T cell subsets." *Proc Natl Acad Sci U S A* 102(6): 2010-2015.

Wills-Karp, M., J. Santeliz, et al. (2001). "The germless theory of allergic disease: revisiting the hygiene hypothesis." *Nat Rev Immunol* 1(1): 69-75.

Wilson, M. S., M. D. Taylor, et al. (2010). "Helminth-induced CD19+CD23hi B cells modulate experimental allergic and autoimmune inflammation." *Eur J Immunol* 40(6): 1682-1696.

Wohlfert, E. and Y. Belkaid (2008). "Role of endogenous and induced regulatory T cells during infections." *J Clin Immunol* 28(6): 707-715.

Wolf, S. D., B. N. Dittel, et al. (1996). "Experimental autoimmune encephalomyelitis induction in genetically B cell-deficient mice." *J Exp Med* 184(6): 2271-2278.

Wong, S. C., A. L. Puaux, et al. (2010). "Macrophage polarization to a unique phenotype driven by B cells." *Eur J Immunol* 40(8): 2296-2307.

Wykes, M., J. Poudrier, et al. (1998). "Regulation of cytoplasmic, surface and soluble forms of CD40 ligand in mouse B cells." *Eur J Immunol* 28(2): 548-559.

Xiu, Y., C. P. Wong, et al. (2008). "B lymphocyte depletion by CD20 monoclonal antibody prevents diabetes in nonobese diabetic mice despite isotype-specific differences in Fc gamma R effector functions." *J Immunol* 180(5): 2863-2875.

Yanaba, K., J. D. Bouaziz, et al. (2008). "A regulatory B cell subset with a unique CD1dhiCD5+ phenotype controls T cell-dependent inflammatory responses." *Immunity* 28(5): 639-650.

Yang, C. H., L. Tian, et al. (2008). "Immunological mechanisms and clinical implications of regulatory T cell deficiency in a systemic autoimmune disorder: roles of IL-2 versus IL-15." *Eur J Immunol* 38(6): 1664-1676.

Yang, M., L. Sun, et al. (2010). "Novel function of B cell-activating factor in the induction of IL-10-producing regulatory B cells." *J Immunol* 184(7): 3321-3325.

Yazdanbakhsh, M., P. G. Kremsner, et al. (2002). "Allergy, parasites, and the hygiene hypothesis." *Science* 296(5567): 490-494.

Yen, D., J. Cheung, et al. (2006). "IL-23 is essential for T cell-mediated colitis and promotes inflammation via IL-17 and IL-6." *J Clin Invest* 116(5): 1310-1316.

Zaccone, P., Z. Fehervari, et al. (2003). "Schistosoma mansoni antigens modulate the activity of the innate immune response and prevent onset of type 1 diabetes." *Eur J Immunol* 33(5): 1439-1449.

11

Regulation of Oligodendrocyte Differentiation: Relevance for Remyelination

Olaf Maier

Institute of Cell Biology and Immunology, University of Stuttgart
Germany

1. Introduction

A major distinguishing feature of the vertebrate nervous system is the formation of myelin sheaths. The myelin sheath has two main functions. First, it electrically insulates the axon thereby enabling saltatory conduction and highly increasing conduction velocity. This also strongly reduces energy consumption since restoration of ion gradients occurs only at the nodes of Ranvier (i.e. at less than 1 % of the axonal surface). Second, the myelin sheath is important for trophic support and protection of the axon (Nave, 2010).

Oligodendrocytes (OLG) are the myelinating cells of the central nervous system (CNS). In contrast to Schwann cells, the myelinating cells of the peripheral nervous system (PNS), OLG form multiple extensions. Each of these extensions forms a myelin sheath after contacting an axon. Due to the synthesis and maintenance of multiple myelin sheaths OLG are highly metabolic active and thus produce large amounts of reactive oxygen species. Moreover, they contain a large amount of iron, which can cause free radical formation. Accordingly, OLG are highly vulnerable to lipid peroxidation and DNA damage due to oxidative stress. It is therefore not surprising that OLG cell death as well as myelin degradation (demyelination) are features of many acute and chronic diseases of the CNS, e.g. trauma, ischemia, spinal cord injury, Alzheimer's Disease and even schizophrenia (McTigue & Tripathi, 2008; Bradl & Lassmann, 2010). Ultimately demyelination results in axonal degeneration and decline of neuronal functions.

Demyelination or dysmyelination (impaired myelin synthesis) are the defining feature of CNS white matter diseases (leukodystrophies). Primary and secondary leukodystrophies can be distinguished. Whereas in primary leukodystrophies, myelin and OLG are directly affected, in secondary leukodystrophies the function of other cells, e.g. astrocytes, is perturbed resulting indirectly in OLG cell death and demyelination. Examples for primary leukodystrophies are Pelizaeus-Merzbacher disease (PMD) and spastic paraplegia type 2 (SPG2), which are characterized by dysmyelination in the CNS (Inoue, 2005), as well as globoid cell leukodystrophy (Krabbe's disease) and metachromatic leukodystrophy. These diseases are caused by impaired degradation of the major myelin lipids galactosylceramide (GalCer) and sulfatide, respectively, and are characterized by progressive demyelination and mental retardation (Wenger et al., 2000; Gieselmann, 2003). The best example for an inherited secondary leukodystrophy is Alexander disease, which is caused by mutation of the astrocytic intermediate filament protein GFAP (Johnson, 2004).

The most common demyelinating diseases are multiple sclerosis (MS) and neuromyelitis optica (NMO), which are both characterized by an autoimmune attack of the immune system on the CNS. Whereas it is generally accepted that, in MS, OLG are the primary target of the immune attack, it has been recently discovered that aquaporin 4, localized in astrocytes, is the primary target in NMO (Roemer et al., 2007; Parratt & Prineas, 2010). The resulting dysfunction and death of astrocytes then causes demyelination and OLG death.

After demyelination the function of the affected area is restored by remyelination, the intrinsic repair mechanism after demyelination. Remyelination of demyelinated axons in the CNS occurs when OLG progenitor cells (OPC) proliferate, migrate to the site of damage, locally differentiate into mature OLG and finally produce new myelin sheaths that are wrapped around the naked axon (C. Zhao et al., 2005). Therefore remyelination largely resembles the developmental myelination process and accordingly knowledge of all steps relevant for developmental OLG differentiation and myelination is essential for potential therapies based on tissue regeneration (Franklin & ffrench-Constant, 2008).

Here I will review main aspects of myelin formation in the CNS starting with the synthesis and transport of myelin components and the morphological differentiation of OLG, which culminates in the formation of multiple myelin sheaths. I will then discuss intrinsic and extrinsic factors that regulate OLG differentiation. Finally, I will address specific aspects of remyelination and will draw attention to differences between developmental myelination and remyelination, e.g. due to changes in the CNS microenvironment.

2. Differentiation of oligodendrocytes

Most aspects of OLG biology have been studied in rodents and in rodent-derived cells. These studies have revealed that the differentiation of OLG is a highly regulated process, in which several stages can be distinguished. During embryonal development neural stem cells in the ventral ventricular zone of the CNS (and later also in more dorsal areas) develop into OPC. These cells are characterized by the expression of the ganglioside A2B5, the chondroitin sulfate proteoglycan NG2 and the platelet-derived growth factor receptor α (PDGFRα; Nishiyama et al., 1999). OPC proliferate and migrate throughout the CNS to their final destination. Around birth the OPC start to differentiate and extend multiple processes. Those branches that do not find an axon retract and OPC that cannot make axonal contact undergo apoptotic cell death. When a process makes contact with an axon, the cell synthesizes myelin components and vast amounts of membrane, which is wrapped several times around the axon. After extrusion of the cytoplasm the formation of the compact myelin sheath is completed (Baumann & Pham-Dinh, 2001; Bradl & Lassmann, 2009). These stages are characterized by the sequential expression of cellular marker molecules. Concomitantly, OPC-specific marker molecules are lost (see Fig. 1).

2.1 Myelin structure and composition

The myelin sheath is not homogeneous. The compact myelin, which is important for the electrical insulation of the axon, can be distinguished from several regions of non-compact myelin (Sherman & Brophy, 2005). These include the adaxonal and abaxonal plasma membranes, which face the axon and the extracellular matrix (ECM), respectively, the radial component, important for energy and metabolite transport within the myelin sheath, and the paranodal loops. These are the main contact sites between myelin and axon and are especially relevant for the functionality as well as structural integrity of the nodes of Ranvier (Tait et al. 2000).

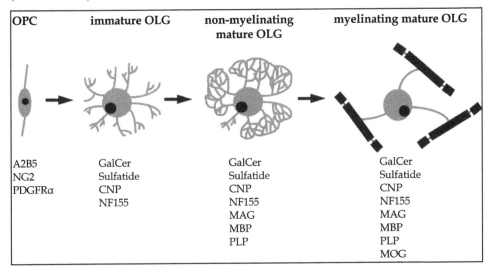

OPC	immature OLG	non-myelinating mature OLG	myelinating mature OLG
A2B5	GalCer	GalCer	GalCer
NG2	Sulfatide	Sulfatide	Sulfatide
PDGFRα	CNP	CNP	CNP
	NF155	NF155	NF155
		MAG	MAG
		MBP	MBP
		PLP	PLP
			MOG

Fig. 1. Schematic representation of OLG developmental stages. Indicated are stages of OLG differentiation ultimately resulting in myelin sheath formation (black) as well as proteins and lipids specific for these developmental stages (adapted from Maier et al., 2005).

To fulfil its function of electrical insulation, the myelin sheath is highly enriched in lipids, which comprise approx. 70 % of its dry weight. The most abundant myelin lipids are cholesterol and the glycosphingolipids GalCer and its sulfated form sulfatide. Cholesterol is essential for myelin formation (Saher et al. 2005) while GalCer and sulfatide are important for the correct formation of the paranodal loops (Dupree et al., 1998; Marcus et al. 2006). The major myelin proteins are proteolipid protein (PLP), its derivative DM20 and myelin basic protein (MBP), which comprise together approx. 80 % of the total myelin proteins (Brunner et al. 1989: Griffiths et al., 1998). PLP/DM20 and MBP are localized in the compact internodal myelin and are required for the compaction of the myelin sheath. Important non-compact myelin proteins are, e.g., 2'3'-cyclic nucleotide 3'-phosphodiesterase (CNP), localized throughout the non-compact myelin, myelin-associated glycoprotein (MAG) in the adaxonal membrane, myelin/oligodendrocyte glycoprotein (MOG) in the abaxonal membrane and the 155 kDa isoform of neurofascin (NF155) in the paranodal loops (Brunner et al., 1989; Schachner & Bartsch, 2000; Tait et al., 2000). For a comprehensive description of myelin composition see, e.g., Baumann & Pham-Dinh, 2001; Aggarwal et al., 2011.

2.2 Synthesis and transport of myelin components

Each OLG myelinates all contacted axons simultaneously and completes the initial wrapping of axons within 12 to 18 hours (Watkins et al., 2008). To achieve this task OLG have to synthesize tremendous amounts of myelin in a very short time (Pfeiffer et al., 1993).

Accordingly, synthesis and transport of myelin components must be highly coordinated in time and space. Moreover, since the composition of the myelin membrane and the membrane of the OLG soma differ significantly, myelin components must be sorted prior to their transport to the myelin sheath. Three main steps required for this polarized transport can be distinguished: i) the sorting of proteins and lipids destined for the different plasma membrane domains, ii) the directed transport towards the different plasma membrane domains along the cytoskeleton and finally iii) the specific targeting to and incorporation into the correct membrane domain. Since these aspects are relevant for the understanding of OLG differentiation, here I will discuss briefly some features of the synthesis and transport of myelin proteins and consequences of incorrect protein synthesis and/or transport, focussing on the major proteins PLP and MBP. Due to space limitations I will not address the directed transport and targeting to the myelin sheath (see, e.g., Krämer et al., 2001, Anitei & Pfeiffer, 2006; Maier et al., 2008)

The exact routes by which transmembrane proteins are transported to the myelin sheath are not well understood and distinct transport pathways towards the myelin sheath have been discussed (Krämer et al., 2001; Anitei & Pfeiffer, 2006; Maier et al., 2008). In general, transmembrane proteins, such as PLP, are synthesized at the endoplasmic reticulum and transported via the Golgi apparatus to the plasma membrane. For PLP there is good evidence that the newly synthesized protein is first transported to the plasma membrane of the cell soma. From there it is internalized and stored in late endosomes before it is finally transported by a transcytotic pathway to the myelin sheath (Trajkovic et al., 2006; Feldmann et al., 2011). Surprisingly, although PLP deletion results in neuronal degeneration, it has only minor effects on myelin formation (Garbern et al. 2002). In contrast, overexpression of PLP causes its accumulation in late endosomes and/or lysosomes together with cholesterol and results in missorting of several membrane markers indicating that major trafficking pathways are affected thereby ultimately interfering with myelination and OLG viability (Simons et al., 2002). Indeed, most cases of PMD are caused by PLP gene duplication resulting in a massive overexpression of PLP demonstrating the relevance of these findings for human disease. In addition, missense mutations in PLP can result in PMD or SPG2 due to the accumulation of PLP in the ER resulting in an unfolded protein response and finally in OLG cell death (Krämer-Albers et al., 2006).

MBP is a multi-functional protein and several isoforms of MBP have been described (Boggs, 2006). In contrast to PLP, MBP is a cytoplasmic protein and is therefore synthesized at free ribosomes in the cytoplasm. Myelin-specific MBP isoforms mediate myelin compaction by interconnecting the cytoplasmic leaflets of the myelin membrane. Accordingly, MBP must have strong adhesive properties. To preclude these adhesive properties taking effect in the cell soma, the MBP messenger RNA (mRNA) is transported into the OLG processes where the protein is synthesized and directly associates with the myelin membrane. To prevent premature MBP protein synthesis the MBP mRNA is incorporated into granules which are transported along microtubules into the OLG branches (Barbarese et al., 1995). This incorporation is mediated by the mRNA binding factor hnRNP A2, which is highly expressed during OLG differentiation (Maggipinto et al., 2004). The importance of correct MBP expression for myelination is demonstrated by the finding that MBP absence causes dysmyelination. This is exemplified by the severe reduction of compact myelin in the so called shiverer mouse due to partial MBP deletion (Roach at al., 1985).

2.3 Morphological differentiation: role of the cytoskeleton

An intact cytoskeleton is essential for all aspects of OLG biology. Both actin filaments and microtubules are essential for the coordinated transport of myelin components to the myelin sheath and the actin cytoskeleton is important for OPC migration. Of particular interest is the role of the cytoskeleton during the morphological differentiation of the OLG.

Each of the multiple branches of the OLG forms a myelin sheath upon axonal contact. One OLG can thus myelinate up to 40 different axons (Pfeiffer et al., 1993). Outgrowth of cellular processes is therefore a fundamental property of OLG and both microtubules and actin filaments are essential to coordinate the morphological changes accompanied with OLG differentiation (Richter-Landsberg, 2008; Bauer et al., 2009). In general, microtubules are especially important for process outgrowth and stabilization whereas actin filaments are more important for the formation of the lamellipodium that initiates the formation of the myelin sheath.

Both depolymerization and stabilization of microtubules perturb the formation of myelin-like membrane sheets *in vitro* indicating that microtubule turnover is required for correct myelination (Benjamins & Nedelkoska, 1994). Nevertheless, a stable microtubular cytoskeleton is required to promote outgrowth and maintenance of cellular processes during OLG differentiation. Indeed, acetylated tubulin, indicative for stable microtubules is present in OLG branches. Moreover, microtubules can be stabilized by associated proteins such as MAP2c and tau (Richter-Landsberg & Gorath, 1999). Tau, in particular, has been implicated in stabilization of microtubules in OLG branches. Whereas OPC express tau isoforms with three microtubule binding domains, differentiating OLG predominantly express tau isoforms containing four microtubule binding domains, which may promote microtubule stability. Moreover, phosphorylation of tau is decreased during OLG differentiation, thereby promoting interaction of tau with microtubules and microtubule stabilization (Richter-Landsberg, 2008). In addition to stabilizing proteins, microtubules are modulated by proteins that promote their disassembly. One prominent protein that mediates microtubule disassembly is stathmin. Accordingly, stathmin expression is downregulated during OLG differentiation (Liu et al., 2003).

Similar to microtubules actin filaments are important for outgrowth and stabilization of OLG extensions. The actin cytoskeleton has been especially implicated in the formation of the lamellipodium, which initiates the enwrapment of the axon. Important regulators of actin cytoskeleton dynamics are proteins of the Rho family of GTPases (Ridley, 2006). Indeed, several members of this family, namely RhoA, Rac and Cdc42 have been implicated in OLG process outgrowth and myelination (Liang et al., 2004, Thurnherr et al., 2007, Rajasekharan et al., 2009). Activation of both Rac and Cdc42 promotes myelination, whereas activation of RhoA inhibits OLG differentiation. An important downstream effector of Rho GTPases that has been implicated in OLG process outgrowth and myelination is the neuronal Wiskott Aldrich Syndrome Protein (nWASP) (Bacon et al. 2007). Activation of nWASP, e.g. by Cdc42, can activate the Arp2/3 complex, which acts as a nucleating factor for actin filament polymerization thereby promoting the formation of the actin network required for lamellipodium formation (Ridley, 2006).

Not surprisingly, several myelin components are interacting with the cytoskeleton thereby facilitating the coordination of the myelination process. Of particular relevance are the cytoplasmic myelin proteins CNP and MBP (Dyer & Benjamins, 1989). CNP can interact with both actin filaments and microtubules and acts as a microtubule assembly protein (De Angelis et al., 1996; Lee et al., 2005). Consequently, CNP is essential for OLG arborization and membrane expansion during myelination. Although cytoplasmic, CNP is anchored to the plasma membrane by isoprenylation and inhibition of CNP isoprenylation perturbs arborization and OLG differentiation (Lee et al., 2005; Smolders et al., 2010). Similar to CNP, MBP can interact with both actin filaments and microtubules and is important for cytoskeleton integrity in OLG. Dephosphorylated MBP, which is predominantly localized in myelin, stabilizes microtubules and enhances microtubule polymerization (Galiano et al., 2006). Moreover, dephosphorylated MBP can act as membrane anchoring protein for actin filaments (Boggs, 2006).

3. Regulation of oligodendrocyte differentiation

OLG differentiation is a highly regulated multistep process. Here I will discuss intrinsic and extrinsic factors that regulate OLG differentiation and myelination. Although the understanding of the interplay between the intrinsic and extrinsic factors that orchestrate OLG myelination is far from complete, I will also address how these factors can initiate and modulate signaling pathways implicated in OLG differentiation.

3.1 Intrinsic factors

In culture, OPC synthesize myelin components and form myelin-like membrane sheets in absence of CNS-derived factors suggesting that differentiation into mature OLG is an intrinsic property of these cells. Differentiation is predominantly regulated on the level of gene transcription and protein translation and much progress has been made in the characterization of these intrinsic factors for OLG differentiation. However, it is still far from understood how the function of these intrinsic factors is coordinated to mediate OLG differentiation.

On the level of gene transcription promoting and repressing transcription factors of OLG differentiation have been identified. Transcription factors that promote differentiation of OPC into mature OLG are, e.g., Olig1, Olig2 and Nkx2.2 and Sox10 (Liu & Casaccia, 2010; Miron et al., 2011). Especially relevant for the initiation of OLG differentiation is the concomitant expression of Olig2 and Nkx2.2 (Zhou et al., 2001). Most transcription factors that promote differentiation are, however, expressed in all stages of OLG development indicating that their presence is not sufficient to induce OLG differentiation. Indeed, several transcription factors that are expressed in OPC, such as Hes5, Id2, Id4, Sox5 and Sox6, strongly inhibit OLG differentiation (Liu & Casaccia, 2010; Miron et al., 2011). Blocking the expression of these inhibitory factors is essential to promote OLG differentiation and there is increasing evidence that this is achieved by epigenetic mechanisms.

In principle, epigenetic inhibition of gene expression can be achieved by two major mechanisms: i) repression of transcription by DNA or histone modification and ii) inhibition of protein translation by microRNAs (miRNAs). Both mechanisms are operational during OLG differentiation. The predominant modification of histones relevant for OLG differentiation is deacetylation, which inhibits gene transcription. Indeed, activity of histone deacetylases is essential for OPC generation and their development into mature OLG. Histone deacetylases can, e.g., bind to the promoter region of OLG differentiation repressors such as Hes5 and Id4 thereby preventing their expression and thus promoting OLG differentiation (Liu & Cassacia, 2010; Copray et al., 2011). In addition, expression of other proteins can be regulated by histone deacetylation. Thus, the expression of stathmin is repressed by this mechanism during OLG differentiation (Liu et al., 2003) thereby promoting microtubule polymerization and stabilization of the outgrowing OLG branches.

MiRNAs are small non-coding RNAs of approximately 23 nucleotides that are processed from larger precursor RNAs by the RNaseIII enzymes Dicer and Drosha. By binding to the 3′ untranslated region of mRNAs one miRNA can inhibit the translation of multiple mRNAs (Bartel, 2004). Expression of Dicer increases during OLG differentiation and conditional knockout of Dicer in OLG results in dys- or demyelination depending on the stage of Dicer repression (Dugas et al., 2010; X. Zhao et al., 2010). In these studies miR219 and miR338 have been identified as important regulators of OLG differentiation. Both miR219 and miR338 can directly suppress the inhibiting transcription factors Sox6 and Hes5 thereby promoting OLG differentiation (Dugas et al., 2010; X. Zhao et al., 2010). An additional target of miR219 is the PDGFRα, (Dugas et al., 2010), which, although important for OPC proliferation and migration, inhibits OLG differentiation (see next section).

3.2 Extrinsic factors

Although *in vitro* OLG can form myelin-like membranes in the absence of axons, there is ample evidence that *in vivo* myelination is coordinated by the presence of axons. However, in contrast to the PNS, where axonal expression of neuregulin-1 type III determines the myelination by Schwann cells (Taveggia et al., 2005), no master regulator for myelination in the CNS has been identified. It is more likely that several factors act together to initiate and promote myelination in the CNS. In general, signals modulating OLG differentiation can be divided into two classes: long-range signals such as growth factors and short-range signals such as ECM and cell adhesion molecules (see Table 1 for important factors regulating OLG behavior). Since the differentiation into a myelinating phenotype is an intrinsic property of OLG while myelination of the axon has to be tightly controlled, it is perhaps not surprising that many axonal factors inhibit OLG differentiation. Here I will address some of the exogenous factors that modulate myelination and subsequently discuss how these signals may be integrated to result in the induction and modulation of myelin formation.

3.2.1 Modulation of oligodendrocyte differentiation by neurons

During embryonic development neurons prevent premature differentiation of OPC. For this purpose they express inhibitory proteins at the axonal surface, e.g. the polysialylated form of the neural cell adhesion molecule (PSA-NCAM), which is a general inhibitor of cell adhesion (Charles et al., 2000). In addition, neurons express molecules that can directly inhibit OLG differentiation. Examples are Jagged and the Leucine-rich repeats and Ig domain-containing, neurite outgrowth inhibitor (Nogo) receptor-interacting protein-1 (LINGO-1). Jagged is the axonal ligand of the Notch receptor in the OLG membrane and activation of the Notch signaling pathway interferes with OLG development (S. Wang et al., 1998). LINGO-1 is part of the Nogo-66 receptor complex in the axonal membrane and interaction of this receptor complex with OLG proteins such as Nogo-A and MAG can inhibit axonal growth. Conversely, inactivation of LINGO-1 promotes myelination suggesting that LINGO-1 is a key inhibitor of OLG differentiation (Mi et al., 2005). Since LINGO-1 is also expressed by OLG, homophilic LINGO-1 interactions may also interfere with OLG development.

An important factor for the induction of OLG differentiation is the electrical activity of neurons (Demerens et al., 1996) most likely by the release of adenosine which may activate purinergic receptors at the OLG surface (Stevens et al., 2002). Very recently it has been shown that also the neurotransmitter glutamate, released at the synapse upon action potentials, can promote OLG differentiation (Wake et al., 2011).

It is likely that *in vivo* the direct contact of an OLG extension with the axon is important to initiate OLG myelination. The best candidate for an axonal molecule required to induce myelination is the ECM molecule laminin-2, since laminin-2 deficiency causes myelination defects in mice and humans (Chun et al., 2003; Colognato et al., 2005). In addition, neuregulin-1 promotes OLG differentiation (Z. Wang et al., 2007). Other molecules that may be involved in the interaction between OLG and axon and thus promote OLG maturation are gangliosides, which can bind to MAG at the OLG cell surface (Yang et al., 1996).

3.2.2 Modulation of oligodendrocyte differentiation by astrocytes

The intimate relationship of OLG with astrocytes is demonstrated by the formation of gap junctions between these cell types (Orthmann-Murphy et al., 2008). In addition to the direct exchange of molecules via these cell-cell interaction sites, astrocytes modulate OLG function by the release of growth factors and by the deposition of ECM molecules.

Astrocytes are the primary source of growth factors in the CNS (Moore et al., 2011). Among these are, e.g., PDGF-AA and fibroblast growth factor-2 (FGF-2), which mediate proliferation and migration of OPC (Milner et al., 1997; Baron et al., 2000). PDGF-AA is also important for OLG survival in presence of laminin-2 (Baron et al., 2003). However, both PDGF-AA and FGF-2 inhibit OLG differentiation at least *in vitro* (Noble et al., 1988; Bansal & Pfeiffer, 1994). Moreover, astrocytes inhibit OLG maturation during CNS development by secretion of bone morphogenetic proteins (BMP), which are strong suppressors of OLG differentiation (See et al., 2004). Besides these inhibitory factors, however, several factors secreted by astrocytes promote OLG differentiation and myelination. Prominent examples are insulin-like growth factor-1 (IGF-1), leukemia inhibitory factor (LIF) and ciliary neurotrophic factor (CNTF) (McMorris et al., 1986; Stankoff et al., 2002). Interestingly, electrical activity of axons causes the release of LIF from astrocytes (Ishibashi et al., 2005), providing a link between neuronal and astrocytic modulation of myelination. Moreover, astrocytes affect OLG function by synthesizing ECM-molecules, such as fibronectin and tenascin C (Price & Hines, 1985; Götz et al., 1997). Fibronectin promotes proliferation and migration of OPC (Milner et al., 1996; Baron et al., 2002), which is important during embryonal development. However, fibronectin impairs morphological differentiation of OLG *in vitro* (Buttery & ffrench-Constant, 1999; Maier et al., 2005). Similarly, tenascin C inhibits process outgrowth and myelin membrane formation of OLG (Czopka et al., 2009).

Factor	Predominant source	Effect on OLG
Soluble Factors		
Adenosine	neurons	promotes differentiation
Glutamate	neurons	promotes differentiation
PDGF-AA	astrocytes	promotes migration and proliferation; inhibits differentiation
FGF-2	astrocytes	promotes migration and proliferation; inhibits differentiation
IGF-1	astrocytes	promotes differentiation
CNTF	astrocytes	promotes differentiation
LIF	astrocytes	promotes differentiation
BMP	astrocytes	inhibits differentiation
Membrane proteins		
LINGO-1	neurons	inhibits differentiation
Jagged	neurons	inhibits differentiation
PSA-NCAM	neurons	inhibits interaction with axon
Neuregulin-1	neurons	promotes myelination
ECM molecules		
Laminin-2	neurons	promotes differentiation
Fibronectin	astrocytes	promotes migration and proliferation; inhibits differentiation
Tenascin C	astrocytes	inhibits migration and differentiation
Other factors		
Electrical activity	neurons	promotes differentiation

Table 1. Neuronal and astrocytic factors that regulate OLG behaviour and differentiation

3.2.3 Modulation of oligodendrocyte signaling pathways by extrinsic factors

It is obviously essential that the signals supplied by these extrinsic factors are integrated at the OLG cell surface, followed by signal transduction into the cell and modulation of signaling pathways resulting in OLG differentiation. Here I will focus on two main aspects that are important to coordinate signaling pathways in the developing OLG. First, the interaction of ECM molecules, in particular laminin-2 and fibronectin, with receptors on the OLG cell surface and the modulation of these interactions by growth factors. Second, the multiple roles of the Src-family non-receptor tyrosine kinase Fyn in OLG maturation.

ECM molecules such as laminin-2 and fibronectin interact predominantly with integrin receptors in the plasma membrane. Integrins are heterodimeric proteins consisting of one α- and one β-subunit. OLG express a limited number of integrins, namely αvβ1-, αvβ3-and αvβ5-integrins, which bind to ECM-molecules containing an RGD-motif such as fibronectin and vitronectin, and α6β1-integrin, which can bind to laminin-2. Proliferation and migration of OPC, stimulated by PDGF, are mediated by activation of αvβ1 and αvβ3-integrins, implicating RGD-containing ECM-molecules in these processes (Milner et al., 1996; Baron et al., 2002). The importance of α6β1 integrin for myelination was indicated by applying antagonists of the β1-subunit, which inhibit myelination *in vitro* and *in vivo* (Buttery and ffrench-Constant, 1999; Relvas et al., 2001). However, the OLG-specific knockout of the β1-subunit does not cause demyelination (Benninger et al., 2006) indicating that another laminin-2 receptor is present in the OLG membrane. Indeed, dystroglycan has been identified as a receptor for laminin-2, which is required for myelination (Colognato et al., 2007). The β1-subunit in OLG is, however, important for cell survival *in vivo* (Benninger et al., 2006). Interestingly, in presence of laminin-2 the PDGFRα dissociates from αv-containing integrins and instead interacts with α6β1-integrin causing a change in signaling from cell proliferation to cell survival (Baron et al., 2003). Similarly, laminin-2 causes the interaction of the neuregulin receptor erbB2 with α6β1-integrin. This causes a switch in neuregulin signaling from cell proliferation towards cell survival and differentiation (Colognato et al., 2004). These examples show how integrins coordinate short range (ECM-mediated) and long range (growth factors, cytokines) signals, which are both required to regulate cell behaviour.

Although it is still far from understood how the signals received at the plasma membrane are further processed to promote OLG differentiation, several signaling pathways have been identified. For example, binding of laminin-2 to α6β1-integrin promotes OLG differentiation and myelination by the activation of integrin-linked kinase (Chun et al., 2003). Moreover, activated α6β1 integrin binds to the Src family kinase Fyn and this interaction is important for the modulation of the PDGF and neuregulin signaling pathways described above and thus for OLG survival and differentiation (Colognato et al., 2004). Indeed, Fyn has been identified as a key regulator of OLG differentiation. The relevance of Fyn for myelination is exemplified by the finding that the OLG-specific knockout of Fyn results in hypomyelination *in vivo* (Biffiger et al., 2000). Fyn has been implicated in various aspects of OLG biology ranging from migration to myelination. Importantly, Fyn kinase activity is activated by interaction with cell adhesion molecules such as NCAM120 and contactin in the OLG membrane which may interact with axonal proteins thereby initiating myelination (Krämer et al, 1999). Moreover, Fyn can act as a bridge between integrins or other membrane receptors and the cytoskeleton and, depending on the developmental stage of the OLG and the corresponding expression of potential interaction partners, Fyn may bind to different proteins thereby explaining its diverse roles in OLG differentiation. In OPC, binding of PDGF to its receptor PDGFRα results in recruitment of Fyn and modulation of the actin cytoskeleton thereby increasing OPC migration (Miyamoto et al., 2008). Later in OLG development, integrin signaling via Fyn promotes morphological differentiation by activating Rac and Cdc42 and inactivating RhoA, again implicating modulation of the actin cytoskeleton in this process (Liang et al., 2004). Interestingly, LINGO-1 suppresses OLG differentiation and myelination by inactivation of Fyn kinase thereby activating RhoA signaling pathways (Mi et al., 2005). Besides modulating the actin cytoskeleton, Fyn can also affect the microtubular network via binding to tau thereby stabilizing microtubules and thus promoting process outgrowth and OLG differentiation (Klein et al., 2002).

4. Remyelination

Remyelination as the natural regenerative mechanism after a demyelinating insult is the basis of the functional recovery of the affected neurons (Bruce et al., 2010). Since mature OLG are incapable to myelinate nude axons (Crang et al., 1998; Watkins et al., 2008), remyelination requires the de novo differentiation of OPC. Importantly, OPC, characterized by the expression of NG2 and PDGFRα, are present throughout the adult CNS (Polito and Reynolds, 2006) and remyelination is usually very effective after transient demyelination. However, the new myelin sheaths are frequently shorter and thinner than the original sheaths thus giving rise to so-called shadow plaques (Franklin and ffrench-Constant, 2008). Moreover, in chronic diseases, such as MS, remyelination is often incomplete and ultimately fails in most patients resulting in increased neurodegeneration and progressive disease. A main goal for the treatment of chronic demyelinating diseases is therefore to increase the remyelination of the affected axons and thus at least partially restore axonal function.

Two main strategies are followed to improve remyelination: promotion of the endogenous remyelinating capacity and transplantation of exogenous stem cells or progenitor cells. Cell transplantation studies are predominantly performed in animals suffering from dysmyelination, such as the shiverer mouse, or by chemically induced demyelination to ensure that the observed myelination is due to the transplanted cells. In such studies it has been shown that several cell types are able to (re)myelinate CNS axons, such as neural stem cells, Schwann cell precursor cells, olfactory ensheathing cells and OPC (J. Yang et al., 2009). Of these, fetal OPC, possibly derived from induced stem cells, are probably suited best for CNS remyelination (Franklin, 2002; Tepavcevic & Blakemore, 2005). One problem in studying the potential of exogenous OPC to differentiate and (re)myelinate axons after transplantation is that endogenous OPC inhibit the migration and survival of transplanted OPC (O'Leary and Blakemore, 1997). Accordingly, endogenous OPCs have to be eliminated, e.g. by X-ray treatment (Hinks et al., 2001), which may cause conditions that differ from those in most demyelinating diseases. Several other obstacles in cell transplantation are: i) finding a cell source that is abundant enough to repopulate the CNS without causing ethical problems, ii) the delivery of the cells to the CNS and iii) their migration through the CNS to the demyelinated areas.

Irrespective of these considerations, the most useful strategy depends predominantly on the disease one wants to treat. Thus in primary inherited leukodystrophies, such as PMD, the most useful therapy would be the transplantation of allogeneic OPC. In contrast, in MS endogenous OPC are present in and around chronic demyelinated lesions indicating that the environment that these OPC encounter is not permissive for differentiation (Wolswijk, 1998). It is therefore unlikely that transplanted cells will be able to sufficiently migrate and differentiate under these conditions. Irrespective of the cellular source it is therefore essential to modulate the environment resulting in conditions that are permissive for remyelination.

4.1 Inhibitors of remyelination in the diseased CNS

Although remyelination does occur in MS and can be very efficient in a subset of MS patients even after a long disease course (Patrikios et al., 2006; Patani et al., 2007), remyelination eventually fails in most patients. Two obvious potential reasons for remyelination failure are axonal loss or depletion of the endogenous OPC pool. Although such a scenario cannot be excluded in some cases, it is unlikely to be the predominant reason for remyelination failure since in most lesions axons are still preserved and OPC are present in or around the lesion site, often in close proximity of a demyelinated axon. This strongly suggests that inhibitory factors are present in the lesion area that impair OLG differentiation and remyelination. Indeed, in MS a block of OLG differentiation in chronic lesions has been observed (Kuhlmann et al., 2008). This impaired remyelination is characterized by the accumulation of OPC that remain in an undifferentiated stage resulting in a failure to generate myelinating OLG (Goldschmidt et al., 2009). In general, disease-dependent and disease-independent factors can be distinguished that may affect remyelination and in this section I will summarize several of these factors.

The demyelinated axons themselves may repress the interaction with OLG branches and thus their remyelination by the expression of inhibitory cell adhesion molecules. Nude axons in chronic MS-lesions re-express PSA-NCAM, which inhibits OLG differentiation during development (Charles et al., 2000, 2002). Similarly, there is good evidence that expression of LINGO-1 in the lesion area inhibits efficient remyelination (Mi et al., 2007). Moreover, OPC functions may be changed in demyelinating diseases. It has, e.g., been shown that stathmin levels are increased in MS patients, which may contribute to reduced OLG differentiation and remyelination failure in MS lesions (Liu et al., 2005).

Several changes in the environment surrounding the recruited OPC may contribute to the inhibition of cell differentiation. Most relevant in the context of demyelinating diseases is that myelin components strongly inhibit OLG differentiation and (re-)myelination, which is at least partially due to inactivation of Fyn kinase activity (Kotter et al., 2006; Baer et al, 2009). Accordingly, it is essential that the myelin debris that is present in the lesion due to the demyelination process is efficiently removed to allow OPC differentiation and thus remyelination to proceed. Clearance of myelin debris is mediated predominantly by activated microglia, the resident immune cells of the CNS, and macrophages that have entered the CNS parenchyma from the periphery (Neumann et al., 2009). However, it should be kept in mind that microglia can act as antigen presenting cells after ingestion of myelin debris and thus may activate myelin-specific T-cells that have entered the CNS. Moreover, reactive microglia can produce proinflammatory cytokines and reactive oxygen species. Therefore activated microglia may actually enhance the demyelination process (Lassmann & van Horssen, 2011).

In addition to activation of microglia, demyelination results in the activation of astrocytes. Depending on the signals that these astrocytes receive, their activation can be beneficial or detrimental for the remyelination process (Williams et al., 2007). Activated astrocytes secrete growth factors and ECM molecules, e.g. PDGF-AA, FGF-2 and fibonectin, which promote proliferation of OPC and their recruitment to the lesion area. Other factors secreted by astrocytes can promote differentiation of these OPC to mature OLG (see section 3.2.2). However, some of these astrocyte-derived factors can have opposing effects. The chemokine CXCL1, e.g., can stimulate OPC proliferation but also acts as a stop signal for OPC migration (Tsai et al., 2002; Filipovic & Zecevic, 2008). Since in MS, astrocytes surrounding chronic lesions can secrete CXCL1 they may therefore repress the recruitment of OPC to the lesion site (Omari et al., 2006). Moreover, the persistent presence of fibronectin and other ECM molecules, e.g. chondroitin sulfates and hyaluronic acid, can impair OLG differentiation and may, together with astrocyte proliferation, result in the formation of a glial scar thus impairing the remyelination process (Kotter et al., 2011; Miron et al., 2011). This is particularly the case in chronic demyelination when repair mechanisms have failed. In this respect, it has been speculated that the formation of a glial scar is the consequence rather than the cause of remyelination failure (Franklin & Kotter, 2008).

The major disease-independent factor that impedes remyelination is age. In general, regenerative mechanisms are less efficient in old animals compared to young animals and this has also been observed for remyelination. This age-related effect is predominantly due to impaired recruitment of the OPC to the lesion area and a delay in their subsequent differentiation to myelinating OLG (Sim et al., 2002). There may be several reasons for this effect. First, OPC themselves may be less efficient in migration and differentiation. Indeed, the response to growth factors differs in adult OPC compared neonatal OPC possibly delaying the recruitment of OPC into lesion areas (Lin et al., 2009; Cui et al., 2010). Furthermore, histone deacetylates are less active in OPC of adult animals. This can impair the repression of inhibitory transcription factors, which is required for OLG differentiation (Shen et al., 2008) and thus result in a delay of OLG differentiation. It should, however, be mentioned that adult OPC are highly efficient in myelination of nude axons when transplanted into the CNS of shiverer mice indicating that the intrinsic myelinating capacity of adult OPC is not reduced compared to neonatal OPC provided they are in an environment that is permissive for myelination (Windrem et al., 2004). It is therefore more likely that age-related changes in the CNS environment result in a delay of OLG differentiation. One likely cause for impaired OLG differentiation in demyelinating diseases is that adult microglia and macrophages are less efficiently recruited to the lesion area resulting in a delayed clearing of myelin debris (Neumann et al., 2009). Accordingly, the prolonged presence of myelin in the lesion prevents OLG differentiation and may even close the therapeutic window in which remyelination can proceed (Kotter et al., 2011).

4.2 Initiation and promotion of remyelination

Although present throughout the CNS, adult OPC do not differentiate spontaneously into myelinating OLG implying that they are in a quiescent stage. Accordingly, OPC have to be activated by extrinsic factors, which are most likely derived from activated microglia and astrocytes, as these cells are highly sensitive to injury-induced environmental changes. Similar to developmental myelination, several stages of OPC activation can be distinguished during remyelination, starting with OPC proliferation and migration to the lesion site followed by cell differentiation (Franklin & ffrench-Constant, 2008).

Major progress in the elucidation of the requirements for remyelination has been done in MS and animal models of MS. In MS, the immune system attacks the OLG resulting in demyelination and neurodegeneration and virtually all components of the innate and adaptive immune system have been implicated in the demyelination and/or neurodegeneration in MS lesions (Gandhi et al., 2009; Kasper & Shoemaker, 2010). Interestingly and perhaps paradoxically, there is increasing evidence that inflammation is also important for remyelination. First, remyelination is abundant in immunologically active MS lesions whereas it is rarely observed in chronic, immunologically less active lesions (Goldschmidt et al., 2009). Second, genome studies of remyelination have revealed that pro-inflammatory cytokines are important for OLG regeneration. Indeed, the pro-inflammatory cytokine tumor necrosis factor (TNF) is important for remyelination after cuprizone-induced demyelination (Arnett et al., 2001, 2003). Third, as mentioned above, activated microglia and macrophages are required to clear the myelin debris from the lesion area, which is a prerequisite for remyelination. Interestingly, clearing of myelin debris by microglia can be enhanced by infiltrating myelin-specific T cells (Nielsen et al., 2009). Fourth, T cells and microglia can promote OLG proliferation and differentiation by producing neurotrophic factors such as brain derived neurotrophic factor (BDNF; Hohlfeld et al. 2006; Neumann et al., 2009). Indeed, T cells are required for efficient remyelination (Bieber et al., 2003).

Although inflammation can promote remyelination and the immune response might therefore be beneficial for neuroregeneration in MS, MS is predominantly an inflammatory disease (Lassmann & van Horssen, 2011). Maintaining an acute inflammatory milieu in order to improve remyelination may therefore be harmful to the patient. Nevertheless, immunomodulation may be a promising immediate approach to promote remyelination. Indeed, glatiramer acetate and FTY720 (fingolimod), two compounds that are approved for MS therapy, may promote remyelination. Glatiramer acetate, a polypeptide resembling MBP, alters the T cell response in MS from a pro-inflammatory Th1 to an anti-inflammatory Th2 phenotype. Interestingly, these glatiramer acetate-specific Th2 cells produce IGF-1 and BDNF and promote oligodendrogenesis and myelin repair in chemically induced demyelination (Skihar et al., 2009). The sphingosine-1-phosphate analogue FTY720 is used predominantly to inhibit the egress of T cells from secondary lymphoid organs. In addition, FTY720 can promote OLG differentiation (Miron et al., 2010) and as FTY720 can enter the CNS parenchyma it may thus directly promote remyelination.

Another direct approach to promote remyelination might be the injection of adult stem cells. Indeed, intracerebal or intraventricular injection of stem cells results in effective myelination in various models of demyelination. However, due to the multiple focal lesions in MS a systemic application is probably required. It is therefore promising that intravenous administration of adult neural and bone-marrow derived stem cells can enhance remyelination and ameliorate symptoms in experimental autoimmune encephalomyelitis (EAE), the animal model of MS (Pluchino et al., 2003; J. Yang et al., 2009). However, there is some evidence that this effect is predominantly due to the immunomodulatory function of stem cells (Pluchino et al., 2005) and it is still a matter of debate whether stem cells can indeed translocate into the CNS parenchyma and directly myelinate demyelinated axons (Franklin and ffrench-Constant, 2008; Franklin & Kotter, 2008).

Since OPC are present in chronic MS lesions but fail to differentiate the most relevant approach to improve remyelination will be to change the environment within the lesion from inhibitory to permissive for myelination. This would largely increase the therapeutic window in which remyelination can occur and thus would be expected to protect axons from further degeneration. Also in this field some promising results have been obtained. Of particular interest is the observation that the inhibitory effect of myelin components on OLG differentiation due to inactivation of Fyn can be antagonized by pharmacological inhibition of the RhoA signaling pathway (Baer et al., 2009). Moreover, suppression of the OLG differentiation inhibitor LINGO-1 by a specific antagonist stimulates OLG differentiation and promotes remyelination and axonal integrity in EAE (Mi et al., 2007, 2009).

5. Conclusion

OLG differentiation and myelination are extremely complex and highly regulated processes and disturbance of myelination is associated with various CNS diseases. Understanding of OLG differentiation is essential to establish neuroprotective therapies that are based on remyelination. Of particular relevance to develop such therapies is a profound knowledge of the intrinsic and extrinsic factors that coordinate myelination. The role of astrocytes and microglia are of special interest in view of their ambiguous role in neurodegenerative diseases. Here the challenge will be to minimize their role in neurodegeneration and maximize their role in neuroprotection and regeneration. A promising approach may therefore be to modulate astrocytes in such a way that the release of pro-myelinating factors is increased whereas the release of molecules detrimental for myelination is reduced. Concerning microglia it will be important to promote their capacity to efficiently clear the myelin debris in the lesions while at the same time minimizing their harmful effects since the presence of myelin debris is arguable the most important inhibitory factor for remyelination.

Much progress has been made to improve remyelination in model systems. Nevertheless currently no therapy directly aimed at improving remyelination exists and it is therefore now the question how this knowledge can be translated into therapeutic approaches. The most effective approach to achieve remyelination therapy will certainly depend on the diseases to treat. The first diseases, in which it is realistic to directly improve remyelination with cell-based therapies, will most likely be leukodystrophies, such as PMD. For chronic MS it is less likely that cell transplantation is a realistic treatment option. Here the promotion of the endogenous remyelination capacity is more promising, which will largely depend on the generation of a permissive environment for OLG differentiation. The progress that has been made in the last decade makes one cautiously optimistic that therapies based on remyelination are becoming a feasible scenario for the treatment of MS-patients.

6. References

Aggarwal, S.; Yurlova, L. & Simons, M. 2011. Central nervous system myelin: structure, synthesis and assembly. *Trends in Cell Biology*, Vol.21, No.10 (October 2011), pp. 585-593. ISSN: 0962-8924.

Anitei, M. & Pfeiffer, S.E. (2006). Myelin biogenesis: sorting out protein trafficking. *Current Biology*, Vol.16, No.11 (June 2006), pp. R418-R421. ISSN: 0960-9822.

Arnett, H.A.; Mason, J.; Marino, M.; Suzuki, K.; Matsushima, G.K. & Ting, J.P. (2001). TNFα promotes proliferation of oligodendrocyte progenitors and remyelination. *Nature Neuroscience*, Vol.4, No.11 (November 2001), pp. 1116-1122. ISSN: 1097-6256.

Arnett, H.; Wang, Y.; Matsushima, G.K.; Suzuki, K. & Ting, J.P. (2003). Functional genomic analysis of remyelination reveals importance of inflammation in oligodendrocyte regeneration. *Journal of Neuroscience*, Vol.23, No.30 (October 2003), pp. 9824-9832. ISSN: 0270-6474.

Bacon, C.; Lakics, V.; Machesky, L. & Rumsby, M. (2007). N-WASP regulates extension of filopodia and processes by oligodendrocyte progenitors, oligodendrocytes, and Schwann cells - implications for axon ensheathment at myelination. *Glia*, Vol.55, No.8 (June 2007), pp. 844-858. ISSN: 0894-1491.

Baer, A.S.; Syed, Y.A.; Kang, S.U.; Mitteregger, D.; Vig, R.; ffrench-Constant, C.; Franklin, R.J.; Altmann, F.; Lubec, G. & Kotter, M.R. (2009). Myelin-mediated inhibition of oligodendrocyte precursor differentiation can be overcome by pharmacological modulation of Fyn-RhoA and protein kinase C signalling. *Brain*, Vol.132, No.2 (February 2009), pp. 465-481. ISSN: 0006-8950.

Bansal, R. & Pfeiffer, S. (1994). Inhibition of protein and lipid sulfation in oligodendrocytes blocks biological responses to FGF-2 and retards cytoarchitectural maturation, but not developmental lineage progression. *Developmental Biology*, Vol. 162, No. 2 (April 1994), pp. 511-524. ISSN: 0012-1606.

Barbarese, E.; Koppel, D.E.; Deutscher, M.P.; Smith, C.L.; Ainger, K.; Morgan, F. & Carson, J.H. (1995). Protein translation components are colocalized in granules in oligodendrocytes. *Journal of Cell Science*, Vol.108, No.8 (August 1995), pp. 2781-2790. ISSN: 0021-9533.

Baron, W.; Metz, B.; Bansal, R.; Hoekstra, D. & de Vries, H. (2000). PDGF and FGF-2 signaling in oligodendrocyte progenitor cells: regulation of proliferation and differentiation by multiple intracellular signaling pathways. *Molecular and Cellular Neuroscience*, Vol.15, No.3 (March 2000), pp. 314-329. ISSN: 1044-7431.

Baron, W.; Shattil, S.J. & ffrench-Constant, C. (2002). The oligodendrocyte precursor mitogen PDGF stimulates proliferation by activation of $\alpha v \beta 3$ integrins. *The EMBO Journal*, Vol.21, No.8 (April 2002), pp. 1957-1966. ISSN: 0261-4189.

Baron, W.; Decker, L.; Colognato, H. & ffrench-Constant, C. (2003). Regulation of integrin growth factor interactions in oligodendrocytes by lipid raft microdomains. *Current Biology*, Vol.13, No.2 (January 2003), pp. 151-155. ISSN: 0960-9822.

Bartel, D.P. (2004). MicroRNAs: Genomics, biogenesis, mechanism, and function. *Cell*, Vol.116, No.2 (January 2009), pp. 281-297. ISSN: 0092-8674.

Bauer, N.G.; Richter-Landsberg, C. & ffrench-Constant, C. (2009). Role of oligodendroglial cytoskeleton in differentiation and myelination. *Glia*, Vol.57, No.16 (December 2009), pp. 1691-1705. ISSN: 0894-1491.

Baumann, N. & Pham-Dinh, D. (2001). Biology of oligodendrocyte and myelin in the mammalian central nervous system. *Physiological Reviews*, Vol.81, No.2 (April 2001), pp. 871-927, ISSN: 0031-9333.

Benjamins, J.A. & Nedelkoska, L. (1994). Maintenance of membrane sheets by cultured oligodendrocytes requires continuous microtubule turnover and Golgi transport. *Neurochemical Research*, Vol. 19, No.5 (May 1994), pp. 631-639. ISSN: 0364-3190.

Benninger, C.; Colognato, H.; Thurnherr, T.; Franklin,R.J.; Leone, D.P.; Atanasoski, S.; Nave, K.A.; ffrench-Constant, C.; Suter, U. & Relvas, J.B. (2006). β1-integrin signalling mediates premyelinating oligodendrocyte survival but is not required for myelination and remyelination. *Journal of Neuroscience*, Vol.26, No.29 (July 2006), pp. 7665-7673. ISSN: 0270-6474.

Bieber, A.J.; Kerr, S. & Rodriguez, M. (2003). Efficient central nervous system remyelination requires T cells. *Annals of Neurology*, Vo.53, No.3 (May 2003), pp. 680-684. ISSN: 0364-5134.

Biffiger, K.; Bartsch, S.; Montag, D.; Aguzzi, A.; Schachner M. & Bartsch, U. (2000). Severe hypomyelination of the murine CNS in the absence of myelin-associated glycoprotein and Fyn tyrosine kinase. *Journal of Neurosience*, Vol. 20, No.19 (October 2000), pp. 7430-7437. ISSN: 0270-6474.

Boggs, J.M. (2006). Myelin basic protein: a multifunctional protein. *Cellular and Molecular Life Sciences*, Vol.63, No.17 (September 2006), pp. 1945-1961. ISSN: 1420-682X.

Bradl, M. & Lassmann, H. (2010). Oligodendrocytes: biology and pathology. *Acta Neuropathologica*, Vol.119, No.1 (January 2010), pp. 37-53. ISSN: 0001-6322.

Bruce, C.C.; Zhao, C. & Franklin, R.J. (2010). Remyelination - An effective means of neuroprotection. *Hormones and Behavior*, Vol.57, No.1 (January 2010), pp. 56-62. ISSN: 0018-506X.

Brunner, C.; Lassmann, H.; Waehneldt, T.V.; Matthieu, J.M. & Linington, C. (1989). Differential ultrastructural localization of myelin basic protein, myelin/oligodendroglial protein, and 2',3'-cyclic nucleotide 3'-phosphodiesterase in the CNS of adult rats. *Journal of Neurochemistry*, Vol.52, No.1 (January 1989), pp. 296-304. ISSN: 0022-3042.

Buttery, P.C. & ffrench-Constant, C. (1999). Laminin-2/integrin interactions enhance myelin membrane formation by oligodendrocytes. *Molecular and Cellular Neuroscience*, Vol.14, No.3 (September 1999), pp. 199-212. ISSN: 1044-7431.

Charles, P.; Hernandez, M.P.; Stankoff, B.; Aigrot, M.S.; Colin, C.; Rougon, G.; Zalc, B. & Lubetzki, C. (2000). Negative regulation of central nervous system myelination by polysialylated-neural cell adhesion molecule. *Proceedings of the National Academy of Sciences of the USA*, Vol.97, No.13 (June 2000), pp. 7585-7590. ISSN: 0027-8424.

Charles, P.; Reynolds, R.; Seilhean, D.; Rougon, G.; Aigrot, M.S.; Niezgoda, A.; Zalc, B. & Lubetzki, C. (2002). Re-expression of PSA-NCAM by demyelinated axons: an inhibitor of remyelination in multiple sclerosis? *Brain*, Vol.125, No. 9 (September 2002), pp. 1972-1979. ISSN: 0006-8950.

Chun, S.J.; Rasband, M.N.; Sidman, R.L.; Habib, A.A. & Vartainen, T. (2003). Integrin-linked kinase is required for laminin-2 induced oligodendrocyte cell spreading and CNS myelination. *Journal of Cell Biology*, Vol.163, No.2 (October 2003), pp. 397-408. ISSN: 0021-9525.

Colognato, H.; Baron, W.; Avellana-Adalid, V.; Relvas, J.B.; Baron-Van Evercooren, A.; Georges-Labouesse, E. & ffrench-Constant, C. (2002). CNS integrins switch growth factor signalling to promote target-dependent survival. *Nature Cell Biology*, Vol. 4, No.11 (November 2002), pp. 833-841. ISSN: 1465-7392.

Colognato, H.; Ramachandrappa, S.; Olsen, I.M. & ffrench-Constant, C. (2004). Integrins direct Src family kinases to regulate distinct phases of oligodendrocyte development. *Journal of Cell Biology*, Vol.167, No.2 (October 2004), pp. 365-375. ISSN: 0021-9525.

Colognato, H.; ffrench-Constant, C. & Feltri, M. (2005). Human diseases reveal novel roles for neural laminins. *Trends in Neurosciences*, Vol.28, No.9 (September 2005), pp. 480-486. ISSN: 0166-2236.

Colognato, H.; Galvin, J.; Wang, Z.; Relucio, J.; Nguyen, T.; Harrison, D.; Yurchenco, P.D. & ffrench-Constant, C. (2007). Identification of dystroglycan as a second laminin receptor in oligodendrocytes, with a role in myelination. *Development*, Vol.134, No.9 (May 2007), pp. 1723-1736. ISSN: 1011-6370.

Copray, S.; Huynh, J.L.; Sher, F.; Casaccia-Bonnefil, P. & Boddeke, E. (2009). Epigenetic mechanisms facilitating oligodendroyte development, maturation, and aging. *Glia*, Vol. 57, No.15 (November 2009), pp.1579-1587. ISSN: 0894-1491.

Crang, A.J.; Gilson, J. & Blakemore, W.F. (1998). The demonstration by transplantation of the very restricted remyelinating potential of post-mitotic oligodendrocytes. *Journal of Neurocytology*, Vol.27 (August 1998), No.7, pp. 541-553. ISSN: 0300-4864.

Cui, Q.L.; Fragoso, G.; Miron, V.E.; Darlington, P.J.; Mushynski, W.E.; Antel, J. & Almazan, G. (2010). Response of human oligodendrocyte progenitors to growth factors and axon signals. *Journal of Neuropathology and Experimental Neurology*, Vol. 69, No.9 (September 2010), pp. 930-944. ISSN: 0022-3069.

Czopka, T.; von Holst, A.; Schmidt, G.; ffrench-Constant, C. & Faissner, A. (2009). Tenascin C and tenascin R similarly prevent the formation of myelin membranes in a RhoA-dependent manner, but antagonistically regulate the expression of myelin basic protein via a separate pathway. *Glia*, Vol.57, No.16, (December 2009), pp. 1790-1801. ISSN: 0894-1491.

De Angelis, D.A. & Braun, P.E. (1996) 2',3'-Cyclic nucleotide 3'-phosphodiesterase binds to actin-based cytoskeletal elements in an isoprenylation-independent manner. *Journal of Neurochemistry*, Vol.67, No.3 (September 1996), pp. 943-951. ISSN: 0022-3042.

Demerens, C.; Stankoff, B.; Logak, M.; Anglade, P.; Allinquant, B.; Couraud, F.; Zalc, B. & Lubetzki, C. (1996). Induction of myelination in the central nervous system by electrical activity. *Proceeding of the National Academy of Sciences of the USA*, Vol.93, No.18 (September 1996), pp. 9887-9892. ISSN: 0027-8424.

Dugas, J.C.; Cuellar, T.L.; Scholze, A.; Ason, B.; Ibrahim, A.; Emery, B.; Zamanian, J.L.; Foo, L.C.; McManus, M.T. & Barres, B.A. (2010). Dicer1 and miR-219 are required for normal oligodendrocyte differentiation and myelination. *Neuron*, Vol.65, No.5 (March 2010), pp. 597-611. ISSN: 0896-6273.

Dupree, J.L.; Coetzee, T.; Blight, A.; Suzuki, K. & Popko, B. (1998). Myelin galactolipids are essential for proper node of Ranvier formation in the CNS. *Journal of Neuroscience*, Vol.18, No.5 (March 1998), pp. 1642-1649. ISSN: 0270-6474.

Dyer, C.A. & Benjamins, J.A. (1989). Organization of oligodendroglial membrane sheets. I: Association of myelin basic protein and 2',3'-cyclic nucleotide 3'-phosphohydrolase with cytoskeleton. *Journal of Neuroscience Research*, Vol. 24, No.2 (October 1989), pp. 201-211. ISSN: 0360-4012.

Feldmann, A.; Amphornrat, J.; Schönherr, M.; Winterstein, C.; Möbius, W.; Ruhwedel, T.; Danglot, L.; Nave, K.A.; Galli, T.; Bruns, D.; Trotter, J. & Krämer-Albers, E.M. (2011). Transport of the major myelin proteolipid protein is directed by VAMP3 and VAMP7. *Journal of Neuroscience*, Vol.31, No.15 (April 2011), pp. 5659-5672. ISSN: 0270-6474.

Filipovic, R. & Zecevic, N. (2008). The effect of CXCL1 on fetal oligodendrocyte progenitor cells. *Glia*, Vol.56, No.1 (January 2008), pp. 1-15. ISSN: 0894-1491.

Franklin, R.J. (2002). Remyelination of the demyelinated CNS: the case for and against transplantation of central, peripheral and olfactory glia. *Brain Research Bulletin*, Vol.57, No.6 (April 2002), pp. 827-832. ISSN: 0361-9230.

Franklin, R.J.M. & ffrench-Constant, C. (2008). Remyelination in the CNS: from biology to therapy. *Nature Reviews. Neuroscience*, Vol.9, No. 11 (November 2008), pp. 839-855. ISSN: 1471-0048.

Franklin, R.J. & Kotter, M.R. (2008). The biology of CNS remyelination: the key to therapeutic advances. *Journal of Neurology*, Vol.255, Suppl. 1 (March 2008), pp. 19-25. ISSN: 0340-5354.

Galiano, M.R.; Andrieux, A.; Deloulme, J.C.; Bosc, C.; Schweitzer, A.; Job, D. & Hallak, M.E. (2006). Myelin basic protein functions as a microtubule stabilizing protein in differentiated oligodendrocytes. *Journal of Neuroscience Research*, Vol. 84, No.3 (August 2006), pp. 534-541. ISSN: 0360-4012.

Gandhi, R.; Laroni, A. & Weiner, H.L. (2010). Role of the innate immune system in the pathogenesis of multiple sclerosis. *Journal of Neuroimmunology*, Vol.221, No.1-2 (April 2010), pp. 7-14. ISSN: 0165-5728.

Garbern, J.Y.; Yool, D.A.; Moore, G.J.; Wilds, I.B.; Faulk, M.W.; Klugmann, M.; Nave, K.A.; Sistermans, E.A.; van der Knaap, M.S.; Bird, T.D.; Shy, M.E.; Kamholz, J.A. & Griffiths I.R. (2002). Patients lacking the major CNS myelin protein, proteolipid protein 1, develop length-dependent axonal degeneration in the absence of demyelination and inflammation. *Brain*, Vol.125, No.3 (March 2002), pp. 551-561. ISSN: 0006-8950.

Gieselmann, V. (2003). Metachromatic leukodystrophy: recent research developments. *Journal of Child Neurology*, Vol.18, No.9 (September 2003), 591-594. ISSN: 0883-0738.

Goldschmidt, T.; Antel, J.; König, F.B.; Brück, W. & Kuhlmann T. (2009). Remyelination capacity of the MS brain decreases with disease chronicity. *Neurology*, Vol. 72, No.22 (June 2009), pp. 1914-1921. ISSN: 0028-3878.

Götz, M.; Bolz, J.; Joester, A. & Faissner, A. (1997). Tenascin-C synthesis and influence on axonal growth during rat cortical development. *European Journal of Neuroscience*, Vol. 9, No.3 (March 1997), pp. 496–506. ISSN: 0953-816X.

Giffiths, I.; Klugmann, M.; Andersen, T.; Thomson, C.; Vouykouklis. D. & Nave, K.A. (1998). Current concepts of PLP and its role in the nervous system. *Microscopy Research and Technique*, Vol.41, No.5 (June 1998), pp. 345-358. ISSN: 1059-910X.

Hinks, G.L.; Chari, D.M.; O'Leary, M.T.; Zhao, C.; Keirstead, H.S.; Blakemore, W.F. & Franklin, R.J. (2001). Depletion of endogenous oligodendrocyte progenitors rather than increased availability of survival factors is a likely explanation for enhanced survival of transplanted oligodendrocyte progenitors in X-irradiated compared to normal CNS. *Neuropathology and Applied Neurobiology*, Vol.27, No.1 (February 2001), pp. 59–67. ISSN: 0305-1846.

Hohlfeld, R.; Kerschensteiner, M.; Stadelmann, C.; Lassmann, H. & Wekerle, H. (2006). The neuroprotective effect of inflammation: implications for the therapy of multiple sclerosis. *Neurological Sciences*, Vol.27, Suppl.1 (March 2006), pp. 1-7. ISSN: 1590-1874.

Inoue, K. (2005). PLP1-related inherited dysmyelinating disorders: Pelizaeus-Merzbacher disease and spastic paraplegia type 2. *Neurogenetics*, Vol.6, No.1 (February 2005), pp. 1-6. ISSN: 1364-6745.

Ishibashi, T.; Dakin, K.A.; Stevens, B.; Lee, P.R.; Kozlov, S.V.; Stewart, C.L. & Fields, R.D. (2006). Astrocytes promote myelination in response to electrical impulses. *Neuron*, Vol.49, No.6 (March 2006), pp. 823-832. ISSN: 0896-6273.

Johnson, A.B. (2004). Alexander disease: a leukodystrophy caused by a mutation in GFAP. *Neurochemical Research*, Vol.29, No.5 (May 2004), pp. 961-964. ISSN: 1573-6903.

Kasper, L.H. & Shoemaker, J. (2010). Multiple sclerosis immunology. The healthy immune system vs. the MS immune system. *Neurology*, Vol.74, Suppl. 1 (January 2010), pp. 2-8. ISSN: 0028-3878.

Klein, C.; Krämer, E.M.; Cardine, A.M.; Schraven, B.; Brandt, R. & Trotter, J. (2002). Process outgrowth of oligodendrocytes is promoted by interaction of Fyn kinase with the cytoskeletal protein Tau. *Journal of Neuroscience*, Vol. 22, No.3 (February 2002), pp. 698-707. ISSN: 0270-6474.

Kotter, M.R.; Li, W.W.; Zhao, C. & Franklin, R.J.M. (2006). Myelin impairs CNS remyelination by inhibiting oligodendrocyte precursor cell differentiation. *Journal of Neuroscience*, Vol.26, No.1 (January 2006), pp. 328-332. ISSN: 0270-6474.

Kotter, M.R.; Stadelmann, C. & Hartung, H.P. (2011). Enhancing remyelination in disease – can we wrap it up? *Brain*, Vol.134, No.7 (July 2011), pp. 1882-1900. ISSN: 0006-8950.

Krämer, E.M.; Klein, C.; Koch, T.; Boytinck, M. & Trotter, J. (1999). Compartmentation of Fyn kinase with glycosylphosphatidylinositol-anchored molecules in oligodendrocytes facilitates kinase activation during myelination. *Journal of Biological Chemistry*, Vol.274, No.41 (October 1999), pp. 29042-29049. ISSN: 0021-9258.

Krämer, E.M.; Schardt, A. & Nave, K.A. (2001). Membrane traffic in myelinating oligodendrocytes. *Microscopy Research and Technique*, Vol.52, No.6 (March 2001), pp. 656-671, ISSN: 1059-910X.

Krämer-Albers, E.M.; Gehrig-Burger, T.; Thiele, C.; Trotter, J. & Nave, K.A. (2006). Perturbed interactions of mutant proteolipid protein/DM20 with cholesterol and lipid rafts in oligodendroglia: implications for dysmyelination in spastic paraplegia. *Journal of Neuroscience*, Vol.26, No.45 (November 2006), pp. 11743-11752. ISSN: 0270-6474.

Kuhlmann, T.; Miron, V.; Cui, Q.; Wegner, C.; Antel, J. & Brück, W. (2008). Differentiation block of oligodendroglial progenitor cells as a cause for remyelination failure in chronic multiple sclerosis. *Brain*, Vol.131, No.7 (July 2008) pp. 1749-1758. ISSN: 0006-8950.

Lassmann, H. & van Horssen, J. (2011) The molecular basis of neurodegeneration in multiple sclerosis. *FEBS Letters*, Vol.585, No.23 (December 2011), pp. 3715-3723. ISSN: 0014-5793.

Lee, J.; Gravel, M.; Zhang, R.; Thibault, P. & Braun, P.E. (2005). Process outgrowth in oligodendrocytes is mediated by CNP, a novel microtubule assembly protein. *Journal of Cell Biology*, Vol.170, No.4 (August 2005), pp. 661-673. ISSN: 0021-9525.

Liang, X.; Draghi, N.A. & Resh, M.D. (2004). Signaling from integrins to Fyn to Rho family GTPases regulates morphologic differentiation of oligodendrocytes. *Journal of Neuroscience*, Vol.24, No.32 (August 2004), pp. 7140-7149. ISSN: 0270-6474.

Lin, G.; Mela, A; Guilfoyle, E.M. & Goldman, J.E. (2009). Neonatal and adult O4(+) oligodendrocyte lineage cells display different growth factor responses and different gene expression patterns. *Journal of Neuroscience Research*, Vol.87, No.15 (November 2009), pp. 3390-3402. ISSN: 0360-4012.

Liu, J.; Muggironi, M.; Marin-Husstege, M. & Cassaccia-Bonnefil, P. (2003). Oligodendrocyte process outgrowth in vitro is modulated by epigenetic regulation of cytoskeletal severing proteins. *Glia*, Vol.44, No.3 (December 2003), pp. 264-274. ISSN: 0894-1491.

Liu, J.; Stadelmann, C.; Moscarello, M.; Bruck, W.; Sobel, A.; Mastronardi, F.G. & Cassaccia-Bonnefil. P. (2005). Expression of stathmin, a developmentally controlled cytoskeleton-regulating molecule, in demyelinating disorders. *Journal of Neuroscience*, Vol.25, No.3 (January 2005), pp. 737-747. ISSN: 0270-6474.

Liu, J. & Casaccia, P. (2010). Epigenetic regulation of oligodendrocyte identity. *Trends in Neurosciences*, Vol.33, No.4 (April 2010), pp. 193-201. ISSN: 0166-2236.

Maggipinto, M.; Rabiner C.; Kidd, G.J.; Hawkins, A.J.; Smith, R. & Barbarese, E. (2004). Increased expression of the MBP mRNA binding protein hnRNP A2 during oligodendrocyte differentiation. *Journal of Neuroscience Research*, Vol.75, No.5 (March 2004), pp. 614-623. ISSN: 0360-4012.

Maier, O.; van der Heide, T.; van Dam, A.M.; Baron, W.; de Vries, H. & Hoekstra, D. (2005). Alteration of the extracellular matrix interferes with raft-association of neurofascin in oligodendrocytes. Potential significance for multiple sclerosis? *Molecular and Cellular Neuroscience*, Vol.28, No.2 (February 2005), pp. 390-401. ISSN: 1044-7431.

Maier, O.; Hoekstra, D. & Baron, W. (2008). Polarity development in oligodendrocytes: sorting and trafficking of myelin components. *Journal of Molecular Neuroscience*, Vol.35. No.1 (May 2008), pp. 35-53. ISSN: 0895-8696.

Marcus, J.; Honigbaum, S.; Shroff, S.; Honke, K.; Rosenbluth, J. & Dupree, J.L. (2006). Sulfatide is essential for the maintenance of CNS myelin and axon structure. *Glia*, Vol.53, No.4 (March 2006), pp. 372-381. ISSN 0894-1491.

McMorris, F.A.; Smith, T.M.; DeSalvo, S. & Furlanetto, R.W. (1986). Insulin-like growth factor I/somatomedin C: a potent inducer of oligodendrocyte development. *Proceedings of the National Academy of Sciences of the USA*, Vol.83, No.3 (February 1996), pp. 822-826. ISSN: 0027-8424.

McTigue, D.M. & Tripathi, R.B. (2008). The life, death, and replacement of oligodendrocytes in the adult CNS. *Journal of Neurochemistry* Vol.107, No.1 (October 2008), pp. 1-19. ISSN: 0022-3042.

Mi, S.; Miller, R.H.; Lee, X.; Scott, M.L.; Shulag-Morskaya, S.; Shao, Z.; Chang, J.; Thill, G.; Levesque, M.; Zhang, M.; Hession, C.; Sah, D.; Trapp, B.; He, Z.; Jung, V.; McCoy, J.M. & Pepinsky, R.B. (2005). LINGO-1 negatively regulates myelination by oligodendrocytes. *Nature Neuroscience*, Vol.8, No.6 (June 2005), pp. 745-751. ISSN: 1097-6256.

Mi, S.; Hu, B.; Hahm, K.; Luo, Y.; Kam Hui, E.S.; Yuan, Q.; Wong, W.M.; Wang, L.; Su, H.; Chu, T.H.; Guo, J.; Zhang, W.; So, K.F.; Pepinsky, B.; Shao, Z.; Graff, C.; Garber, E.; Jung, V.; Wu, E.X. & Wu, W. (2007). LINGO-1 antagonist promotes spinal cord remyelination and axonal integrity in MOG-induced experimental autoimmune encephalomyelitis. *Nature Medicine*, Vol.13, No.10 (October 2007), pp. 1228-1233. ISSN: 1078-8956.

Mi, S.; Miller, R.H.; Tang, W.; Lee, X.; Hu, B.; Wu, W.; Zhang, Y.; Shields, C.B.; Zhang, Y.; Miklasz, S.; Shea, D.; Mason, J.; Franklin, R.J.; Ji, B.; Shao, Z.; Chédotal, A.; Bernard, F.; Roulois, A.; Xu, J.; Jung, V. & Pepinsky, B. (2009). Promotion of central nervous system remyelination by induced differentiation of oligodendrocyte precursor cells. *Annals of Neurology*, Vol. 65, No. 3 (March 2009), pp. 304-315. ISSN: 0364-5134.

Milner, R.; Edwards, G.; Streuli, C. & ffrench-Constant, C. (1996). A role in migration for the αvβ1 integrin expressed on oligodendrocyte precursors. *Journal of Neuroscience*, Vol.16, No.22 (November 1996), pp. 7240-7252. ISSN: 0270-6474.

Milner, R.; Anderson, H.J.; Rippon, R.F.; McKaym J.S.; Franklin R.J.; Marchionni, M.A.; Reynolds, R. & ffrench-Constant, C. (1997). Contrasting effects of mitogenic growth factors on oligodendrocyte precursor cell migration. *Glia*, Vol.19, No.1 (January 1997), pp. 85-90. ISSN: 0894-1491.

Miron, V.E.; Ludwin, S.K.; Darlington, P.J.; Jarjour, A.A.; Soliven, B.; Kennedy, T.E. & Antel, J.P. (2010). Fingolimod (FTY720) enhances remyelination following demyelination of organotypic cerebellar slices. *American Journal of Pathology*, Vol.176, No.6, (June 2010), pp. 2682-2694. ISSN: 0002-9440.

Miron, V.E.; Kuhlmann, T. & Antel, J.P. (2011). Cells of the oligodendroglial lineage, myelination, and remyelination. *Biochimica et Biophysica Acta. Molecular Basis of Disease*, Vol.1812, No.2 (February 2011), pp. 184-193. ISSN: 0925-4439.

Miyamoto, Y; Yamauchi, J. & Tanoue, A. (2008). Cdk5 phosphorylation of WAVE2 regulates oligodendrocyte progenitor cell migration through nonreceptor tyrosine kinase Fyn. *Journal of Neuroscience*, Vol. 28, No.33 (August 2008), pp. 8326-8337. ISSN: 0270-6474.

Moore, C.S.; Abdullah, S.L.; Brown, E.; Arulpragasam, A. & Crocker, S.J. (2011). How factors secreted from astrocytes impact myelin repair. *Journal of Neuroscience Research*, Vol. 89, No.1 (January 2011), pp. 13-21. ISSN: 0360-4012.

Nave, K.H. (2010). Myelination and support of axonal integrity by glia. *Nature*, Vol.468, No. 7321 (November 2010), pp. 244-252. ISSN: 0028-0836.

Neumann, H.; Kotter, M.R. & Franklin, R.J.M. (2009). Debris clearance by microglia: an essential link between degeneration and regeneration. *Brain*, Vol.1323, No.2 (February 2009), pp. 288-295. ISSN: 0006-8950.

Nielsen, H.H.; Ladeby, R.; Fenger, C.; Toft-Hansen, H.; Babcock, A.A.; Owens, T. & Finsen, B. (2009) Enhanced microglial clearance of myelin debris in T cell-infiltrated central nervous system. *Journal of Neuropathology and Experimental Neurology*, Vol.68, No.8 (August 2009), pp. 845-856. ISSN: 0022-3069.

Nishiyama, A.; Lin, X.H.; Giese, N.; Heldin, C.H. & Stallcup, W.B. (1996). Colocalization of NG2 proteoglycan and PDGF α-receptor on O-2A progenitor cells in the developing rat brain. *Journal of Neuroscience Research*, Vol.43, No. 3 (February 1996), pp. 299-314. ISSN: 0360-4012.

Noble, M.; Murray, K.; Stroobant, P.; Waterfield, M.D. & Riddle, P. (1988). Platelet-derived growth factor promotes division and motility and inhibits premature differentiation of the oligodendrocyte/type-2 astrocyte progenitor cell. *Nature*, Vol.333, No.6173 (June 1988), pp. 560-562. ISSN: 0028-0836.

O'Leary, M.T. & Blakemore, W.F. (1997). Oligodendrocyte precursors survive poorly and do not migrate following transplantation into the normal adult central nervous system. *Journal of Neuroscience Research*, Vol.48, No.2 (April 1997), pp. 159-167. ISSN: 0360-4012.

Omari, K.M.; John, G.; Lango, R.; Raine, C.S. (2006). Role for CXCR2 and CXCL1 on glia in multiple sclerosis. *Glia*, Vol.53, No. 1 (January 2006), pp. 24-31. ISSN: 0894-1491.

Orthmann-Murphy, J.L.; Abrams, C.K. & Scherer, S.S. (2008). Gap junctions couple astrocytes and oligodendrocytes. *Journal of Molecular Neuroscience*, Vol.35, No.1 (May 2008), pp. 101-116. ISSN: 0895-8696.

Parratt, J.D. & Prineas, J.W. (2010) Neuromyelitis optica: a demyelinating disease characterized by acute destruction and regeneration of perivascular astrocytes. *Multiple Sclerosis Journal*, Vol.16., No.10 (October 2010), pp. 1156-1172. ISSN: 1352-4585.

Patani, R.; Balaratnam, M.; Vora, A. & Reynolds, R. (2007). Remyelination can be extensive in multiple sclerosis despite a long disease course. *Neuropathology and Applied Neurobiology*, Vol.33, No.3 (June 2007), pp. 277-287. ISSN: 0305-1846.

Patrikios, P.; Stadelmann, C.; Kutzelnigg, A.; Rauschka, H.; Schmidbauer, M.; Laursen, H.; Sorensen, P.S.; Brück, W.; Lucchinetti, C. & Lassmann, H. (2006). Remyelination is extensive in a subset of multiple sclerosis patients. *Brain*, Vol.129, No.12 (December 2006), pp. 3165-3172. ISSN: 0006-8950.

Pfeiffer, S.E.; Warrington, A.E. & Bansal, R. (1993). The oligodendrocyte and its many cellular processes. *Trends in Cell Biology*, Vol.3, No.6 (June 1993), pp. 191-197. ISSN: 0962-8924.

Pluchino, S.; Quattrini, A.; Brambilla, E.; Gritti, A.; Salani, G.; Dina, G.; Galli, R.; Del Carro, U.; Amadio, S.; Bergami, A.; Furlan, R.; Comi, G.; Vescovi, A.L. & Martino, G. (2003). Injection of adult neurospheres induces recovery in a chronic model of multiple sclerosis. *Nature*, Vol.422, No.6933 (April 2003), pp. 688-694. ISSN: 0028-0836.

Pluchino, S.; Zanotti, L.; Rossi, B.; Brambilla, E.; Ottoboni, L.; Salani, G.; Martinello, M.; Cattalini, A.; Bergami, A.; Furlan, R.; Comi, G.; Constantin, G. & Martino, G. (2005). Neurosphere-derived multipotent precursors promote neuroprotection by an immunomodulatory mechanism. *Nature*, Vol.436, No.7048 (July 2005), pp. 266-271. ISSN: 0028-0836.

Polito, A. & Reynolds, R. (2006). NG2-expressing cells as oligodendrocyte progenitors in the normal and demyelinated adult central nervous system. *Journal of Anatomy*, Vol. 207, No.6 (December 2006), pp. 707-716. ISSN: 1469-7580.

Price, J. & Hines, R.O. (1985). Astrocytes in culture synthesize and secrete a variant form of fibronectin. *Journal of Neuroscience*, Vol.5, No.8 (August 1985), pp. 2205-2211. ISSN: 0270-6474.

Rajasekharan, S.; Baker, K.A.; Horn, K.E.; Jarjour, A.A; Antel, J.P. & Kennedy TE. (2009). Netrin 1 and Dcc regulate oligodendrocyte process branching and membrane extension via Fyn and RhoA. *Development*, Vol.136, No.3 (February 2009), pp. 415-426. ISSN: 1011-6370.

Relvas, J.B.; Setzu, A.; Baron, W.; Buttery, P.C.; LaFlamme, S.E.; Franklin, R.J. & ffrench-Constant, C. (2001). Expression of dominant-negative and chimeric subunits reveals an essential role for β1 integrin during myelination. *Current Biology*, Vol.11, No.13 (July 2001), pp. 1039-1043. ISSN: 0960-9822.

Richter-Landsberg, C. & Gorath, M. (1999). Developmental regulation of alternatively spliced isoforms of mRNA encoding MAP2 and tau in rat brain oligodendrocytes during culture maturation. *Journal of Neuroscience Research*, Vol.56, No. 3 (May 1999), pp. 259-270. ISSN: 0360-4012.

Richter-Landsberg, C. (2008). The cytoskeleton in oligodendrocytes. Microtubule dynamics in health and disease. *Journal of Molecular Neuroscience*, Vol. 35, No. 1 (May 2008), pp. 55-63. ISSN: 0895-8696.

Ridley, A.J. (2006). Rho GTPases and actin dynamics in membrane protrusions and vesicle trafficking. *Trends in Cell Biology*, Vol.16, No.10 (October 2006), pp. 522-529. ISSN: 0962-8924.

Roach, A.; Takahashi, N.; Pravtcheva, D.; Ruddle, F. & Hood, L.E. (1985). Chromosomal mapping of mouse myelin basic protein gene and structure and transcription of the partially deleted gene in shiverer mutant mice. *Cell*, Vol. 42, No.1 (August 1985), pp. 149-155. ISSN: 0092-8674.

Roemer, S.F.; Parisi, J.E.; Lennon, V.A.; Benarroch, E.E.; Lassmann, H.; Bruck, W.; Mandler, R.N.; Weinshenker, B.G.; Pittock, S.J.; Wingerchuk, D.M. & Lucchinetti, C.F. (2007). Pattern-specific loss of aquaporin-4 immunoreactivity distinguishes neuromyelitis optica from multiple sclerosis. *Brain*, Vol.130, No. 5 (May 2007), pp. 1194-1205. ISSN: 0006-8950.

Saher, G.; Brügger, B.; Lappe-Siefke, C.; Möbius, W.; Tozawa, R.; Wehr, M.C.; Wieland, F.; Ishibashi, S. & Nave, K.A. (2005). High cholesterol level is essential for myelin membrane growth. *Nature Neuroscience*, Vol.8, No.4 (April 2005), pp. 468-475. ISSN: 1097-6256.

Schachner, M. & Bartsch, U. (2000). Multiple functions of the myelin-associated glycoprotein MAG (siglec-4) in formation and maintenance of myelin. *Glia*, Vol.29, No.2 (January 2000), pp. 154-165. ISSN: 0894-1491.

See, J.; Zhang, X.; Eraydin, N.; Mun, S.B.; Mamontov, P.; Golden, J.A. & Grinspan, J.B. (2004). Oligodendrocyte maturation is inhibited by bone morphogenetic protein. *Molecular and Cellular Neuroscience*, Vol.26, No.4 (August 2004), pp. 481-492. ISSN: 1044-7431.

Shen, S.; Sandoval, J.; Swiss, V.A.; Li, J.; Dupree, J.; Franklin, R.J. & Casaccia-Bonnefil, P. (2008). Age-dependent epigenetic control of differentiation inhibitors is critical for remyelination efficiency. *Nature Neuroscience*, Vol.11, No.9 (September 2008), pp. 1024-1034. ISSN: 1097-6256.

Sherman, D.L. & Brophy, P.J. (2005). Mechanisms of axon ensheathment and myelin growth. *Nature Reviews Neuroscience*, Vol.6, No.9 (September 2005), pp. 683-690. ISSN: 1471-0048.

Sim, F.J.; Zhao, C.; Penderis, J. & Franklin, R.J. (2002). The age-related decrease in CNS remyelination efficiency is attributable to an impairment of both oligodendrocyte progenitor recruitment and differentiation. *Journal of Neuroscience*, Vol.22, No.7 (April 2002), pp. 2451-2459. ISSN: 0270-6474.

Simons, M.; Krämer, E.M.; Macchi, P.; Rathke-Hartlieb, S.; Trotter, J.; Nave, K.A. & Schulz, J.B. (2002). Overexpression of the myelin proteolipid protein leads to accumulation of cholesterol and proteolipid protein in endosomes/lysosomes: implications for Pelizaeus-Merzbacher disease. *Journal of Cell Biology*, Vol.157, No.2 (April 2002), pp. 327-336. ISSN: 0021-9525.

Skihar, V.; Silva, C.; Chojnacki, A.; Döring, A.; Stallcup, W.B.; Weiss, S. & Yong, V.W. (2009). Promoting oligodendrogenesis and myelin repair using the multiple sclerosis medication glatiramer acetate. *Proceedings of the National Academy of Sciences of the USA*, Vol.106, No.42 (October 2009), pp. 17992-17997. ISSN: 0027-8424.

Smolders, I.; Smets, I.; Maier, O.; vandeVen, M.; Steels, P. & Ameloot, M. (2010). Simvastatin interferes with process outgrowth and branching of oligodendrocytes. *Journal of Neuroscience Research*, Vol. 88, No.15 (November 2010), pp. 3361-3375. ISSN: 0360-4012.

Stankoff, B.; Aigrot, M.S.; Noel, F.; Wattilliaux, A.; Zalc, B. & Lubetzki, C. (2002). Ciliary neurotrophic factor (CNTF) enhances myelin formation: a novel role for CNTF and CNTF-related molecules. *Journal of Neuroscience*, Vol.22, No.21 (November 2002), pp. 9221-9227. ISSN: 0270-6474.

Stevens, B.; Porta, S.; Haak, L.L.; Gallo, V. & Fields, R.D. (2002) Adenosine: a neuron-glial transmitter promoting myelination in the CNS in response to action potentials. *Neuron*, Vol.36, No.5 (December 2002), pp. 855-868. ISSN: 0896-6273.

Tait, S.; Gunn-Moore, F.; Collinson, J.M.; Huang, J.; Lubetzki, C.; Pedraza, L.; Sherman, D.L.; Colman, D.R. & Brophy, P.J. (2000). An oligodendrocyte cell adhesion molecule at the site of assembly of the paranodal axo-glial junction. *Journal of Cell Biology*, Vol.150, No.3 (August 2000), pp. 657-666. ISSN: 0021-9525.

Taveggia, C.; Zanazzi, G.; Petrylak, A.; Yano, H.; Rosenbluth, J.; Einheber, S.; Xu, X.; Esper, R.M.; Loeb, J.A.; Shrager, P.; Chao, M.V.; Falls, D.L.; Role, L. & Salzer, J.L. (2005). Neuregulin-1 type III determines the ensheathment fate of axons. *Neuron*, Vol.47, No.5 (September 2005), pp. 681-694. ISSN: 0896-6273.

Tepavcevic, V. & Blakemore, W.F. (2005). Glial grafting for demyelinating disease. *Philosophical Transactions of the Royal Society of London. Series B, Biological Sciences*, Vol.360, No.1461 (September 2005), pp. 1775-1795. ISSN: 0962-8436.

Thurnherr, T.; Benninger, Y.; Wu, X.; Chrostek, A.; Krause, S.M.; Nave, K.A.; Franklin, R.J.; Brakebusch, C.; Suter, U. & Relvas, J.B. (2006). Cdc42 and Rac1 signaling are both required for and act synergistically in the correct formation of myelin sheaths in the CNS. *Journal of Neuroscience*, Vol.26, No.40, pp. 10110-10119. ISSN: 0270-6474.

Trajkovic, K.; Dhaunchak, A.S.; Goncalves, J.T.; Wenzel, D.; Schneider, A.; Bunt, G.; Nave, K.A. & Simons, M. (2006). Neuron to glia signaling triggers myelin membrane exocytosis from endosomal storage sites. *Journal of Cell Biology*, Vol.172, No.6 (March 2006), pp.937-948. ISSN: 0021-9525.

Tsai, H.H.; Frost, E.; To,V.; Robinson, S.; ffrench-Cosntant, C.; Geertman, R.; Ransohoff, R.M & Miller, R.H. (2002). The chemokine receptor CXCR2 controls positioning of oligodendrocyte precursors in developing spinal cord by arresting their migration. *Cell*, Vol.110, No.3 (August 2002), pp. 373-383. ISSN: 0092-8674.

Wake, H.; Lee, P.R. & Fields, R.D. (2011). Control of local protein synthesis and initial events in myelination by action potentials. *Science*, Vol.333, No.6049 (September 2011), pp. 1647-1651. ISSN 0036-8075.

Wang, S.; Sdrulla, A.D.; diSibio, G.; Bush, G.; Nofziger, D.; Hicks, C.; Weinmaster, G. & Barres, B.A. (1998). Notch receptor activation inhibits oligodendrocyte differentiation. *Neuron*, Vol.21, No.1 (July 1998), pp. 63-75. ISSN: 0896-6273.

Wang, Z.; Colognato, H. & ffrench-Constant, C. (2007). Contrasting effects of mitogenic growth factors on myelination in neuron- oligodendrocyte co-cultures. *Glia*, Vol.55, No.5 (April 2007), pp. 537-545. ISSN: 0894-1491.

Watkins, T.A.; Emery, B.; Mulinyawe, S. & Barres, B.A. (2008). Distinct stages of myelination regulated by γ-secretase and astrocytes in a rapidly myelinating CNS coculture system. *Neuron*, Vol. 26, No.4 (November 2008), pp. 555-569. ISSN: 0896-6273.

Wenger, D.A.; Rafi, M.A.; Luzi, P.; Datto, J. & Costantino-Ceccarini, E. (2000). Krabbe disease: genetic aspects and progress toward therapy. *Molecular Genetics and Metabolism*, Vol.70, No.1 (May 2000), pp. 1-9. ISSN: 1096-7192.

Williams, A.; Piaton, G. & Lubetzki, C. (2007). Astrocytes – friends or foes in multiple sclerosis? *Glia*, Vol.55, No.13 (October 2007), pp. 1300-1312. ISSN: 0894-1491.

Windrem, M.S.; Nunes, M.C.; Rashbaum, W.K.; Schwartz, T.H.; Goodman, R.A.; McKhann, G. 2nd; Roy, N.S. & Goldman, S.A. (2004). Fetal and adult human oligodendrocyte progenitor cell isolates myelinate the congenitally dysmyelinated brain. *Nature Medicine*, Vol.10, No.1 (January 2004), pp. 93-97. ISSN: 1078-8956.

Wolswijk, G. (1998). Chronic stage multiple sclerosis lesions contain a relatively quiescent population of oligodendrocyte precursor cells. *Journal of Neuroscience*, Vol.18, No. 2 (January 1998), pp. 601-609. ISSN: 0270-6474.

Yang, J.; Rostami, A. & Zhang, G.X. (2009). Cellular remyelination therapy in multiple sclerosis. *Journal of the Neurological Sciences*, Vol.276, No. 1-2 (January 2009), pp. 1-5. ISSN: 0022-510X.

Yang, L.J.; Zeller, C.B.; Shaper, N.L.; Kiso, M.; Hasegawa, A.; Shapiro, R.E. & Schnaar, R.L. (1996). Gangliosides are neuronal ligands for myelin-associated glycoprotein. *Proceedings of the National Academy of Sciences of the USA*, Vol.93, No.2 (January 1996), pp. 814-818. ISSN: 0027-8424.

Zhao, C.; Fancy, S.P.; Magy, L.; Urwin, J.E. & Franklin, R.J. (2005). Stem cells, progenitors and myelin repair. *Journal of Anatomy*, Vol.207, No. 3 (September 2005), pp. 251-258. ISSN: 1469-7580.

Zhao, X.; Han, X.; Yu, Y.; Ye, F.; Chen, Y.; Hoang, T.; Xu, X.; Mi, Q.S.; Xin, M.; Wang, F.; Appel, B. & Lu, Q.R. (2010). MicroRNA-mediated control of oligodendrocyte differentiation. *Neuron*, Vol.65, No.5 (March 2010), pp. 612-626. ISSN: 0896-6273.

Zhou, Q.; Choi, G. & Anderson, D.J. (2001). The bHLH transcription factor Olig2 promotes oligodendrocyte differentiation in collaboration with Nkx2.2. *Neuron*, Vol. 31, No.5 (September 2001), pp. 791-807. ISSN: 0896-6273.

Permissions

The contributors of this book come from diverse backgrounds, making this book a truly international effort. This book will bring forth new frontiers with its revolutionizing research information and detailed analysis of the nascent developments around the world.

We would like to thank Dr. Jagat R. Kanwar, for lending his expertise to make the book truly unique. He has played a crucial role in the development of this book. Without his invaluable contribution this book wouldn't have been possible. He has made vital efforts to compile up to date information on the varied aspects of this subject to make this book a valuable addition to the collection of many professionals and students.

This book was conceptualized with the vision of imparting up-to-date information and advanced data in this field. To ensure the same, a matchless editorial board was set up. Every individual on the board went through rigorous rounds of assessment to prove their worth. After which they invested a large part of their time researching and compiling the most relevant data for our readers. Conferences and sessions were held from time to time between the editorial board and the contributing authors to present the data in the most comprehensible form. The editorial team has worked tirelessly to provide valuable and valid information to help people across the globe.

Every chapter published in this book has been scrutinized by our experts. Their significance has been extensively debated. The topics covered herein carry significant findings which will fuel the growth of the discipline. They may even be implemented as practical applications or may be referred to as a beginning point for another development. Chapters in this book were first published by InTech; hereby published with permission under the Creative Commons Attribution License or equivalent.

The editorial board has been involved in producing this book since its inception. They have spent rigorous hours researching and exploring the diverse topics which have resulted in the successful publishing of this book. They have passed on their knowledge of decades through this book. To expedite this challenging task, the publisher supported the team at every step. A small team of assistant editors was also appointed to further simplify the editing procedure and attain best results for the readers.

Our editorial team has been hand-picked from every corner of the world. Their multi-ethnicity adds dynamic inputs to the discussions which result in innovative outcomes. These outcomes are then further discussed with the researchers and contributors who give their valuable feedback and opinion regarding the same. The feedback is then collaborated with the researches and they are edited in a comprehensive manner to aid the understanding of the subject.

Apart from the editorial board, the designing team has also invested a significant amount of their time in understanding the subject and creating the most relevant covers. They scrutinized every image to scout for the most suitable representation of the subject and create an appropriate cover for the book.

The publishing team has been involved in this book since its early stages. They were actively engaged in every process, be it collecting the data, connecting with the contributors or procuring relevant information. The team has been an ardent support to the editorial, designing and production team. Their endless efforts to recruit the best for this project, has resulted in the accomplishment of this book. They are a veteran in the field of academics and their pool of knowledge is as vast as their experience in printing. Their expertise and guidance has proved useful at every step. Their uncompromising quality standards have made this book an exceptional effort. Their encouragement from time to time has been an inspiration for everyone.

The publisher and the editorial board hope that this book will prove to be a valuable piece of knowledge for researchers, students, practitioners and scholars across the globe.

List of Contributors

Jill Koshiol
National Cancer Institute, USA

Melinda Butsch Kovacic
Cincinnati Children's Hospital Medical Center, USA

Curtis J. Pritzl, Young-Jin Seo and Bumsuk Hahm
Departments of Surgery and Molecular Microbiology & Immunology, University of Missouri – Columbia, USA

Luis Llorente
Department of Immunology and Rheumatology, Instituto Nacional de Ciencias Médicas y Nutrición Salvador Zubirán, Mexico City, Mexico

Judit Anton-Remirez
Rehabilitation Service, Complejo Hospitalario de Navarra, Pamplona, Navarra, Spain

Jesus Feliu
Hematology Service, Complejo Hospitalario de Navarra, Pamplona, Navarra, Spain

Carlos Panizo
Hematology Service, Clínica Universidad de Navarra, Pamplona, Navarra, Spain

Ricardo García-Muñoz and María Pilar Rabasa
Hematology Service, Hospital San Pedro, Logroño, La Rioja, Spain

Rupinder K. Kanwar and Jagat R. Kanwar
Nanomedicine-Laboratory of Immunology and Molecular Biomedical Research (LIMBR), Centre for Biotechnology and Interdisciplinary Biosciences (BioDeakin), Institute for Technology & Research Innovation, Deakin University, Geelong, Australia
Technology Precinct, Waurn Ponds, Geelong, Victoria, Australia

Anton G. Kutikhin
Kemerovo State Medical Academy, Russian Federation

Pietro Fagiolino
Centro de Monitoreo de Fármacos, Universidad de la República, Montevideo, Uruguay

Sandra Orozco-Suárez, Iris Feria-Romero and Israel Grijalva
Unidad de Investigación Médica en Enfermedades Neurológicas, Mexico

Dario Rayo, Jaime Diegopérez and Ma.Ines Fraire
Hospital de Pediatria, CMN Siglo XXI, Mexico

Justina Sosa
Hospital de Especialidades, CM "La Raza",IMSS.México D.F., Mexico

Lourdes Arriaga
Unidad de Investigación en Inmunoquímica,Hospital de Especialidades, CMN Siglo XXI, IMSS México D.F., Mexico

Mario Alonso Vanegas
Instituto Nacional de Neurología y Neurocirugía,"Manuel Velasco Suárez", México D.F., Mexico

Luisa Rocha
Departamento de Farmacobiología, Centro de Investigacion y de Estudios Avanzados, Sede Sur, Mexico

Bonnan Mickael and Cabre Philippe
Service de Neurologie, Centre Hospitalier Universitaire Zobda Quitman, Fort-de-France, French West Indies

Maria de los Angeles Robinson-Agramonte
International Center for Neurological Restoration, Cuba

Carlos Alberto Goncalves
Federal University of Rio Grande del Sur. Porto Alegre, Brazil

Alina González-Quevedo
Institute of Neurology and Neurosurgery, Cuba

M. Denizot, J. J. Hoarau and P. Gasque
GRI, Immunopathology and Infectious Disease Research Grouping (IRG, GRI), University of La Reunion, Reunion Island

J. W. Neal
Neuropathology Laboratory, Dept. of Histopathology, Cardiff University Medical School, UK

Susanne Sattler and Fang-Ping Huang
Imperial College London, UK

Luciën E.P.M. van der Vlugt, Leonie Hussaarts and Hermelijn H. Smits
Leiden University Medical Center, The Netherlands

Olaf Maier
Institute of Cell Biology and Immunology, University of Stuttgart, Germany